Oral Pathology in Clinical Dental Practice

Oral Pathology
IN CLINICAL DENTAL PRACTICE

Robert E. Marx, DDS

Professor of Surgery and Chief
Division of Oral and Maxillofacial Surgery
Miller School of Medicine
University of Miami
Miami, Florida

QUINTESSENCE PUBLISHING

Berlin, Barcelona, Chicago, Istanbul, London, Milan, Moscow, New Delhi,
Paris, Prague, São Paulo, Seoul, Singapore, Tokyo, Warsaw

Dedication

This book is dedicated to all those dentists who have picked up on diseases and conditions that have led to an early diagnosis and treatment, thus saving their patients from disease progression, deformity, and at times, even death.

It is also dedicated to those dentists who may have missed the early signs or obvious diseases while focusing exclusively on the dentition. It is hoped that this book will provide examples and guidance as well as the encouragement to be a diagnostician before being a treatment provider.

Library of Congress Cataloging-in-Publication Data

Names: Marx, Robert E., author.
Title: Oral pathology in clinical dental practice / Robert E. Marx.
Description: Hanover Park, IL : Quintessence Publishing Co. Inc., [2017]
|
Includes bibliographical references. | Description based on print
version
record and CIP data provided by publisher; resource not viewed.
Identifiers: LCCN 2017028350 (print) | LCCN 2017028970 (ebook) | ISBN
9780867157673 (ebook) | ISBN 9780867157642 (hardcover)
Subjects: | MESH: Mouth--pathology | Jaw--pathology | Face--pathology |
Mouth
Mucosa--pathology | Mouth Diseases--pathology | Jaw Diseases--pathology
Classification: LCC RK301 (ebook) | LCC RK301 (print) | NLM WU 140 | DDC
617.5/22 dc23
LC record available at https://lccn.loc.gov/2017028350

QUINTESSENCE PUBLISHING
USA

Quintessence Publishing Co, Inc
4350 Chandler Drive
Hanover Park, IL 60133
www.quintpub.com

5 4 3 2 1

Editor: Leah Huffman
Design: Erica Neumann
Production: Sue Robinson

Printed in the USA

Contents

Preface

Dentists and their dental hygiene team historically have been the great identifiers of oral diseases—not only the common ones of dental caries and periodontal inflammation but also those of oral cancers, serious infections, systemic diseases, and many more. I have personally seen astute "pickups" by referring dentists that have identified serious conditions that actually saved lives. The early recognition of an abnormality, no matter how trivial it may seem at first, can result in a better chance for cure or control and treatments that reduce deformities and disabilities.

On the other hand, I have also treated individuals in whom a denture was made incorporating the expansion of a tumor and several times a history consisting of repeated dental restorations around a fungating cancer. Although this other side of the coin is less common, it is a reality.

This book was written to encourage the early recognition of oral disease and guide the dentist and dental hygiene team in how to recognize certain conditions and what path to take that will most benefit the patient. It also reviews each condition/disease in a concise manner so as to keep them up to date on how the disease develops, who is most likely to present with it, the clinical and radiographic appearance, a reasonable differential diagnosis, a brief overview of the most common microscopic appearance, and, importantly, a suggested course of action—that is, when to observe and for how long, when to refer and to whom, when to biopsy, and when to order tests and for what, etc.

It is hoped that the descriptions and representative photographs as well as the guidance for each disease will help each dentist and dental hygiene team member become a complete oral health care professional and in doing so save a life or two.

1

Recognizing Abnormalities and Pathologic Conditions

This book is the progeny of a previous two-volume comprehensive oral and maxillofacial pathology text written by this author and pathologist Diane Stern. The original volumes included detailed workups, differential diagnoses, and treatments aimed at treatment providers, predominantly oral and maxillofacial surgeons. However, it is usually the practicing restorative dentist or another specialist that recognizes an abnormality or a pathologic condition during the patient visit. It is for these practitioners that this text is provided. Although it discusses the final treatment of each lesion, it more importantly advances a "suggested course of action" that the recognizing practitioner should consider.

The recognition of abnormalities and pathologic conditions requires a three-pronged approach of "listen-look-plan" and is within the training and scope of every dentist.

Listen

The "listen" part begins with the patient's *chief complaint*. If you listen carefully, the patient may actually tell you his or her diagnosis, which you can either confirm or refute or use to lead you to the next phase of recognition, the *history of present illness* (HPI). In the HPI, one should attempt to ascertain when the complaint began, whether it has increased in size or involved other areas, what makes it better or worse, what may have started it, and whether it has been treated before. The third phase of the "listen" part is the *past medical history* (PMH), which is best accomplished by an intake PMH form. The dental provider can use this form to ask more detailed questions about any admitted conditions. In addition, a short, focused, verbal PMH pertinent to dental providers should include the following 10 important, directed questions:

1. Do you have any medical conditions you take medicine for?
2. What medications do you take?
3. Do you take any blood thinners?
4. Do you take a medicine for osteopenia or osteoporosis?
5. Have you ever had a cancer anywhere in your body?
6. Have you taken medicines for cancer?
7. Have you received radiation treatments to your mouth area, neck, or throat?
8. Are you allergic to any medications? If so, what type of reaction did you get?
9. Do you have a heart murmur?
10. Have you had any previous surgeries?

Look

The "look" part involves an oral examination that every dentist is well trained to do. The examiner is cautioned to resist the natural inclination to focus on the obvious dental or periodontal needs of the patient and instead look at all areas of the oral cavity. In particular, examine the chief complaint and the dentition last; neither will disappear during your examination. Be sure to look at the more hidden places in the oral cavity such as the posterior lingual mandible, the hamular notch area, and the posterior lateral border of the tongue, which may require a gloved hand pulling the tongue forward. Today it is also prudent to examine the face and neck for obvious skin lesions and masses as well as the patient's overall appearance and gait.

The second phase of "look" involves what can be done to find out more about the lesion if one is found. That is, is it painful to touch? Does it blanch on palpation? Is it firm, hard, doughy, or soft? Does it have a specific color? Is it movable of fixed? Is it ulcerated, blistered, raised, or flat?

Plan

The "plan" part involves a decision that each dental provider must make: Is this abnormality or pathologic condition something I have the training and experience to diagnose and treat, or is this something I should refer to another individual provider? It is hoped that the "suggested course of action" included with each presentation within this text provides a guideline to answer that question.

2

Red and White Lesions

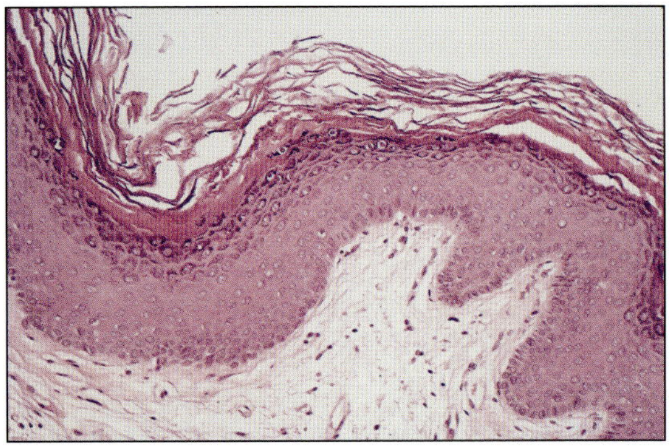

► Wavy strands of keratin above keratinocytes showing a normal progression of maturity without atypia.

Benign Hyperkeratosis

Nature of disease

A thickening of the mucosal epithelium with the production of orthokeratin without epithelial dysplasia.

Predilections

Occurs mostly in adults related to either mechanical irritation or a chemical reaction or unrelated to any observable cause. There is no sex or racial predilection. It may also be idiopathic.

Clinical features

A white patch referred to as *leukoplakia*. It is usually asymptomatic. It is often slightly elevated and may be thickened but will not be indurated.

Radiographic presentation

None.

Differential diagnosis

As a patch of clinical leukoplakia, it must be distinguished from premalignant dysplasia, carcinoma in situ, verrucous carcinoma, and invasive carcinoma. Additionally, lichen planus and *Candida* infection may be considered.

Microscopic features

A thicker-than-normal keratinocyte layer with a surface of lightly eosinophilic, wavy orthokeratin. The keratinocytes will appear to be normal without mitotic figures or nuclear pleomorphism.

Suggested course of action

Remove any obvious mechanical irritation (eg, denture irritations, toothbrush trauma, patient habits, etc) and/or chemical reaction (eg, irritating mouthwashes, certain spices or flavoring agents, etc). If there is no response or resolution within 2 weeks or if no obvious cause is noted, a biopsy is indicated.

Treatment

It is a relief to patients to hear that their benign hyperkeratosis lesion is not considered to be a cancer. However, incisional and even excisional biopsy cannot predict either regrowth or a sampling error that may result in a squamous cell carcinoma developing later. Therefore, a 6-month recall schedule is recommended even though no specific treatment is required.

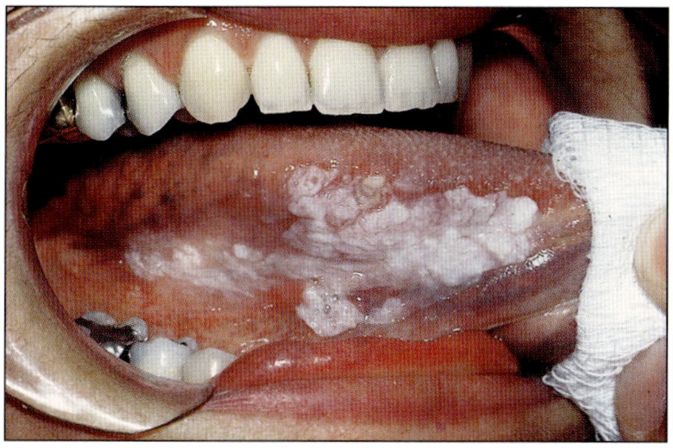

► Leukoplakia.

Leukoplakia

Nature of disease

A white patch on the oral mucosa. Three conditions can present as a clinically apparent white patch: acanthosis/hyperkeratosis, *Candida*, or fibrin.

Predilections

Can occur at any age but is more often seen in adults. There is no sex or racial predilection.

Clinical features

A white patch of oral mucosa most commonly noted on the buccal mucosa, lateral border of the tongue, or floor of the mouth.

Radiographic presentation

None.

Differential diagnosis

Clinical leukoplakia may only represent an ulcer with a fibrin base or *Candida* and sometimes lichen planus by virtue of its acanthosis and hyperkeratosis. However, after benign hyperkeratosis, the most serious considerations are premalignant dyplasias, carcinoma in situ, verrucous carcinoma, and invasive squamous cell carcinoma.

Microscopic features

The three entities that cause a clinical leukoplakia will appear different:

1. Fibrin: Thin strands of light eosinophilic staining over a wound base with inflammation.
2. *Candida*: Vertically positioned hyphae with prominent periodic acid-Schiff (PAS) or silver staining on an epithelial surface.
3. Acanthosis/hyperkeratosis:
   a. Acanthosis/benign hyperkeratosis: A thickened keratinocyte layer without cellular atypia but with surface keratin.
   b. Premalignant dysplasia: Various degrees of epithelial atypia above an intact basement membrane.
   c. Carcinoma in situ: Severe epithelial dysplasia with nuclear pleomorphism and abnormal mitotic figures from the basal cell layer to the surface.
   d. Verrucous carcinoma: A significant exophytic proliferation as well as a blunted endophytic proliferation of epithelial cells but with an intact basement membrane beneath which most often resides a dense inflammatory response.
   e. Invasive carcinoma: Atypical epithelial cells forming bundles and cords through the basement membrane into the underlying tissues.

→

Leukoplakia *(cont)*

Suggested course of action

Biopsy and/or refer to an oral and maxillofacial surgeon.

Treatment

Treatment will vary according to the biopsy result. For:

- Fibrin: Wound care and treatment of the underlying etiology, as well as observation and surveillance for acanthosis/hyperkeratosis.
- Premalignant dysplasia: Excision with frozen section control.
- Carcinoma in situ: Excision with frozen section control.
- Verrucous carcinoma: Excision with frozen section control.
- Invasive carcinoma: Excision with frozen section control and evaluation for radiotherapy and/or chemotherapy.

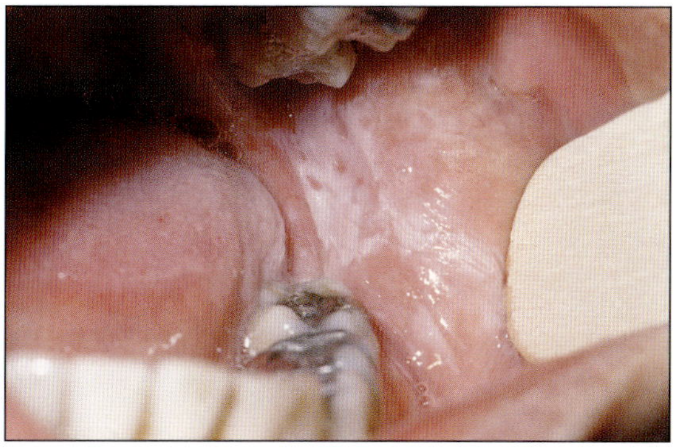

► Smokeless tobacco keratosis from chewing tobacco.

Non–Betel Nut/Slaked Lime Smokeless Tobacco Keratosis

Nature of disease

A reactive nondysplastic hyperkeratosis of the mucosa due to inflammation and stimulation from various smokeless tobacco products.

Predilections

May occur in anyone who uses such products but has a higher incidence in the western United States and the Scandinavian countries due to cultural traditions. More common in men also because of cultural acceptance. No racial predilection is known.

Clinical features

The area corresponding to the placement of the tobacco product (usually the mandibular attached gingiva and mucosa of the vestibule) will appear as an irregular and often leathery white patch referred to as a "snuffle dippers patch." It is usually nonpainful unless the area is inflamed.

Radiographic presentation

None.

Differential diagnosis

The clinician is advised to ask the patient about use of betel nut/slaked lime use versus true smokeless tobacco products. Betel nut/slaked lime keratosis is premalignant, whereas other true tobacco-containing, topical smokeless tobacco products are not. Additionally, clinicians should also consider epithelial dysplasia, carcinoma in situ, invasive squamous cell carcinoma, and even lichen planus and hypertrophic candidiasis.

Microscopic features

Nondysplastic epithelium will be present with a thick layer of pale-staining cells occupying the superficial half of the keratinocyte layer along with significant hyperkeratosis.

Suggested course of action

Confirm that the patch is not the result of betel nut/slaked lime use. Incisional biopsy is indicated to document the absence of dysplasia. Counsel the patient about tobacco cessation, particularly as it relates to erosion of the mucosa and gingiva as well as staining of the teeth.

Treatment

No specific treatment other than cessation of smokeless tobacco use.

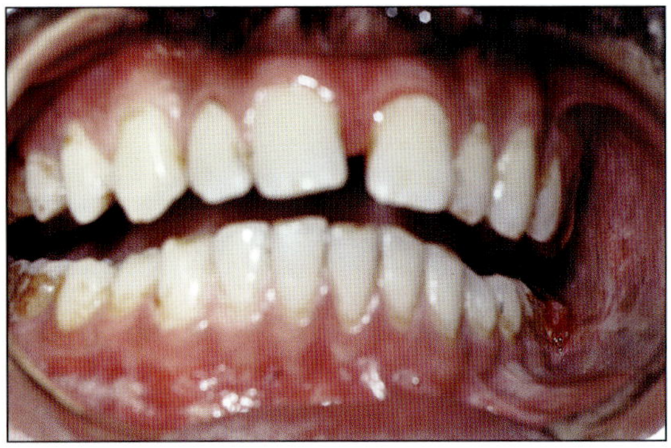

► Trismus, buccal mucosa hyperkeratosis, and fibrosis from betel nut/slaked lime use.

Betel Nut/Slaked Lime Keratosis

Nature of disease

A dysplastic premalignant transformation of mucosal epithelial cells due to the carcinogenic effects of slaked lime. Additionally, the *Areca catechu* chemical in the betel nut often causes a concomitant submucosal fibrosis.

Predilections

Mostly seen in individuals from India, Sri Lanka, and East Asian countries, where the produce is called *quid* or *pan* and used for oral gratification much like chewing gum in the United States.

Clinical features

A white patch is usually seen on either buccal mucosa. There is often a limited jaw opening due to the submucosal fibrosis. Induration around the white patch is common.

Radiographic presentation

None.

Differential diagnosis

The clinician is advised to ask the patient specifically about betel nut/slaked lime use versus use of smokeless tobacco products, as the latter are not carcinogenic to a significant degree. Other considerations include squamous cell carcinoma, actinomycosis, lichen planus, and hypertrophic candidiasis.

Microscopic features

Various degrees of epithelial dysplasia up to invasive carcinoma may be seen together with hyperkeratosis. Dense, poorly cellular collagen is usually seen in the submucosa. Inflammatory cells are variably present.

Suggested course of action

Incisional biopsy to assess for dysplasia or carcinoma or referral to an oral and maxillofacial surgeon.

Treatment

If only premalignant changes are seen on the biopsy, a wide local excision together with skin grafting the defect is accomplished. If invasive carcinoma is identified on the biopsy, a wide local excision and ipsilateral neck dissection is accomplished together with flap reconstruction.

Dyskeratosis Congenita

Nature of disease

A very rare autosomal dominant disorder involving mutations in six genes that code for telomerase, thereby increasing a cell's life span. Forty percent of oral lesions gradually progress to invasive squamous cell carcinoma.

Predilections

Begins in childhood. No sex or racial predilection is known.

Clinical features

Oral lesions of the labial and buccal mucosa will appear white and are frequently thick. Lesions become thicker with age. Skin telangiectasias are common as well as a smooth dorsal tongue surface from loss of filiform papillae. Atrophic nail beds may also be seen.

Radiographic presentation

None.

Differential diagnosis

In younger individuals, hereditary benign intraepithelial dyskeratosis, white sponge nevus, and pachyonychia congenita are considerations. In adults, lichen planus and squamous cell carcinoma are added to these.

Microscopic features

In early lesions, acanthosis and hyperkeratosis are seen. As lesions age, epithelial dysplasia and squamous cell carcinoma may be seen.

Suggested course of action

Close follow-up observing for clinical suggestions of premalignant or malignant changes (ie, ulceration, induration, pain, increase in size, lymphadenopathy, etc). Biopsy as necessary, or refer to an oral and maxillofacial surgeon.

Treatment

Excision of lesions as they show signs of malignant transformation.

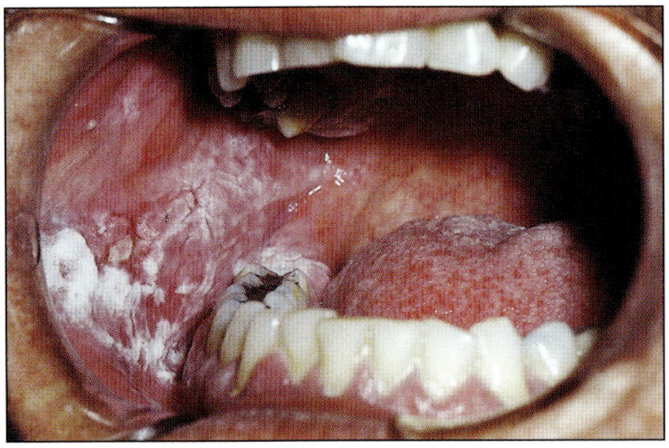

► Erythroleukoplakia representing carcinoma in situ.

Epithelial Dysplasia/Carcinoma in Situ

Nature of disease

Premalignant alterations in the epithelium from genetic alterations in the basal cell layer due to either carcinogens, human papillomaviruses, heredity, or errors in cellular division.

Predilections

Mostly seen in adults but may be rarely seen in patients with congenital dysplastic syndromes. No sex or racial predilection is known. More commonly seen on the lateral border of the tongue or floor of the mouth.

Clinical features

A white or red-white surface lesion without induration. Pain is not usually present. Ulceration is not present unless a focal area of invasive carcinoma exists within the lesion.

Radiographic presentation

None.

Differential diagnosis

Benign hyperkeratosis, lichen planus, and candidiasis should be considered along with invasive squamous cell carcinoma.

Microscopic features

The basement membrane should be intact, and a variable degree of inflammation is seen beneath the basement membrane. The epithelium will show varying degrees of nuclear pleomorphism and cell size and a lack of cellular maturation from the basement membrane to the surface. Mitotic figures and individual cell keratinization may also be seen.

Suggested course of action

Suspicious lesions should be biopsied or referred to an oral and maxillofacial surgeon for evaluation, biopsy, and treatment.

Treatment

After confirmation by biopsy, a wide local excision with frozen section assessment of margins is accomplished. If multiple sections of the main specimen identify an area of invasive squamous cell carcinoma, the area is re-treated with a re-excision and a neck dissection is considered after a metastatic workup is accomplished.

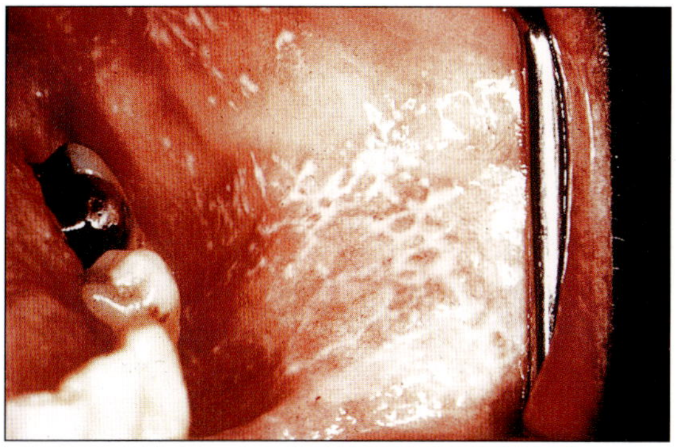

► Striaform lichen planus.

Hypertrophic and Striaform Lichen Planus

Nature of disease

A mild T cell–mediated autoimmune disease that attacks the basal cell layer and basement membrane at the interface between the epithelium and the subjacent connective tissue.

Predilections

Adults over 40 years of age. No sex or racial predilection is known. Mostly seen on the buccal mucosa but may also be seen on the tongue and attached gingiva.

Clinical features

The striaform type presents as asymptomatic, lacy white lines referred to as *Wickham striae*. The hypertrophic type presents as an asymptomatic, irregular white hyperkeratotic patch.

Radiographic presentation

None.

Differential diagnosis

The striaform type is distinctive but may resemble hereditary benign intraepithelial dyskeratosis or candidiasis. The hypertrophic type appears most like clinical leukoplakia, and therefore epithelial dysplasia, carcinoma in situ, proliferative verrucous leukoplakia, verrucous carcinoma, and invasive squamous cell carcinomas should be considered.

Microscopic features

Both will show acanthosis with hyperkeratosis and a bandlike infiltrate subjacent to the basement membrane consisting of mostly (≥90%) lymphocytes as well as a disrupted basement membrane.

Suggested course of action

Clinically apparent striaform lichen planus requires reassurance to the patient of the usual mild and nonprogressive nature of the disease as well as its nonpremalignant biology. Hypertrophic lichen planus requires an incisional or excisional biopsy to rule out more serious diseases.

Treatment

No specific treatment is required.

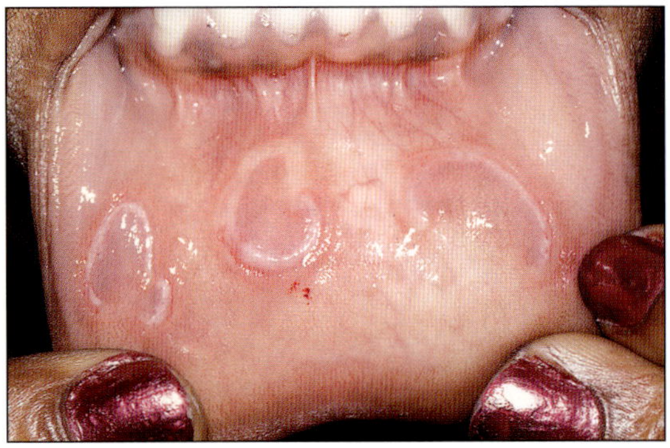

► Mucous patches from secondary syphilis.

Secondary Syphilis (Mucous Patches)

Nature of disease

The systemic second phase of an infection caused by *Treponema pallidum*.

Predilections

In adults, secondary syphilis is a systemic progression from a primary syphilis lesion known as a *chancre*. In newborns, secondary syphilis arises from transplacental transmission from an infected mother to the fetus, and thus the child is born with secondary syphilis. No sex or racial predilection is known.

Clinical features

In adults, the lesions will appear as asymptomatic, flat, red-white lesions or patches of erythema with a pale peripheral ring. In newborns and children, *T pallidum* usually causes developmental disturbances such as the classic triad of mulberry molars, notched incisors, and tapered incisors (screwdriver teeth) known as *Hutchinson's triad*. Additionally, saber-shaped shins, rhagades, interstitial keratitis, and a saddle nose deformity may variably be seen.

Radiographic presentation

None.

Differential diagnosis

Mucous patches of secondary syphilis will appear similar to candidiasis and lichen planus. Erythema multiforme may also be considered if skin lesions are present.

Microscopic features

Biopsies of mucous patches will usually show a plasma cell infiltration among a proliferation of small blood vessels.

Suggested course of action

Suspected cases should be referred to an infectious disease specialist and/or submitted for serologic testing for a VDRL (Venereal Disease Research Lab) test and an FTA (fluorescent treponemal antibody) absorption test.

Treatment

Secondary syphilis is usually treated with one dose of 1.2 to 2.4 million units of benzathine penicillin intramuscularly. In penicillin-allergic patients, doxycycline 100 mg orally twice daily for 14 days or oral erythromycin 500 mg four times daily for 14 days can be substituted.

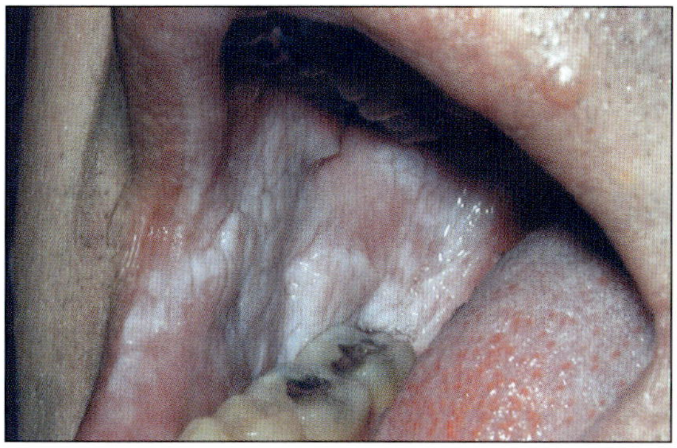

► Thin, soft white patch characteristic of hereditary benign intraepithelial dyskeratosis.

Hereditary Benign Intraepithelial Dyskeratosis

Nature of disease

A very rare autosomal dominant condition involving a racial mix of Native American, black African, and white Caucasian races traced to a single female ancestor in the late 1800s.

Predilections

No sex or specific racial predilection. Seen shortly after birth.

Clinical features

Buccal mucosal lesions are most prominent but may occur on all oral mucosal surfaces except the dorsum of the tongue. The lesions are soft white lesions without induration or ulceration. In older individuals, the lesions become more extensive and may appear folded. Conjunctival lesions that appear bubbling and foamy may be seen as well.

Radiographic presentation

None.

Differential diagnosis

The oral lesions will appear similar to white sponge nevus, lichen planus, and pachyonychia congenita.

Microscopic features

The epithelium will be acanthotic with intracellular edema, giving the cell an eosinophilic waxy appearance. The basal cells and submucosal connective tissue will appear normal.

Suggested course of action

Reassure the patient of the benign nature of the condition and that it is not premalignant.

Treatment

None required.

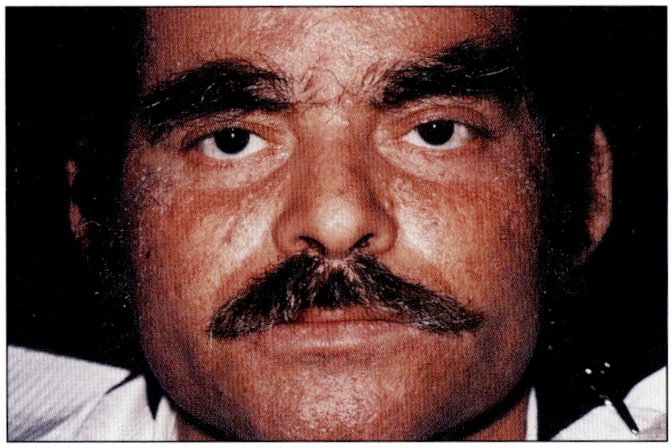

► Multiple small hyperkeratotic papules that overproduce and shed keratin in keratosis follicularis.

Keratosis Follicularis (Darier-White Disease)

Nature of disease

An inherited autosomal dominant trait that causes a defect in the gene that regulates keratin production and the maturation of epithelial cells.

Predilections

Clinically first seen in late childhood and the early teen years. There is no sex or racial predilection.

Clinical features

Early cases will show papules over the face, chest, and back and less commonly on the oral mucosa. As the individual matures, the papules become shiny and brown and then black and produce a distinctive foul odor. Mature oral lesions will be seen as closely grouped papules, giving the mucosa a cobblestone appearance.

Radiographic presentation

None.

Differential diagnosis

Pachyonychia congenita, aggressive acanthosis nigricans, and the palmar and plantar hyperkeratosis finding in Papillon-Lefèvre syndrome are the few conditions in which such dramatic skin hyperkeratosis occurs.

Microscopic features

Acanthosis and prominent hyperkeratosis often forming a villous-like appearance accompany a suprabasilar split similar to that seen in pemphigus. Within the area of the split, rounded epithelial cells with a dark basophilic nucleus surrounded by a pale halo, known as *corps ronds*, are seen.

Suggested course of action

Suspected cases should be referred to a dermatologist.

Treatment

There is no curative treatment. However, isotretinoin (Accutane, Roche) 0.5 to 2.0 mg/kg daily given in two doses reduces the number and size of papules. Additional frequent cleansing with chlorhexidine or 6% salicylic acid can control the excessive keratin and foul odor.

Pachyonychia Congenita

Nature of disease

A rare autosomal dominant condition caused by mutations in the K6a, K16, and K17 keratins that mostly affect nail beds and to a lesser extent the oral mucosa. Pachyonychia congenita is seen within two syndromes: Jadassohn-Lewandowsky syndrome and Jackson-Lawler syndrome.

Predilections

Clinical signs are already present at birth and slowly progress. No sex or racial predilection is known.

Clinical features

Oral lesions are limited and will mostly appear as asymptomatic, soft white patches on the buccal mucosa or the tongue. The most prominent presentation is seen on the fingernails and toenails as a discolored thickening and peeling of the nail that reveals a thickened nail bed underneath.

Radiographic presentation

None.

Differential diagnosis

Because of the nail bed involvement, the clinician should consider skin fungal conditions and systemic fungal diseases as well as proliferative verrucous leukoplakia (PVL), which also produces white oral lesions and disrupted fingernail and toenail formation. If the nail bed involvement is subtle, lichen planus, white sponge nevus, and hereditary benign intraepithelial dyskeratosis may be considered.

Microscopic features

Acanthosis and hyperparakeratosis devoid of dysplasia will be seen.

Suggested course of action

Suspected cases should be referred to a dermatologist. However, if PVL is a strong consideration or if the white patch is either ulcerated or indurated, an incisional biopsy or referral to an oral and maxillofacial surgeon is recommended.

Treatment

No treatment other than local nail care is indicated.

Incontinentia Pigmenti

Nature of disease
An inherited autosomal dominant chromosomal deletion that is lethal in males but survivable in females.

Predilections
Present in females only and begins in infancy. No racial predilection is known.

Clinical features
White, verrucous, asymptomatic oral and skin lesions with occasional vesicle formation. Orally, oligodontia is sometimes seen. Ocular nystagmus and strabismus are also frequently seen. Seizure disorders are rare. Some skin lesions will be brown in color.

Radiographic presentation
None.

Differential diagnosis
The white oral and skin lesions may resemble an early case of keratosis follicularis or pachyonychia congenita. Systemic candidiasis or lichen planus with oral and skin lesions may also be considered.

Microscopic features
White patches will show acanthosis and hyperkeratosis. Discolored lesions will show melanin pigment within macrophages and free melanin in the dermis, hence the name *incontinentia pigmenti.*

Suggested course of action
Suspected cases should be referred to a dermatologist and/or a geneticist.

Treatment
No treatment is required.

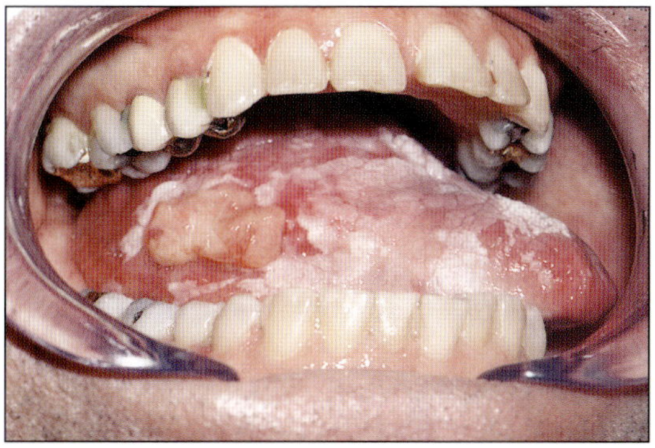

► Early PVL of tongue: Field development of lesion.

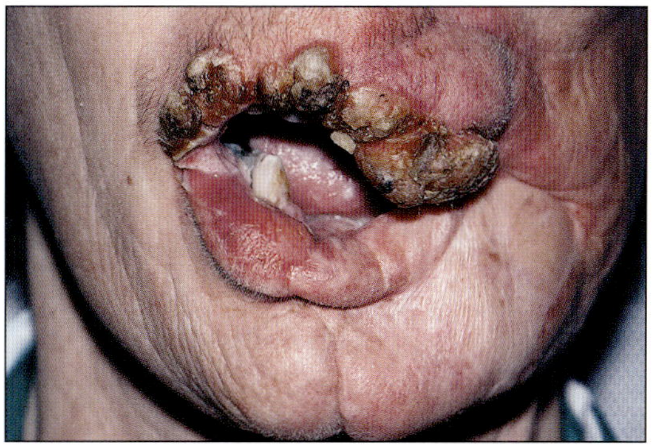

► Later stage of PVL with widespread involvement of invasive squamous cell carcinoma.

Proliferative Verrucous Leukoplakia (PVL)

Nature of disease

A relentless progression from benign-appearing leukoplakia of only hyperkeratosis through to verrucous hyperplasia, verrucous carcinoma, invasive squamous cell carcinoma, and a final stage of an extremely aggressive and treatment-resistant squamous cell carcinoma.

Predilections

Adults over 50 years. Affects women more than men. Unrelated to tobacco products and high-risk human papillomaviruses. No racial predilection is known.

Clinical features

Depending on the stage and advancement of this disease, it may appear as a large surface area of leukoplakia or multiple exophytic verrucous lesions or a large tumor mass. As many as 90% of patients will have a skin and/or nail fungal condition as well as oral candidiasis.

Radiographic presentation

None until its later stages, when it invades bone to produce an irregular osteolysis.

Differential diagnosis

In its early and intermediate stages, PVL will appear similar to candidiasis and lichen planus. As it progresses, verrucous carcinoma unrelated to PVL and hypertrophic candidiasis may be considered. In its aggressive late stage, invasive squamous cell carcinoma unrelated to PVL and high-grade mucoepidermoid carcinoma and other high-grade cancers are considerations.

Microscopic features

Early stages will show a range from normal-appearing epithelium to varying degrees of dysplasia. A peculiar bulbous endophytic protrusion of epithelium with an intact basement membrane is often seen. In intermediate stages, a verrucous proliferation is noted. In later stages, an invasive squamous cell carcinoma with abundant mitotic figures is seen.

Suggested course of action

Suspicious cases should undergo an incisional biopsy and/or referral to an oral and maxillofacial surgeon.

Treatment

Initially, areas of clinical involvement are excised and skin grafted. Follow-up chemoprevention is not curative but slows down the progression of the disease. Oral nystatin swish and spit, oral-systemic griseofulvin 250 mg twice daily, and tocopherol 100 mcg daily are often used as chemoprevention. Advanced cases are treated with resection and sometimes chemotherapy or radiotherapy, although their value is uncertain.

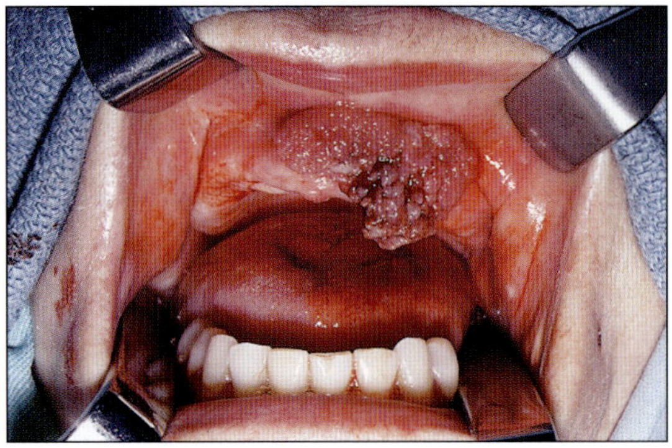

► Exophytic verrucous carcinoma of the anterior maxilla in a patient who smoked one pack of cigarettes per day and did not use smokeless tobacco.

Verrucous Carcinoma

Nature of disease

A noninvasive and nonmetastasizing exophytic proliferation of malignant epithelial cells. Note: Although often attributed to smokeless tobacco use, there is no clear evidence that smokeless tobacco other than betel nut/slaked lime causes verrucous carcinoma.

Predilections

Mostly adults over 50 years of age. Slightly more common in males than in females and mostly occurs on the buccal mucosa or gingiva. No racial predilection is known.

Clinical features

Lesions will appear as red-white velvet-textured exophytic masses arising from a broad surface area. Satellite lesions are common. Lesions are asymptomatic without induration or suspicious lymphadenopathy.

Radiographic presentation

None.

Differential diagnosis

Benign hyperkeratosis, squamous papillomas, and invasive squamous cell carcinoma should be considered. Hypertrophic candidiasis and lichen planus may also be considered.

Microscopic features

Bulbous endophytic and exophytic epithelial proliferations are seen together with an intact basement membrane and subjacent inflammation in the mucosa beneath the basement membrane. There are usually clefts with a hyperparakeratinization between the broad exophytic proliferations.

Suggested course of action

Incisional biopsy to include at least one margin and a depth into bleeding submucosa and/or referral to an oral and maxillofacial surgeon.

Treatment

Wide local excision into the submucosa while observing a 1.0- to 1.5-cm margin controlled by frozen sections.

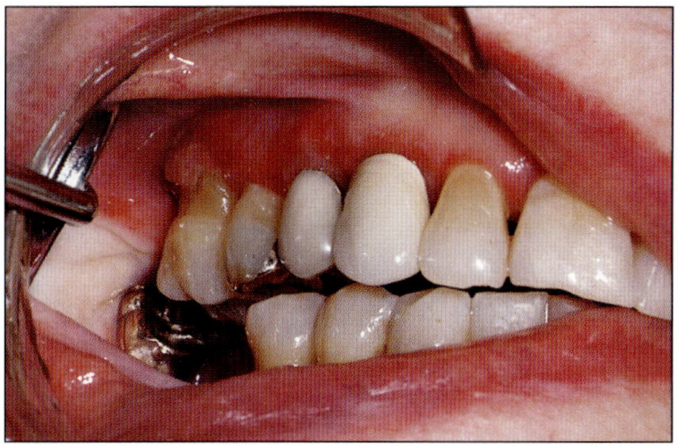

► Reddened oral mucosa and gingiva from the yellow dye (tartrazine) in some Synthroid tablets (AbbVie).

Hypersensitivity Mucositis

Nature of disease
An immune-based inflammatory response to topical or systemic agents.

Predilections
Can occur at any age but is mostly seen in adults taking systemic medications. May also be attributed to some ingredients in dental preparations or to food spices. Systemic medications most well known to cause oral hypersensitivity lesions are thyroid-replacement and anti-hypertension drugs. Topical agents more commonly associated with mucosal reactions are common flavoring and nickel-containing materials. No sex or racial predilection is known.

Clinical features
Lesions will be flat, erythematous patches with mild to moderate pain. Certain acidic juices and spices may incite a higher level of pain.

Radiographic presentation
None.

Differential diagnosis
Painful, red oral mucosal lesions suggest pemphigus, erosive lichen planus, and pemphigoid as the most serious considerations. However, a premalignant field dysplasia or field cancer should also be considered.

Microscopic features
There will be a diffuse sub-basement membrane inflammation composed of a mixture of lymphocytes and plasma cells with plasma cells predominating. The basement membrane will be intact and normal.

Suggested course of action
Potential etiologic agents should be reviewed with the patient. If a topical agent is responsible, discontinuation is recommended. If an oral drug is thought to be responsible, a letter of explanation with a referral of the patient to the prescribing physician is recommended.

Treatment
Identification and discontinuation of the offending drug, or use of an alternate drug or dose of the same drug with a different dye coloring in the tablet, as many of these are caused by a specific dye color. Refractory cases are treated with prednisone.

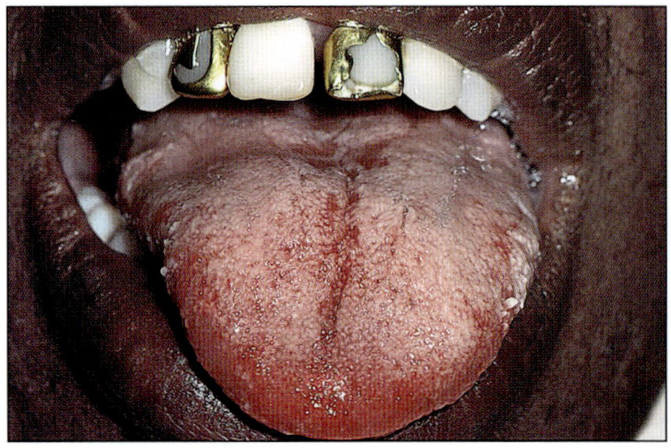

► Hairy leukoplakia in a patient with AIDS.

Hairy Leukoplakia

Nature of disease

An opportunistic infection caused by the Epstein-Barr virus producing focal epithelial proliferation and hyperkeratosis.

Predilections

Seen mostly in adults with some immune compromise. Once thought to be an early sign of HIV/AIDS, it is now known to occur in other immune-compromised patients as well. No sex or racial predilection is known.

Clinical features

Asymptomatic, white hairlike proliferations are mostly seen on the dorsum and/or lateral border of the tongue. There is noted lack of redness and paresthesia.

Radiographic presentation

None.

Differential diagnosis

Although the short hairlike strands and a history of immune compromise will strongly suggest hairy leukoplakia, candidiasis and lichen planus may appear similar, as might condyloma acuminata.

Microscopic features

Exophytic epithelial proliferations with prominent acanthosis and hyperparakeratosis. A noted lack of subjacent inflammation is usually present. Below the parakeratin layers, pale-staining epithelial cells with pyknotic nuclei are prominent.

Suggested course of action

Confirm a history of immune compromise and refer to either an immunologist or an infectious disease specialist. If uncertain, an incisional biopsy will confirm the diagnosis.

Treatment

Occasionally, the areas of hairy leukoplakia are excised. Otherwise, there is no treatment other than treatment of the underlying immune compromise.

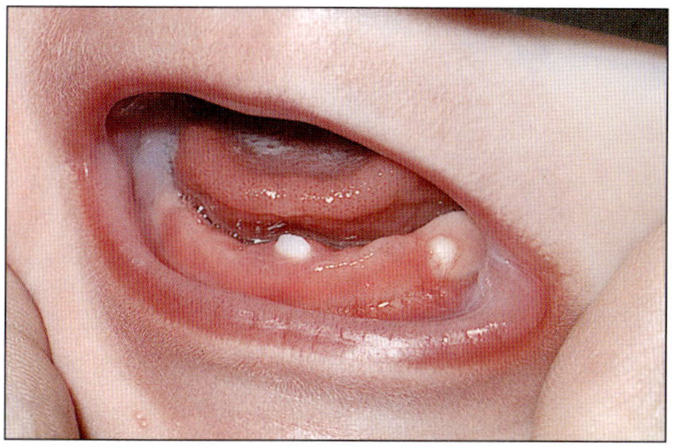

► Small, round white nodule on the posterior alveolar ridge representing a Bohn's nodule.

Dental Lamina Rests/Epithelial Inclusions (Bohn's Nodules and Epstein Pearls)

Nature of disease

Bohn's nodules are white elevations in the edentulous ridge of newborns representing true residual dental lamina remnants or a developing gingival cyst. Epstein pearls are epithelial rests also seen in newborns as white nodules but that arise in the midline of the palate from the fusion of the palatal and nasal processes. Small cysts may develop from these as well.

Predilections

Exclusively newborns less than 1 year of age. No sex or racial predilection is known.

Clinical features

Small, white, asymptomatic expansions of the oral surface in newborns, seen on either the edentulous ridge or the palatal midline.

Radiographic presentation

None.

Differential diagnosis

Other than the early eruption of an expected primary tooth, Bohn's nodules are distinctive. Other than hypertrophy or mucocele development in the palate, Epstein pearls are also quite distinctive.

Microscopic features

If the nodule represents residual rests, it will appear as a collection of odontogenic epithelial cells in a rounded fashion. If the nodule has progressed to a gingival or palatal cyst, there will be a lumen lined by a thin layer of epithelium with focal thickened areas.

Suggested course of action

Reassure parents of the natural involution of the cyst as it erupts into the oral cavity and becomes confluent with the oral epithelium.

Treatment

None required.

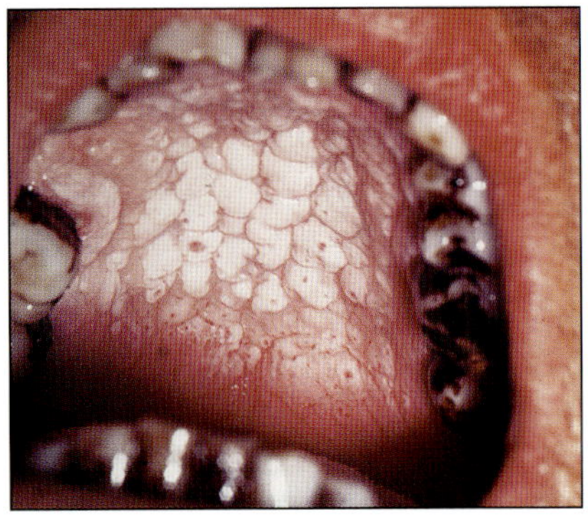

► Nicotine stomatitis from pipe smoking.

Nicotine Stomatitis

Nature of disease

A nonmalignant, nonpremalignant change in the palatal mucosa producing white patches of hyperkeratosis due to the heat from pipe smoking or, more rarely, cigar smoking.

Predilections

Mostly adult men who frequently smoke pipes or, more rarely, adults who smoke cigars. There is no racial predilection.

Clinical features

White patches of thickened epithelium of the palatal mucosa creating a cobblestone appearance with central small red dots representing inflammation at the openings of minor salivary gland ducts.

Radiographic presentation

None.

Differential diagnosis

Nicotine stomatitis is clinically distinctive. However, some cases of candidiasis may appear quite similar.

Microscopic features

Marked acanthosis with hyperkeratosis. Inflammation may also be seen in the submucosa in the clinically red areas.

Suggested course of action

Reassure the individual that the changes are not premalignant. Encourage discontinuation of the smoking habit.

Treatment

None required.

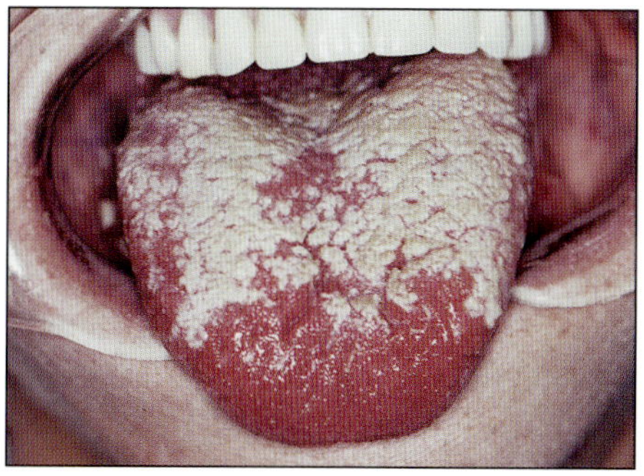

► Thrush.

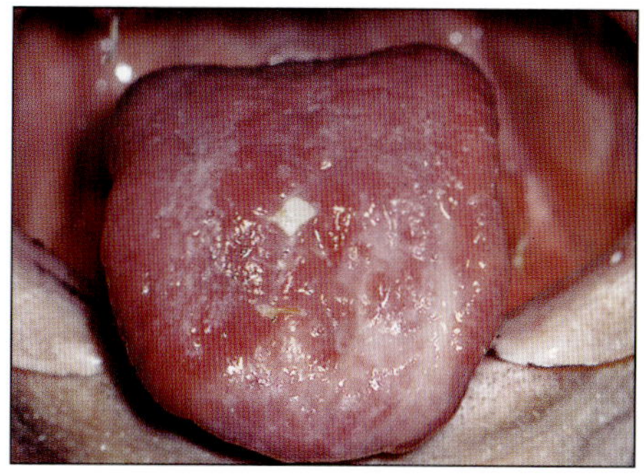

► Atrophic glossitis.

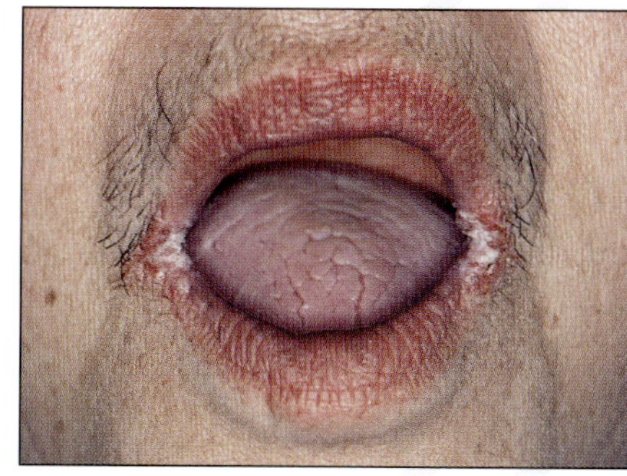

► Angular cheilitis.

Oral Candidiasis

Nature of disease

A fungal (yeast) colonization and/or actual invasive infection by one of the many species of *Candida*, the most common of which is *Candida albicans*.

Predilections

There is no specific age, sex, or racial predilection. However, it is more often seen as an opportunistic infection in someone prone to develop it, including *(1)* children whose immune system is not complete; *(2)* older individuals with age-related reduced immune function; *(3)* patients who were recently on antibiotics; *(4)* patients who underwent radiation therapy; *(5)* patients undergoing chemotherapy; *(6)* patients with diseases that affect the immune system (eg, leukemia, HIV); *(7)* patients with trauma from ill-fitting dentures; and *(8)* patients with warm, moist creases at the commissures of the mouth with reduced occlusal vertical dimension.

Clinical features

There are many clinical presentations of candidiasis:

1. Classic thrush with white *Candida* colonies able to be removed with a tongue depressor
2. Angular cheilitis (perlèche), in which red-white painful lesions on the commissures of the mouth result from a loss of occlusal vertical dimension
3. Median rhomboid glossitis represented by a rhomboid or diamond-shaped, flat red patch on the dorsum of the tongue
4. Hyperplastic candidiasis, which cannot be removed with a tongue depressor and looks similar to leukoplakia
5. Inflammatory hyperplasia under an ill-fitting denture
6. Atrophic glossitis, where the *Candida* has resulted in loss or flattening of the filiform papillae
7. Mucocutaneous candidiasis, which is a severe and more widespread involvement of skin and other mucous membranes
8. Systemic disseminated candidiasis from a candidemia, most often from a central venous line or catheter

Radiographic presentation

None.

Differential diagnosis

In its various presentations, the differential diagnosis will change. The most significant differential is to consider leukoplakia, epithelial dysplasia, squamous cell carcinoma, and lichen planus. →

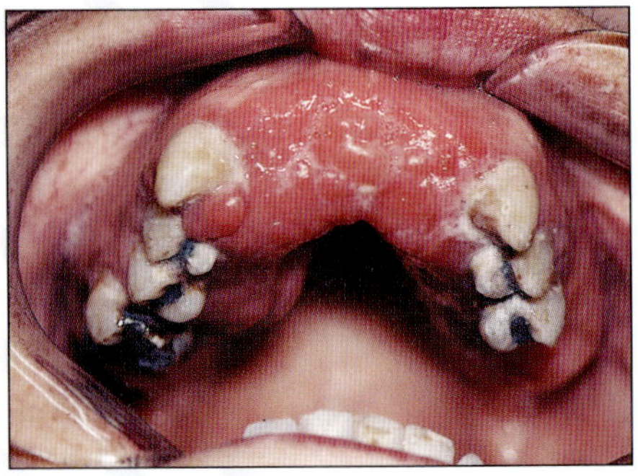

► Inflammatory hyperplasia.

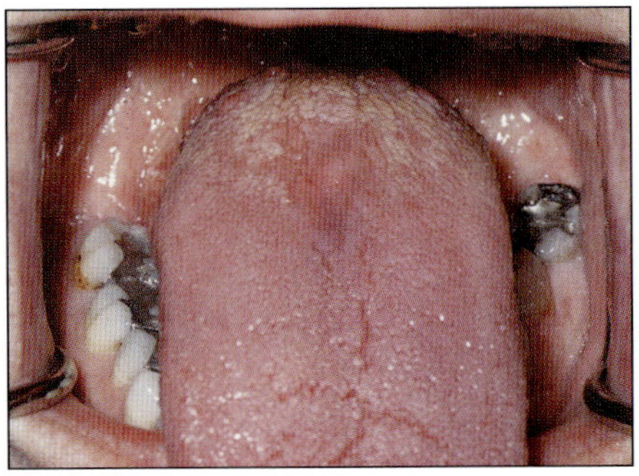

► Median rhomboid glossitis.

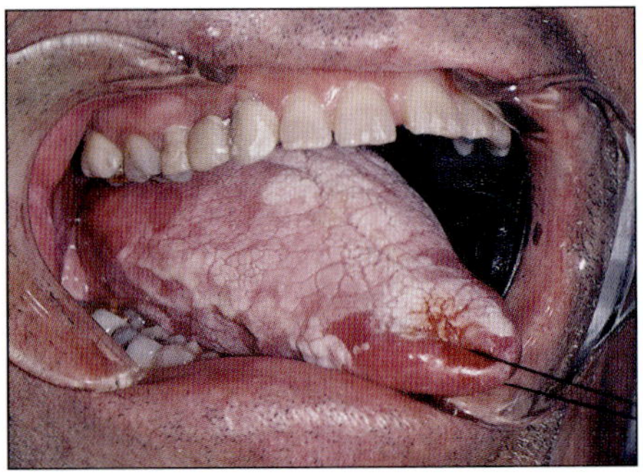

► Hypertrophic candidiasis.

Oral Candidiasis *(cont)*

Microscopic features

Candida are nonseptate hyphae that can be highlighted by a periodic acid-Schiff stain or a silver stain. With these stains, the hyphae will be seen on the mucosal surface and also vertically oriented and burrowing through the epithelial layer. Neutrophils are also often seen within the epithelial layer, presumably in response to the *Candida*. Beneath the basement membrane, a lymphocytic-histiocytic inflammatory infiltrate will be seen.

Suggested course of action

Treat oral lesions initially with oral nystatin suspension 100,000 units/mL using 5-mL swish and spit. Skin and commissure lesions may be treated with nystatin powder. Refractory cases are best referred to an oral medicine specialist or an oral and maxillofacial surgeon.

Treatment

Refractory cases often need systemic as well as topical anti-*Candida* treatment. In such cases, fluconazole 100 mg daily for 5 to 7 days or ketoconazole 200 mg twice daily is used. In the rare systemic or disseminated candidiasis, intravenous micafungin or amphotericin B may be required.

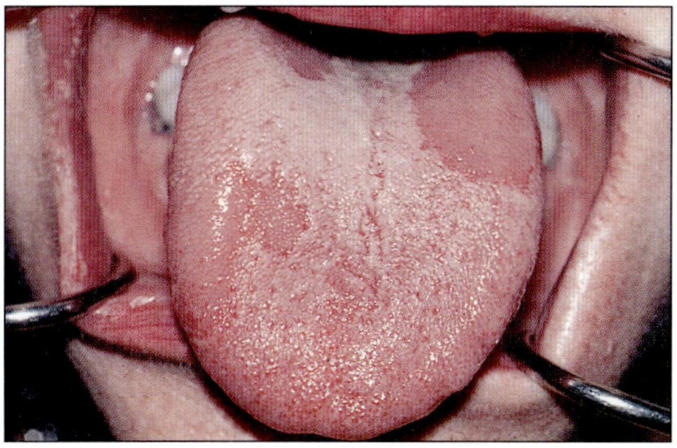

► Benign migratory glossitis.

Benign Migratory Glossitis

Nature of disease

An asymptomatic and innocuous condition involving the tongue in which smooth red areas absent of filiform papillae are contrasted against the textured pale areas of the normal dorsum of the tongue. These red areas will resolve and then appear in another position on the tongue dorsum, hence giving it a migratory appearance over time.

Predilections

Adults mostly. There is no sex or racial predilection.

Clinical features

In a single one-time examination, a portion of the tongue dorsum will appear as normal textured and pale white together with flat, smooth red areas.

Radiographic presentation

None.

Differential diagnosis

Asymptomatic red-white surface lesions on the dorsum of the tongue may be seen in atrophic candidiasis, lichen planus, and, more rarely, in systemic lupus erythematosus and squamous cell carcinoma.

Microscopic features

Narrow, elongated rete pegs are seen between connective tissue papillae that approach a thin surface epithelium. Beneath the basement membrane, an inflammatory infiltrate is usually seen.

Suggested course of action

Reassure the patient of the nonpremalignant nature of benign migratory glossitis and that it does not represent any known systemic disease.

Treatment

None required.

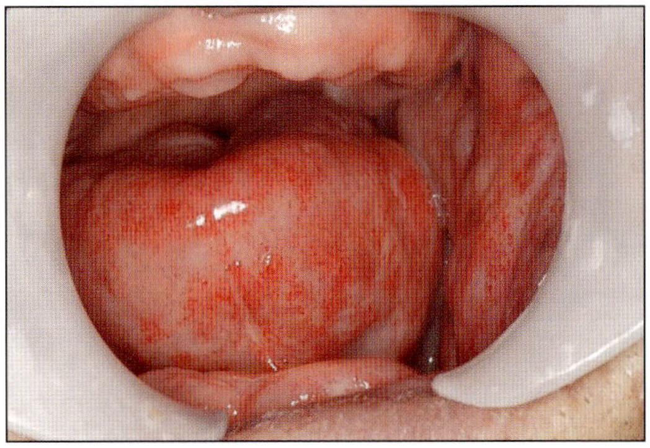

► Acute radiation mucositis.

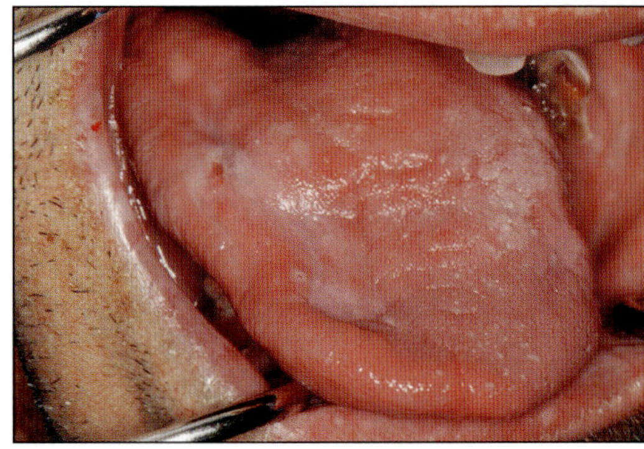

► Chronic radiation mucositis.

Acute and Chronic Radiation Mucositis

Nature of disease

An initial inflammatory condition of the oral mucosa resulting from the cellular injury created by high-dose radiation energy. While the initial phase, usually beginning 3 weeks into a radiotherapy treatment protocol, comprises acute inflammation and hyperemia, this usually subsides about 3 to 4 weeks after completion of radiotherapy into a fibrotic chronic phase.

Predilections

Adults and, more rarely, children who undergo greater than 6,000 cGy of radiotherapy. There is no sex or racial predilection.

Clinical features

In the acute phase, a painful red-white mucosa often with a weeping serous or fibrinous exudate or slough appears. Frequently dysphagia and tender lymphadenopathy are also present. The chronic phase will present as a dry white surface that may have superficial *Candida* infection and may be somewhat firm and contracted.

Radiographic presentation

None.

Differential diagnosis

The acute phase may be identical to a drug-induced mucositis from chemotherapy, which may have been used concomitant with the radiotherapy. Otherwise, consider secondary mucositis from HIV, leukemia, or multiple myeloma. The chronic phase will resemble a chemical burn such as lye ingestion or progressive systemic sclerosis (scleroderma).

Microscopic features

The acute phase will show hyperemia and sludging in most vessels as well as interstitial edema and acute inflammatory cells. The chronic phase will be poorly vascular and poorly cellular with collagen replacing most cellular elements as seen in a scar.

Suggested course of action

During the acute phase, advise the patient to avoid alcohol or acid-containing medicaments and foods. Prescribe "magic mouthwash"—ie, Kaopectate (Chattem) 5 mL, Benadryl (McNeil) 12.5 mg, and dexamethasone 12 mg swish and spit—and/or 2% lidocaine gel to be applied topically before meals and as needed. If secondary infection is suspected (eg, tender lymphadenopathy, significant mucosal pain), also treat with antibiotics: amoxicillin 500 mg three times daily or doxycycline 100 mg daily.

Treatment

No specific curative treatment is known. However, the palliative care discussed above is useful.

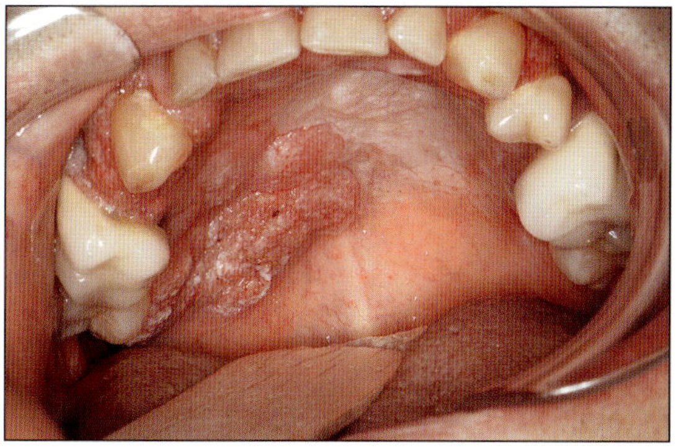

► Widespread surface involvement of dysplasia/carcinoma in situ and invasive carcinoma.

Field Cancerization

Nature of disease

Although smoking and certain human papillomaviruses (HPV) have been linked to oral squamous cell carcinoma, a significant number occur without any apparent carcinogen exposure. One of these is the field cancerization phenomenon in which the normal oral mucosa transforms into squamous cell carcinoma over a wide area and with new lesions developing over time.

Predilections

Adults over 30 years of age, with a slight female predilection. No racial predilection is known.

Clinical features

Pebble-like leukoplakia or erythroplakia over a wide surface area, mostly seen on the gingiva, at the lateral border of the tongue, and on the buccal mucosa. This condition is often painful and does not develop ulcerations or regional lymph node spread until it has been present for some time.

Radiographic presentation

Radiographs are usually normal until late in its course, when bony invasion results in osteolysis.

Differential diagnosis

Proliferative verrucous leukoplakia bears a very close resemblance to field cancerization and is actually another form of it, but one that goes through a verrucous phase (while field cancerization does not). Additionally, lichen planus, candidiasis, and a large isolated T3 squamous cell carcinoma may be considered.

Microscopic features

Field cancerization histopathology is no different than that of isolated dysplasia, carcinoma in situ, and invasive squamous cell carcinoma that represent focal disease, in which atypical epithelial cells with pleomorphic nuclei and mitotic figures occur above an intact basement membrane and then invade through the basement membrane to the subjacent connective tissue, sometimes forming keratin pearls and other times more anaplastic features.

Suggested course of action

Suspicious cases should be photographed for documentation and biopsied. If this cannot be accomplished by the initial examining practitioner, the patient should be referred to an oral and maxillofacial surgeon or a regional cancer center.

Treatment

The lesions present at the time are excised with 1.5-cm margins with frozen section control, and the defect is skin grafted or reconstructed with a tissue flap. A prophylactic neck lymphadenectomy is also usually accomplished. If lymphadenopathy is present, a treatment neck dissection is performed. Close follow-up is observed every 2 to 3 months, with retreatment of new lesions as they arise.

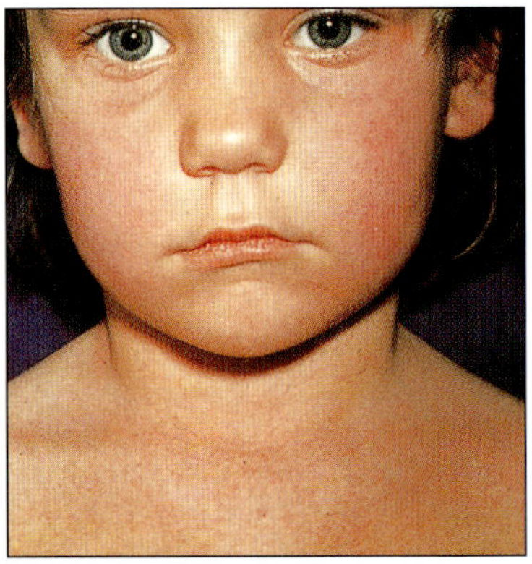

► Red macular skin rash seen in scarlet fever.

Scarlet Fever

Nature of disease

Today, a rare bacterial infection caused by group A beta-hemolytic streptococci (*Streptococcus scarlatina* or *Streptococcus pyogenes*) that produces a unique red macular skin rash and a red swollen tongue by virtue of its erythrotoxin elaboration.

Predilections

Mostly children and young adults. No sex or racial predilection is known.

Clinical features

The child or young adult will present with fever, a sore throat, and headache. The red macular skin rash may appear on the face but will be more prominent in the axillary and groin areas. The tongue will be swollen with reddened fungiform papillae standing out against a white coat on the tongue. This is referred to as "raspberry tongue."

Radiographic presentation

None.

Differential diagnosis

Other infections such as nonspecific streptococcal pharyngitis, infectious mononucleosis, and pseudomembranous pharyngitis should be considered.

Microscopic features

Tissue specimens are rarely taken as they show a nonspecific inflammatory cell infiltrate with prominent endothelial lysis, dilation of small blood vessels, and hyperemia.

Suggested course of action

Throat cultures of suspicious cases should be taken and a referral made to an infectious disease specialist.

Treatment

Penicillin is the drug of choice: either phenoxymethylpenicillin 500 mg orally four times daily for 10 days or one intramuscular dose of benzathine penicillin 1.2 million units. For penicillin-allergic patients, oral erythromycin 500 mg four times daily or 40 mg/kg per day for 10 days for children is prescribed.

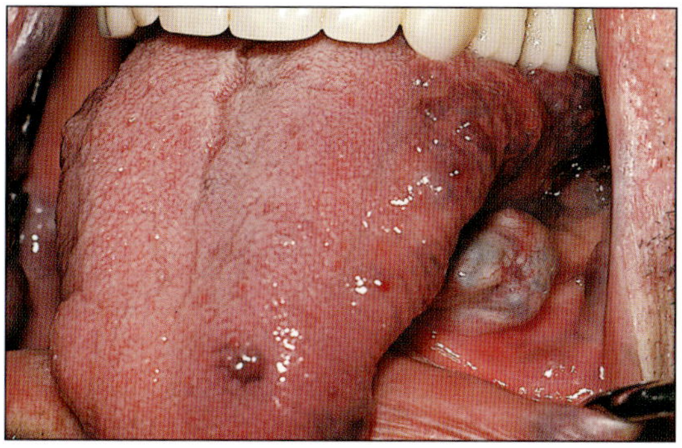

► Classic Kaposi sarcoma.

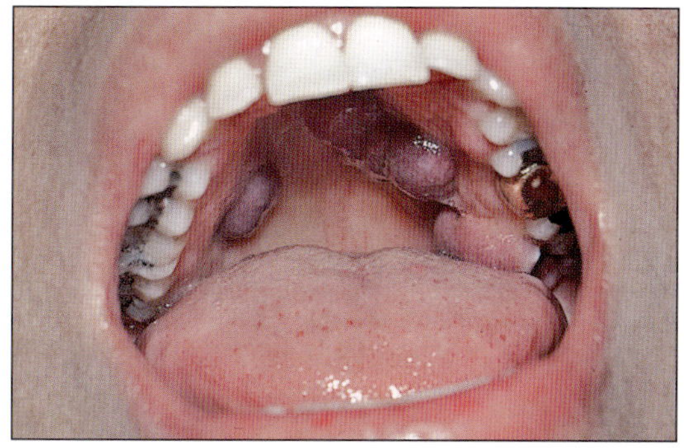

► AIDS-related Kaposi sarcoma.

Kaposi Sarcoma

Nature of disease

A low-grade multifocal vascular malignancy due to a viral infection in an individual with a genetic HLA-DR5 antigen predisposition.

Predilections

There are four types of Kaposi sarcoma:

1. Classic Kaposi sarcoma: This type affects mostly men over 60 years of age and has a strong predilection for those of Greek, Italian, or Jewish ethnicity.
2. African cutaneous Kaposi sarcoma: This type also occurs more commonly in men, specifically men 35 years or older, and is endemic in native black African men.
3. African lymphadenopathic Kaposi sarcoma: This type is endemic in black African children.
4. AIDS-related Kaposi sarcoma: This type is more common in adult men but also can occur in women and children.

Clinical features

The two most common types seen in the United States—classic Kaposi sarcoma and AIDS-related Kaposi sarcoma—appear as bluish-red submucosal or subdermal collections. Some will produce a soft tissue lobulated mass. The African cutaneous type is limited to the skin and is much more infiltrative, producing induration, and will spread rapidly in a proximal direction. The African lymphadenopathic type is a fulminant type involving lymph nodes, salivary glands, and internal organs, often leading to a rapid death.

Radiographic presentation

Usually none unless the mass invades bone; then it is usually only a superficial erosion.

Differential diagnosis

Many cases will mimic an area of ecchymosis from capillary fragility or platelet dysfunction. Those with a mass will suggest an angiosarcoma, rhabdomyosarcoma, hemangioma, lymphangioma, or a low-grade mucoepidermoid carcinoma.

Microscopic features

With some variability, there will be numerous blood-filled channels appearing like slits between spindle cells.

Suggested course of action

Refer to a cancer center or to a medical oncologist for workup.

Treatment

Isolated lesions are treated with intralesional injections of vinblastine 0.1 to 0.5 mg/mL or radiotherapy 1,800 to 2,400 cGy. Systemic treatment is via chemotherapy using vinblastine, etoposide, bleomycin, doxorubicin, and interferon alpha-2 as an adjunct.

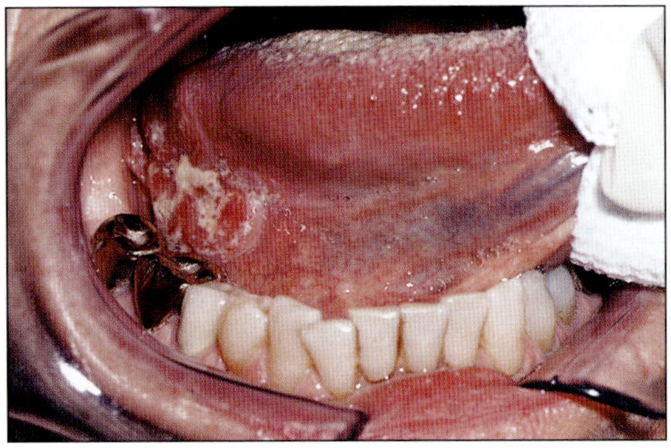

► Squamous cell carcinoma of the lateral border of the tongue.

Oral Squamous Cell Carcinoma

Nature of disease

An invasive epithelial malignancy arising from the basal cells of oral mucosa that may undergo a partial squamous differentiation. Many also develop the ability to metastasize to regional lymph nodes and a few others to distant organs such as the lungs via a vascular route.

Predilections

Adults, with a modest male predilection. More common on the lateral border of the tongue and floor of the mouth. No racial predilection is known. Since 2000, there is a trend toward younger adults (30 to 50 years) and an increased involvement of the tongue, as well as an increased incidence in patients who have never smoked.

Clinical features

May variably appear as a leukoplakia, erythroleukoplakia, erythroplakia, ulcer, verrucoid tissue mass, or indurated mass. Pain may be present but is not common. It may be associated with a palpable painless lymphadenopathy.

Radiographic presentation

If the squamous cell carcinoma invades into bone, it will be seen as an osteolytic area. Extensive invasion may cause a pathologic fracture.

Differential diagnosis

The entities that may be confused with oral squamous cell carcinoma include benign hyperkeratosis, epithelial dysplasias, carcinoma in situ, verrucous carcinoma, lichen planus, and candidiasis.

Microscopic features

Sheets and cords of dysplastic epithelial cells with pleomorphic nuclei, a high nuclear to cytoplasmic ratio, and some mitotic figures. These cells will be seen infiltrating the normal structures below the basement membrane. At times, keratin pearls will be seen. The infiltrations are frequently accompanied by inflammatory cells as well.

Suggested course of action

Note and document the size of the lesion in centimeters. Palpate the neck and document the findings (ie, number, approximate size, and anatomical location of palpable lymph nodes) and then biopsy. Or refer to an oral and maxillofacial surgeon for workup, biopsy, staging, and treatment.

Treatment

Most squamous cell carcinomas are treated with surgery to remove the primary tumor along with a neck dissection of one of many possible types. Lower-staged carcinomas may not require neck dissection. More advanced–staged carcinomas will be followed by radiation therapy or a chemoradiation therapy protocol.

3

Masses Within the Soft Tissues of Oral Mucosa

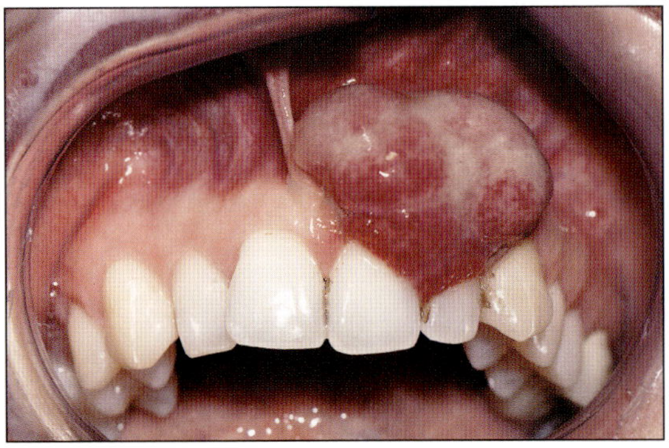

► Pyogenic granuloma.

Pyogenic Granuloma

Nature of disease

An exuberant and proliferative inflammatory response to a local focus of an infection, irritant, or foreign body.

Predilections

Can occur at any age. There is no racial predilection, but there is a small female predilection particularly during pregnancy, in which case it is referred to as a "pregnancy tumor."

Clinical features

A pyogenic granuloma will appear as a soft, fleshy, friable, and easily bleeding mass with a thin and sometimes ulcerated surface. They frequently occur on the interdental papillae but may also occur on the lips, tongue, or buccal mucosa.

Radiographic presentation

None.

Differential diagnosis

Pyogenic granulomas will closely resemble peripheral giant cell proliferations and peripheral ossifying fibromas but more importantly may appear similar to a squamous cell carcinoma or other primary malignancy, including several sarcomas or a metastatic deposit from a malignancy at a distant site.

Microscopic features

Prominent capillary channels containing red blood cells and endothelial cell proliferations are found amid an inflammatory background frequently rich in neutrophils.

Suggested course of action

Review the patient history to confirm or rule out pregnancy in women patients. Excise the mass with 2.0-mm margins, or refer to an oral and maxillofacial surgeon.

Treatment

Pyogenic granulomas are excised down to their base, and any focus of infection, foreign body, or irritating device is removed as well.

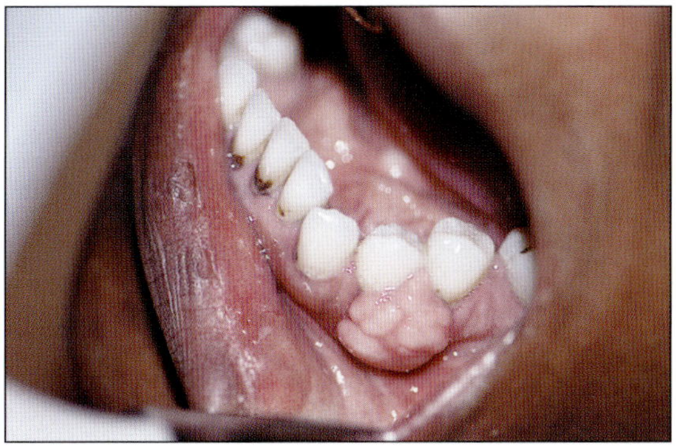

► Peripheral ossifying fibroma arising from the periodontal ligament.

Peripheral Ossifying Fibroma

Nature of disease

A benign, reactive proliferation of fibroblasts from the periodontal ligament that have retained the ability to produce bone.

Predilections

More common in young adults in general and slightly more common in women. No racial predilection is known.

Clinical features

The mass is usually less than 1.5 cm in size and has a pedunculated surface of mature epithelium without ulceration. The mass will be firm and likely will not bleed upon manipulation. It most commonly arises from the interdental papillae.

Radiographic presentation

Most periapical and other similar radiographs will appear normal. Some will identify a widened periodontal ligament space at the crestal surface or a small area of vertical bone loss.

Differential diagnosis

Masses arising out of the gingival crevice may also represent pyogenic granulomas or peripheral giant cell proliferations. However, one should also consider the more serious potential pathologies of a squamous cell carcinoma or a primary malignancy and a metastatic deposit from a malignancy at a distant site.

Microscopic features

Cellular fibrous tissue is seen together with a delicate fibrovascular component, inflammatory cells, and either trabecular bone lined by osteoblasts or round, calcified deposits.

Suggested course of action

Excise with 2.0-mm peripheral margins, including excision of the periodontal ligament structures at its base, or refer to an oral and maxillofacial surgeon.

Treatment

Excision using 2.0-mm peripheral margins and excision of its base.

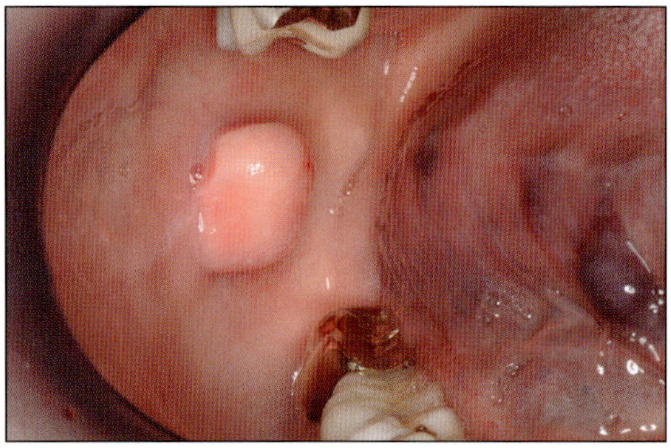

► Fibroma of the buccal mucosa.

Fibroma

Nature of disease

A reactive, benign proliferation of fibroblasts arising from submucosal fibroblasts.

Predilections

No sex or racial predilection is known. In some cases, it has been attributed to cheek or lip biting, which has spawned the term *traumatic fibroma*. However, a clear history of trauma is rare.

Clinical features

A fibroma presents as a firm, broad-based mass with an intact overlying mucosa. The mass is usually found on the buccal mucosa but may also be found on the lips, tongue, or gingiva. The lesion is not painful unless secondarily traumatized.

Radiographic presentation

None.

Differential diagnosis

Most fibromas are clinically distinctive. However, squamous papillomas, some pyogenic granulomas, submucosal salivary gland tumors, and benign soft tissue tumors such as schwannomas may also be considered.

Microscopic features

A densely collagenous stroma with normal-appearing fibroblasts, sparse capillaries, and in some cases a slight inflammatory cell presence is seen.

Suggested course of action

Excise, observing 2.0-mm margins into the submucosa but short of the underlying muscle, or refer to an oral and maxillofacial surgeon.

Treatment

Excision using 2.0-mm margins and into the submucosa shy of the muscular layer or periosteum.

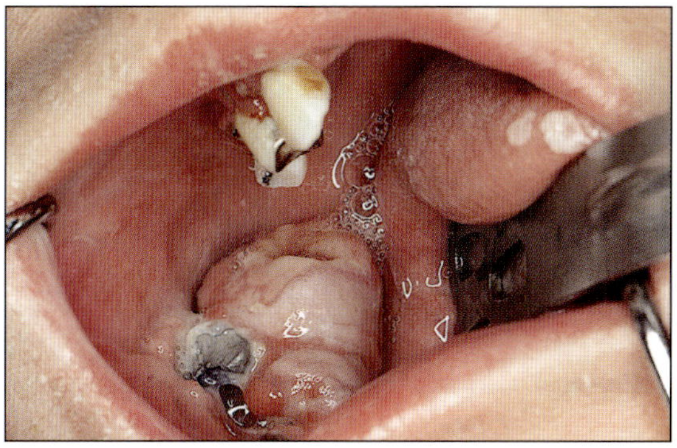

► Peripheral giant cell proliferation.

Peripheral Giant Cell Proliferation

Nature of disease
An inflammatory hyperplasia in which foreign body–type giant cells are seen in the histopathology.

Predilections
Mostly adults. No sex or racial predilection is known.

Clinical features
Lesions will present as a soft, fleshy, friable mass that bleeds easily upon manipulation. Most arise from the gingiva, but unlike the pyogenic granuloma, they may also arise from an edentulous ridge. Many are initiated by a defective dental restoration or a foreign body.

Radiographic presentation
Many peripheral giant cell proliferations will be seen to create a smooth, shallow, cupped-out resorption of the alveolar crest, while others will have no effect on the underlying bone.

Differential diagnosis
A fleshy, bleeding mass at the alveolar crest may also represent a pyogenic granuloma, squamous cell carcinoma, or other primary malignancy, as well as a metastatic deposit from a malignancy at a distant site.

Microscopic features
A fibrous cellular mass with numerous capillaries and an inflammatory infiltrate consisting of mostly plasma cells together with numerous multinucleated giant cells will be seen.

Suggested course of action
Excision observing 2.0-mm peripheral margins to and including the base of the periosteum or periodontal ligament and removal of the initiating factor if identified, or referral to an oral and maxillofacial surgeon.

Treatment
Definitive treatment is excision using 2.0-mm margins to and including the lesion's base and removal of any initiating source.

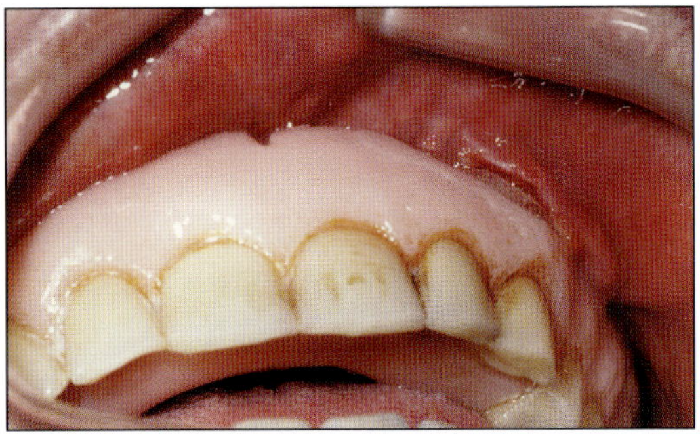

► Epulis fissuratum proliferating around a denture flange.

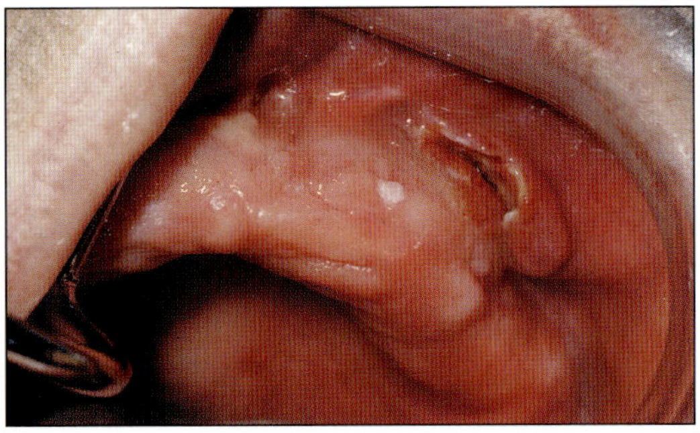

► Epulis fissuratum with the denture removed.

Epulis Fissuratum

Nature of disease

An inflammatory hyperplasia initiated by the traumatic irritation from a denture flange.

Predilections

Mostly adults. No sex or racial predilection is known.

Clinical features

Epulis fissuratums will indeed form a fissure or a groove in the mucosa around a denture flange. The mucosa is usually intact but may at times be ulcerated as it prolapses around the denture flange. Most are painless, but some discomfort may be present as well.

Radiographic presentation

None.

Differential diagnosis

The tissue proliferation and groove will suggest a squamous cell carcinoma as the main consideration. However, a pyogenic granuloma as well as a fistula or soft tissue infection from a periapical abscess, sinusitis, or bone infection should also be considered.

Microscopic features

Fibrous tissue with an inflammatory cell background mostly consisting of lymphocytes and plasma cells. Occasionally, oncocytic changes and proliferations are seen within local minor salivary glands.

Suggested course of action

Excise for biopsy or refer to an oral and maxillofacial surgeon. Remove the offending denture flange and rebase or remake the denture.

Treatment

The redundant epulis is excised to rule out carcinoma and other pathologies considered on the differential diagnosis, followed by a denture flange adjustment and rebase or remake of the appliance.

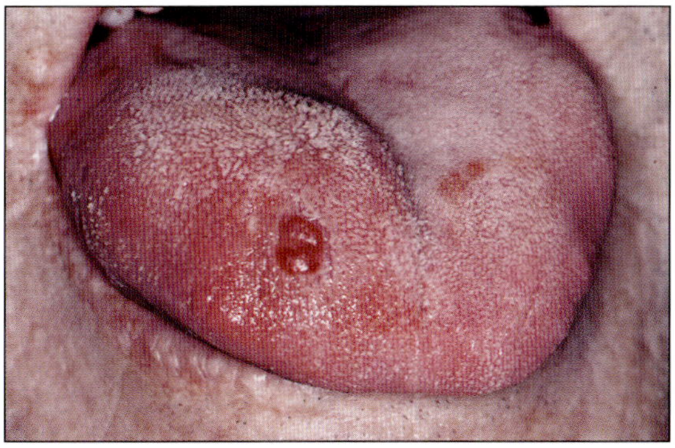

► Traumatic eosinophilic granuloma. The area around the lesion is indurated.

Traumatic Eosinophilic Granuloma

Nature of disease

A rare proliferative and ulcerated lesion whereby theory suggests a reactive response to an injury of tongue or lip muscle in which a histiocytic and eosinophilic infiltration prevents healing.

Predilections

Mostly seen in adults over 30 years of age. No sex or racial predilection is known. Most occur on the dorsum of the tongue, but more rarely they can occur on the lips or buccal mucosa.

Clinical features

Most will present as a lobulated red mass, but others will present as an ulcer with an indurated margin. Most are asymptomatic, but mild pain has been reported in some. Paresthesia or paresis is not observed.

Radiographic presentation

None.

Differential diagnosis

The firm and often indurated nature of a traumatic eosinophilic granuloma as well as a possible history of recurrence after an excision will suggest a squamous cell carcinoma or a rhabdomyosarcoma. Otherwise, a pyogenic granuloma or a granular cell tumor should be considered.

Microscopic features

Degenerating striated muscle fibers will be seen with a significant infiltration of histiocytes and eosinophils.

Suggested course of action

Excision observing 5.0-mm margins into the musculature of the tongue or referral to an oral and maxillofacial surgeon.

Treatment

Excision using 5.0-mm peripheral margins as well as a deep margin should effect a cure. However, traumatic eosinophilic granulomas are known to recur, requiring diligent follow-up.

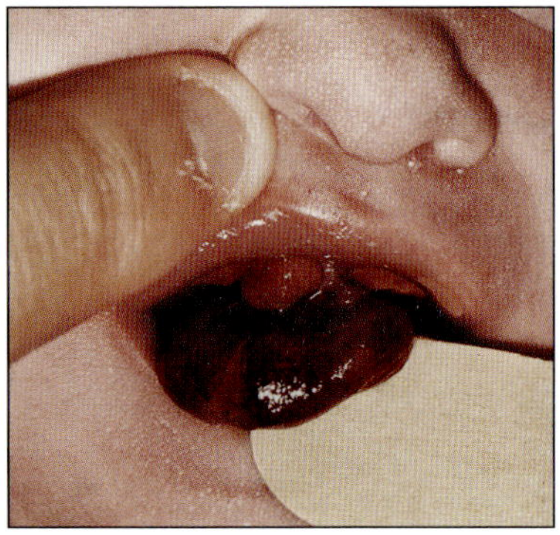

► Congenital epulis of the newborn (a granular cell hamartoma).

Congenital Epulis of the Newborn

Nature of disease

A congenital (present at birth), nonhereditary soft tissue hamartomatous proliferation of granular cells that are likely of neuroectodermal origin.

Predilections

Occurs only in newborns and favors white individuals. There is a strong female predilection. More common in the anterior maxilla (2:1) than the anterior mandible.

Clinical features

At birth, a mass will be present emerging from a short stalk from either the anterior maxillary or anterior mandibular ridge. The mass will range from less than 1 cm to as much as 12 cm, with the average around 3 cm. The surface epithelium will be intact but may be abraded from the child's hands rubbing across it.

Radiographic presentation

None. The mass arises from soft tissues of the alveolar ridge and grows outward, leaving bone unaffected.

Differential diagnosis

Masses in newborns are limited to a few pathologies that may be considered: hemangiomas, lymphangiomas, and rhabdomyosarcomas. Note: Although a melanotic neuroectodermal tumor of infancy may appear similar, it occurs in the first year of life but is not congenital.

Microscopic features

The mass is composed of uniform granular cells with little stroma and an intact, thin epithelial surface without pseudoepitheliomatous hyperplasia. The granules in the granular cells are lysosomes.

Suggested course of action

Refer to an oral and maxillofacial surgeon.

Treatment

Congenital epuli are removed in a straightforward fashion at the level of the stalk.

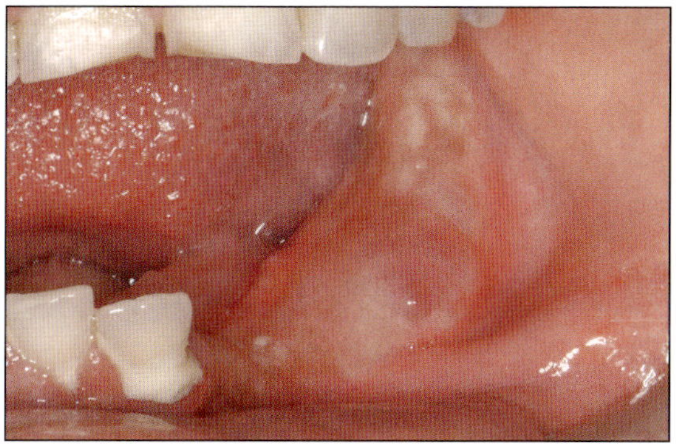

► Peripheral ameloblastoma arising from the soft tissue of the edentulous alveolar ridge.

Peripheral Odontogenic Tumors

Nature of disease

The soft tissue corollary of several central osseous odontogenic tumors. Most are extraosseous ameloblastomas, but others such as the calcifying epithelial odontogenic tumor have also been reported. All are hamartomas rather than true neoplasms. They arise from dental lamina rests (rests of Serres) in the alveolar ridge mucosa. These tumors must be solely confined to soft tissue with no bony component so as to distinguish them from central odontogenic tumors that have grown out of the bone.

Predilections

A rare finding. No age, sex, or racial predilection is known. Most occur in the molar and retromolar area.

Clinical features

Peripheral odontogenic tumors will present as a firm soft tissue mass within the submucosa. The epithelium will be intact, and the mass will be painless.

Radiographic presentation

The radiograph must show an absence within bone to qualify as a peripheral odontogenic tumor. A cupped-out surface remodeling due to the pressure exerted by the mass may be seen.

Differential diagnosis

Firm soft tissue masses particularly in the posterior mandible may represent a mucoepidermoid carcinoma or other minor salivary gland tumor. Otherwise, a peripheral ossifying fibroma or gingival cyst may be considered.

Microscopic features

The histopathology will be indistinguishable from their central bony counterpart.

Suggested course of action

Incisional biopsy or referral to an oral and maxillofacial surgeon.

Treatment

Local excision observing 5.0-mm margins to and including the periosteum.

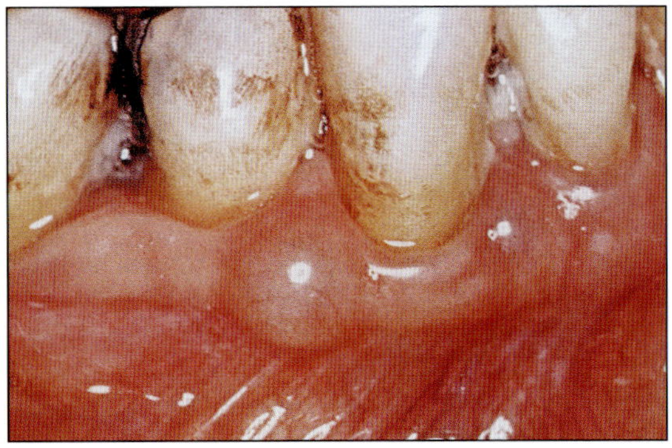

► Gingival cyst.

Gingival Cyst of the Adult

Nature of disease

A rare cyst formation in the attached gingiva arising from dental lamina rests.

Predilections

These cysts occur in adults, as opposed to Epstein pearls/Bohn nodules, which are gingival-mucosal cysts in the newborn. No sex or racial predilection is known.

Clinical features

Usually a painless expansion within the attached gingiva. The expansion is usually less than 1 cm and is not known to cause tooth mobility.

Radiographic presentation

Usually none. However, a cone beam CT scan may show a concave, cupped-out remodeling of either the buccal or lingual cortex due to pressure from cyst expansion.

Differential diagnosis

Expansions in the attached gingiva will suggest underlying pathologies within bone that have broken through the cortex, such as odontogenic keratocysts, lateral periodontal cysts, and small odontogenic tumors. Additionally, lesions such as peripheral ossifying fibromas, peripheral odontogenic tumors, and even some foci of Langerhans cell histiocytosis should be considered.

Microscopic features

Gingival cysts will possess a lumen, a lining of stratified squamous epithelium, and a connective tissue wall similar to that of other odontogenic cysts.

Suggested course of action

Excise the cyst with a pericapsular dissection for diagnosis and resolution, or refer to an oral and maxillofacial surgeon.

Treatment

Gingival cysts are resolved with a straightforward pericapsular excision.

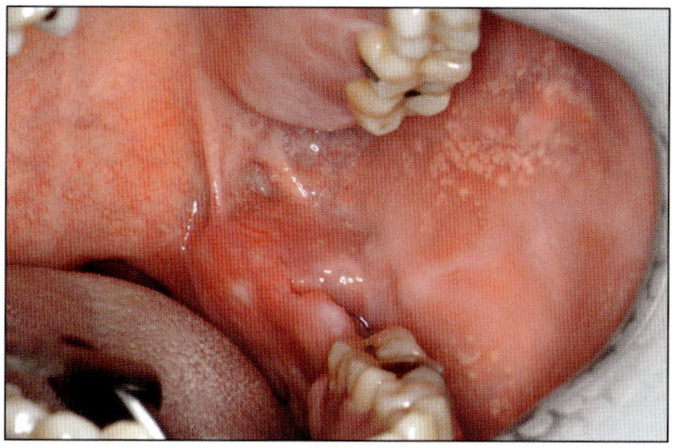

► Low-grade mucoepidermoid carcinoma in the retromolar pad.

Salivary Gland Tumors

Mucoepidermoid Carcinoma of the Oral Mucosa

Nature of disease

A malignant tumor that arises from reserve cells in the ducts of minor salivary glands and partially differentiates into mucus-secreting cells and epidermoid cells.

Predilections

In comparison with other mucosal salivary gland tumors, mucoepidermoid carcinomas have been known to occur more frequently in children and teenagers. However, the majority still develop in adults, with no sex or racial predilection. Most occur in the posterior palatal mucosa, but they also may occur in the lip, tongue, floor of the mouth, or buccal mucosa.

Clinical features

The tissue mass will appear firm or semifirm within the substance of the submucosa. It may be lobulated or noted as having a smooth surface. Ulceration may be present but often is not. In some low-grade mucoepidermoid carcinomas, the mucus production is significant enough to impart a translucent blue color to the mass. Pain or paresthesia is usually not noted.

Radiographic presentation

Most oral mucosal mucoepidermoid carcinomas are low grade and do not invade into bone. Intermediate- and high-grade mucoepidermoid carcinomas will often present with obvious osteolysis in an irregular invasive pattern.

Differential diagnosis

Mucoepidermoid carcinomas of the oral mucosa will appear similar to the other two prominent malignant salivary gland tumors: adenoid cystic carcinoma and polymorphous low-grade adenocarcinoma. If the mucosa is not ulcerated, pleomorphic adenoma should also be considered. If located within the substance of the upper lip, a canalicular adenoma should be considered. →

Mucoepidermoid Carcinoma of the Oral Mucosa *(cont)*

Microscopic features

1. Low-grade mucoepidermoid carcinomas will have well-formed cysts containing mucin. Mucus-secreting cells will be predominant. However, intermediate cells and epidermoid cells will be present as well. However, all cell types are mature and will not show atypia or mitotic figures.
2. Intermediate-grade mucoepidermoid carcinomas will have few if any mucus cysts and will be more solid. Intermediate and epidermoid cells are more numerous, and mucus-secreting cells are more sparse than with low-grade tumors. Some nuclear pleomorphism is usually seen but no mitotic figures.
3. High-grade mucoepidermoid carcinomas are solid without cystic spaces and consist only of intermediate cells and epidermoid cells. Cells will show considerable atypia and some mitotic figures. The absence of any mucus-secreting cells frequently requires the identification of intracellular mucin via a mucicarmine stain for diagnosis.

Suggested course of action

Refer to an oral and maxillofacial surgeon for biopsy and workup.

Treatment

1. Low-grade tumors: Wide local excision observing 1.5-cm margins controlled with frozen sections.
2. Intermediate-grade tumors: Wide local excision observing 2.0-cm margins controlled with frozen sections. Excision of bone is required if imaging identifies bone involvement.
3. High-grade tumor: Very wide excision observing 3.0-cm margins controlled with frozen sections, likely resection of adjacent bone, and an ipsilateral or bilateral neck dissection as per the examination and imaging findings, followed by postoperative radiotherapy.

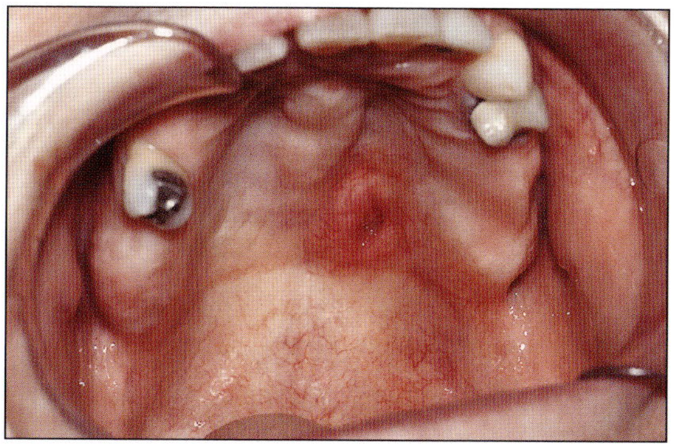

► Adenoid cystic carcinoma of the palate.

Adenoid Cystic Carcinoma of the Oral Mucosa

Nature of disease

A malignant salivary gland tumor that arises from reserve cells in the ductal system of minor salivary glands. It is well known to undergo perineural and intraneural invasion as well as to spread proximally along the involved nerve. It is also well known to grow slowly but metastasize readily and early, giving it a favorable 5-year prognosis but an unfavorable 10-year prognosis.

Predilections

Adults. There is no sex or racial predilection. In the oral mucosa, the most common site is the palate, but it has also been reported to occur in the tongue, lips, and buccal mucosa.

Clinical features

Most present as a painless submucosal mass. The surface may be intact but can also be ulcerated. Paresthesia is variably present, depending on the location of the mass, and may require objective testing to detect early subtle changes. Larger lesions may be painful and can cause facial asymmetry.

Radiographic presentation

In some early cases, no radiographic changes are evident. More commonly, bone erosion and osteolysis are seen with a soft tissue density replacing the bone.

Differential diagnosis

Adenoid cystic carcinomas will present similar to other minor salivary malignancies such as mucoepidermoid carcinomas and polymorphous low-grade adenocarcinomas. If the overlying mucosa is intact, a pleomorphic adenoma should also be considered.

Microscopic features

Small, cuboidal, highly basophilic cells with little if any pleomorphism or mitotic figures are present in all cases. There will also be a mixture of three well-known patterns: cribriform, tubular, and solid. Most tumors contain two or more patterns, with one pattern predominating.

Suggested course of action

Suspected cases should be referred to an oral and maxillofacial surgeon for biopsy and workup.

Treatment

Aggressive surgery is required. In the palate, a hemimaxillectomy up to the skull base is followed by radiotherapy with or without adjunctive chemotherapy. In other soft tissue sites, a wide excision observing 3.0-cm margins and tracing any nerve trunk proximally to clear margins or to the base of the skull is performed, followed by radiotherapy. Note: Neutron or proton beam radiotherapy is more effective than other forms of radiotherapy for adenoid cystic carcinomas.

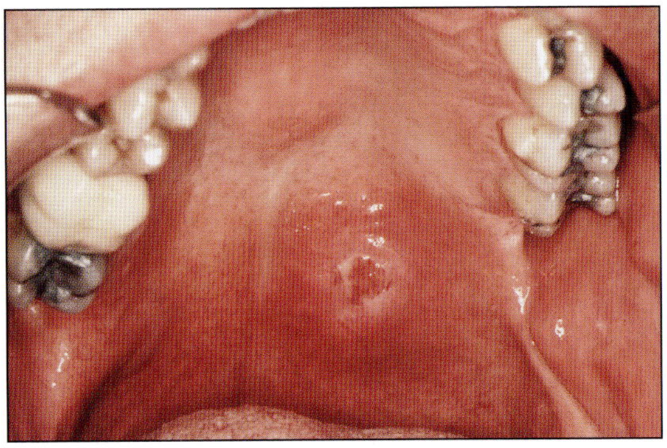

► Polymorphous low-grade adenocarcinoma of the palate.

Polymorphous Low-Grade Adenocarcinoma of the Oral Mucosa

Nature of disease

A low-grade carcinoma arising from reserve cells in the ductal epithelium of minor salivary glands that will be neurotropic but will not exhibit perineural spread.

Predilections

Adults, with a female predilection. No racial predilection is known. Most occur in the posterior palate, but the buccal mucosa and upper lip or base of the tongue have been reported as other sites. This tumor is not known to occur within the major salivary glands.

Clinical features

The tissue mass will be semifirm to firm. The overlying mucosa is usually intact but may be ulcerated at times. The mass will be painless without lobulations.

Radiographic presentation

Most polymorphous low-grade adenocarcinomas are sufficiently low grade that they do not invade into adjacent bone. The few that do will show an erosion of bone and/or localized osteolysis.

Differential diagnosis

Polymorphous low-grade adenocarcinomas will appear similar to the two other prominent salivary gland malignances: adenoid cystic carcinoma and mucoepidermoid carcinoma. If the mucosa is intact, a pleomorphic adenoma should be considered. If it occurs on the upper lip, a canalicular adenoma should also be considered.

Microscopic features

Strands, nests, ducts, and solid cords of cells with pale nuclei and an ill-defined cytoplasm make up this tumor. The stroma is mostly fibrous but may also be myxoid. A cribriform pattern is frequently noted, along with a whorled pattern around small nerves as well as some solid areas.

Suggested course of action

Refer to an oral and maxillofacial surgeon for biopsy and workup.

Treatment

Polymorphous low-grade adenocarcinomas are treated with a wide soft tissue excision, observing 2.0-cm margins controlled with frozen sections. If imaging identifies bone involvement, local bone resection is also accomplished.

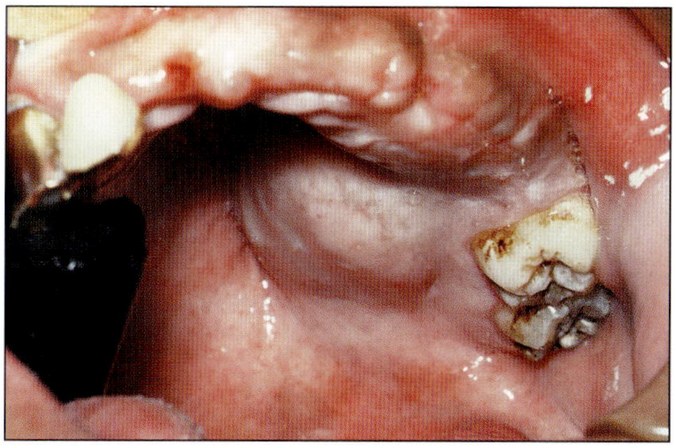

► Pleomorphic adenoma of the palate.

Pleomorphic Adenoma of the Oral Mucosa

Nature of disease

A benign neoplasm that arises from reserve cells within the ductal system of minor salivary glands.

Predilections

Adults. There is no sex or racial predilection. They occur most commonly within the posterior aspect of the palatal submucosa but may also occur in all places where minor salivary glands exist (ie, lips, buccal mucosa, floor of the mouth, etc).

Clinical features

Pleomorphic adenomas of the oral mucosa will present as a firm, movable mass within the submucosa. In its most common location in the palatal submucosa, it may not be mobile due to the restriction of the palatal mucosa itself. The mass is painless and will not be ulcerated unless trauma or a previous biopsy has taken place.

Radiographic presentation

Occasionally, a larger-sized tumor will create a concave, cupped-out thinning of the bony palate due to backpressure from the unyielding palatal soft tissues. Otherwise, no radiographic features are seen.

Differential diagnosis

In the palate, malignant salivary gland tumors such as adenoid cystic carcinomas, mucoepidermoid carcinomas, and polymorphous low-grade adenocarcinomas are the main considerations. In the upper lip, the canalicular adenoma, which is the more common tumor in this location, together with mucous cysts and the same three malignant salivary gland tumors should be considered.

Microscopic features

A diverse array of features may be present from a proliferation of ductal epithelium and myoepithelium. A chondromyxoid matrix is usually seen, foci of hyalinization or keratinization are occasionally seen, and even calcifications may be rarely seen. A collagenous capsule may be present, but it is not a true capsule that contains the tumor. Tumor cells are usually seen within the capsule.

Suggested course of action

Refer to an oral and maxillofacial surgeon.

Treatment

Pleomorphic adenomas cannot be removed for cure by enucleation because of the presence of tumor cells in the capsule. Instead, they require an excision with 1.0-cm margins controlled by frozen sections. In the palate, the palatal periosteum serves as an anatomical barrier. Excision of bone in any location of a pleomorphic adenoma is unnecessary.

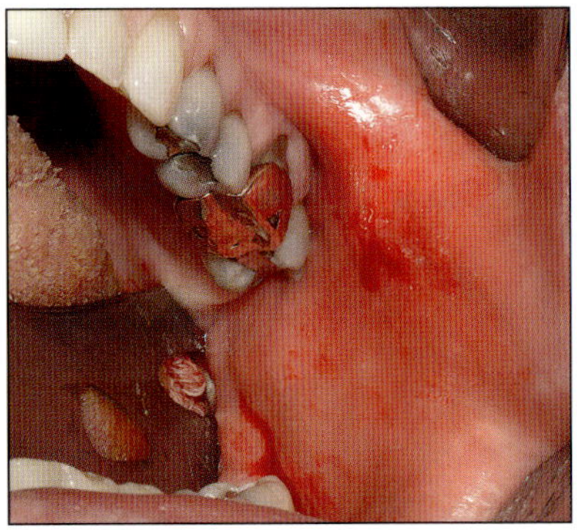

► Basal cell adenoma in the left buccal mucosa.

Basal Cell Adenoma of the Oral Mucosa

Nature of disease

A benign neoplasm arising from the reserve cells in the ductal epithelium of minor salivary glands.

Predilections

Adults over 50 years of age, with a male predilection. Most occur in the parotid gland (70%). However, when they occur in the oral mucosa, the upper lip is the most common site.

Clinical features

Similar to the canalicular adenoma, basal bell adenomas present as small (< 3 cm), round, painless, freely movable masses within the submucosa.

Radiographic presentation

None.

Differential diagnosis

When located on the upper lip, a canalicular adenoma, a mucous cyst, and a pleomorphic adenoma are strong considerations. Malignant salivary gland tumors such as a mucoepidermoid carcinoma and adenoid cystic carcinoma should also be considered.

Microscopic features

Uniform cells with prominent basophilic staining and oval nuclei without pleomorphism or atypia may be seen in either a solid, trabecular, or tubular pattern. The background is a poorly collagenized but hyalinized stroma similar to that seen in canalicular adenomas.

Suggested course of action

Refer to an oral and maxillofacial surgeon for biopsy and treatment.

Treatment

For basal cell adenomas occurring within the oral mucosa, a pericapsular excision or excision with 2.0-mm margins is curative.

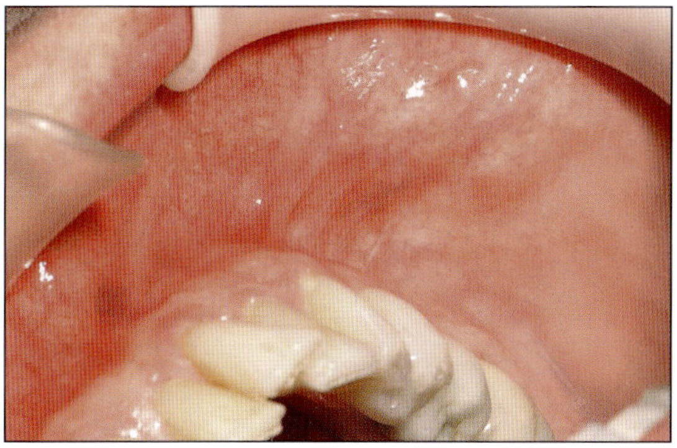

► Canalicular adenoma within the substance of the upper lip.

Canalicular Adenoma

Nature of disease

A benign neoplasm arising from the reserve cells in the ductal epithelium of minor salivary glands.

Predilections

Exclusively involves oral mucosal minor salivary glands. A distinct female predilection and a site predilection for the upper lip (80%) is well known. Most patients are over 50 years of age. No racial predilection is known.

Clinical features

Most are single, round, freely movable masses less than 3 cm in diameter. About 20% are multifocal as separate round, movable masses. The masses are painless, and the overlying mucosa is intact.

Radiographic presentation

None.

Differential diagnosis

Benign considerations include mucous cysts, basal cell adenomas, and pleomorphic adenomas. Additionally, a minor salivary gland sialolith may be considered. Malignant tumor considerations include mucoepidermoid carcinomas and adenoid cystic carcinomas.

Microscopic features

Cuboidal and columnar-shaped cells in a double row forming cords and ductlike formations that are seen connected together in a chainlike fashion against a pale eosinophilic stroma of minimal collagen. There is usually a thin capsule without tumor cells in the capsule.

Suggested course of action

Refer to an oral and maxillofacial surgeon for excisional biopsy and workup for multifocal masses.

Treatment

The single mass or all of the masses representing canalicular adenoma can be excised for cure using a pericapsular dissection.

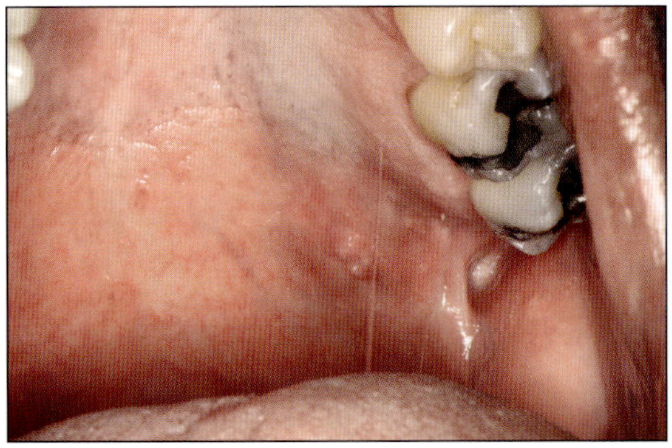

► Low-grade acinic cell carcinoma of the palate.

Acinic Cell Carcinoma of the Oral Mucosa

Nature of disease

Usually a low-grade malignancy arising from the reserve cells of minor salivary gland ductal epithelium. A rare high-grade type occurs as well.

Predilections

Most occur in the parotid gland, but they can also be located in oral sites, especially the palatal and buccal mucosa. Most occur in adults, but rare cases have been reported in children. There is a slight female predilection, with no racial predilection known.

Clinical features

In the oral mucosa, they will appear as a small, lobulated, freely movable mass usually with an intact surface. Like the mucoepidermoid carcinoma, they may have a slight bluish appearance. There is usually no paresthesia noted with this tumor, unless it is the high-grade type.

Radiographic presentation

Most have no radiographic presentation due to their usual low-grade biology. However, the rare high-grade counterpart will show extensive irregular bone resorption.

Differential diagnosis

If the mass has a slight bluish coloration, low-grade mucoepidermoid carcinoma would be the most serious consideration. Otherwise, pleomorphic adenomas, polymorphous low-grade adenocarcinomas, and adenoid cystic carcinomas should be considered.

Microscopic features

Oral mucosal acinic cell carcinomas are often encapsulated at least partially. A solid, papillary, or cystic pattern is created by rounded or polygonal cells with an eosinophilic cytoplasm but a deeply basophilic-staining eccentric nucleus. The cystic spaces are eosinophilic. The tumor cells frequently have coarse, dark-staining granules reminiscent of the zymogen granules seen in the normal parotid acini.

Suggested course of action

Refer to an oral and maxillofacial surgeon for workup and treatment.

Treatment

Excision with 1.5-cm margins controlled with frozen sections is curative. In the rare high-grade acinic cell carcinoma, a resection observing 3.0-cm margins as well as any involved bone followed by radiotherapy is the preferred treatment.

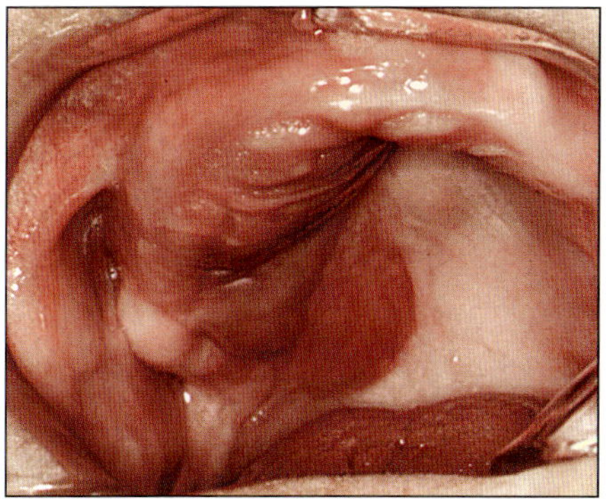

► Extranodal presentation of a non-Hodgkin lymphoma.

Non-Hodgkin Lymphoma

Nature of disease

A proliferation of any one of several types of malignant lymphocyte precursors of the B-cell type or T-cell type.

Predilections

The risk for non-Hodgkin lymphoma increases with age. Extranodal sites, particularly in the palate, pharynx, and buccal mucosa, are more common than in Hodgkin lymphomas. There is no known sex or racial predilection.

Clinical features

In the oral cavity a diffuse, soft, fleshy expansion of the palatal and maxillary mucosa is a common presentation. Others include submucosal masses that may occur with or without cervical lymph node enlargement. Some patients will present with only large, painless neck masses. Many will be seen to have suffered weight loss or will report fatigue.

Radiographic presentation

CT, MRI, and PET scans will identify locations of either nodal or extranodal sites.

Differential diagnosis

Extranodal sites in the palate may be confused with a squamous cell carcinoma or an underlying bone necrosis, such as drug-induced osteonecrosis, osteoradionecrosis, or even an osteomyelitis. Masses within the submucosa will most closely resemble salivary gland tumors and benign schwannomas. Cervical chain lymph node masses may represent a Hodgkin lymphoma, cat-scratch disease, sarcoidosis, or HIV infection. →

Non-Hodgkin Lymphoma *(cont)*

Microscopic features

There are too many types of non-Hodgkin lymphoma to describe each variant. However, the central theme is a sheet of altered lymphocytes that resemble plasma cells instead of lymphocytes in a monotonous pattern where all cells look alike. The distinction for the specific type of non-Hodgkin lymphoma is based on cell size and whether it is a B-cell or T-cell lymphoma. The most recognized types of non-Hodgkin lymphoma are the following:

- Small, lymphocytic B-cell lymphoma
- Extranodal marginal B-cell lymphoma (MALT lymphoma)
- Follicular B-cell lymphoma
- Mantle cell lymphoma
- Diffuse large B-cell lymphoma
- Burkitt lymphoma (small noncleaved cell lymphoma), African type or American type
- Anaplastic large cell lymphoma
- Extranodal natural killer T-cell lymphoma nasal type (previously known as *midline lethal granuloma of the palate*)
- Mycosis fungoides (a peripheral lymphatic lymphoma of the T-cell type)

Note: Large-cell lymphomas generally have a poorer prognosis than small-cell lymphomas.

Suggested course of action

Previously undiagnosed patients suspicious for non-Hodgkin lymphoma should be referred to a hematologist-oncologist. Already diagnosed patients should receive supportive dental and oral care throughout their treatment course.

Treatment

Each type of lymphoma is treated with a different type of specific chemotherapy protocol, with the addition of radiation therapy in selected cases and for selected sites.

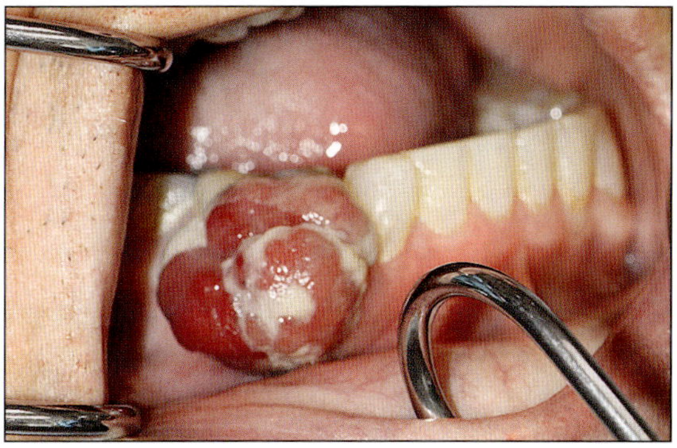

► Breast cancer metastasis to the mandible.

Metastatic Carcinoma Deposits

Nature of disease

A clonal proliferation of malignant cells that have traveled to the jaws or to oral mucosa from a distant site, mostly via venous routes but sometimes via the lymphatics.

Predilections

Most patients have already been diagnosed with a primary malignancy, but some metastatic deposits are from a previously undiagnosed cancer. Breast cancer remains the most common primary site, with an obvious predilection for women, followed by lung cancer with a predilection for men, and then kidney, gastrointestinal tract, prostate, and other cancers. No racial predilection is known. Adults are mostly affected.

Clinical features

Most metastatic deposits in the oral and maxillofacial area are in the mandible, which may cause an expansion, paresthesia, or at times a pathologic fracture. The maxilla is more rarely a site for metastatic deposits, which occur as a sinus or posterior maxillary expansion. Soft tissue metastasis without bone involvement is uncommon (1 to 30 as compared with bone) and occurs mostly as a gingival mass. A common clinical scenario is an isolated mobile tooth that is removed under the diagnosis of advanced periodontal bone loss only to have the metastatic deposit grow out of the socket as a fleshy mass.

Radiographic presentation

Metastases to bone mostly appear as irregular radiolucencies with mild expansion in the mandible. Advanced cases may be associated with a pathologic fracture.

Differential diagnosis

The irregular radiolucency of a metastatic deposit will suggest a primary malignancy, drug-induced osteonecrosis, or osteomyelitis. Osteoradionecrosis is a strong consideration if the patient has previously received tumoricidal doses (> 6,000 cGy) of radiation to the jaws. Soft tissue deposits will be similar to a peripheral giant cell proliferation, a pyogenic granuloma, and a peripheral ossifying fibroma.

Microscopic features

The metastatic deposit will resemble that of the primary site. However, many metastatic deposits are sufficiently undifferentiated that special stains or genetic testing of the cells is needed to ascertain the primary tumor. →

Metastatic Carcinoma Deposits *(cont)*

Suggested course of action

Referral to an oral and maxillofacial surgeon for biopsy and workup.

Treatment

Usually, continued treatment of the primary site is undertaken. In cases of severe pain or a pathologic fracture, resection of the involved area is accomplished as a palliative measure. In cases of painful cancers with a known sensitivity to radiation (ie, plasmacytomas), radiation can be used as a palliative measure.

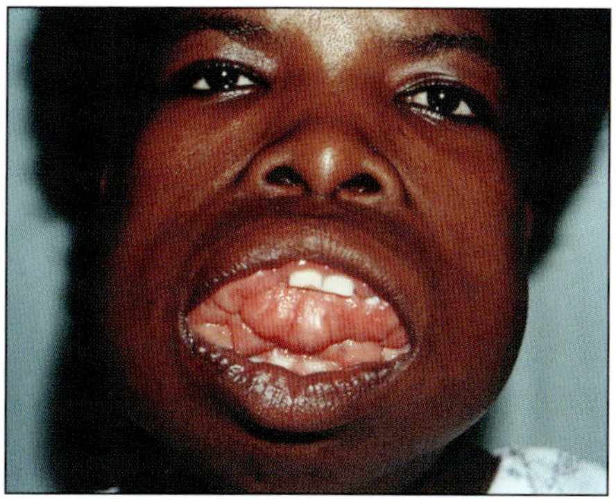

► Hereditary gingival fibromatosis.

Gingival Fibromatosis

Nature of disease

An autosomal dominant genetic trait whereby the gingiva in both jaws undergoes a deposition of dense collagen.

Predilections

Nearly all affected individuals are males of African heritage. Despite its being a genetic trait, it is not congenital. Most patients develop gingival overgrowth in their teenage years.

Clinical features

The gingiva will be enlarged and firm, and the gingival surface will be intact. Many affected patients develop severe gingival enlargement sufficient to cover their dentition. Secondary pseudopockets, gingivitis, and periodontal bone loss related to the encumbrances to oral hygiene are also frequently present.

Radiographic presentation

In longstanding cases, periodontal bone loss is seen; otherwise, bone is not directly affected.

Differential diagnosis

Other diseases that are known to produce a firm gingival enlargement include drug-induced gingival hyperplasia, most commonly seen from phenytoin or cyclosporine use and more rarely from calcium channel blockers; Ramon syndrome, which is cherubism together with gingival fibromatosis; and hereditary neurofibromatosis. Note: Leukemic gingival infiltrates may also cause a gingival enlargement but one that is soft and friable.

Microscopic features

The surface epithelium is normal. However, the subepithelial layers will consist of dense, poorly cellular collagen without inflammation.

Suggested course of action

Suspicious cases should be afforded a prophylaxis, oral hygiene instruction, and routine dental care. A referral to an oral and maxillofacial surgeon for workup and definitive treatment is recommended.

Treatment

Excision via a gingivectomy approach will uncover the teeth and provide for more direct oral hygiene and dental care. Note: The concern about hyperplastic gingival regrowth is replete in older texts but is overstated. Although a tendency for gingival regrowth does exist, the regrowth is much reduced, and in older patients this tendency subsides altogether.

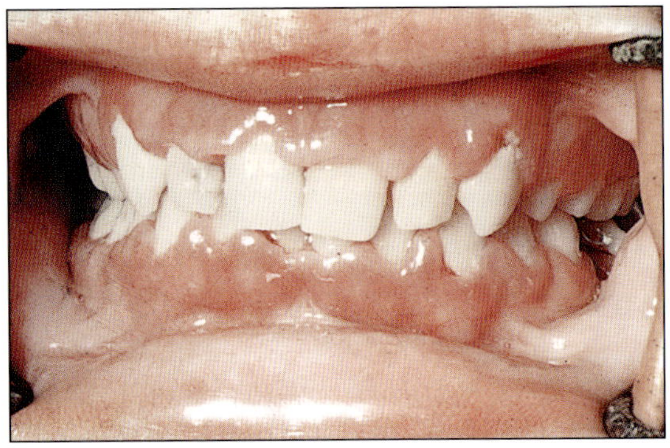

► Friable, soft gingival enlargement seen with a leukemic infiltrate from acute lymphocytic leukemia.

Leukemic Gingival Infiltrate

Nature of disease

A very rare manifestation that may develop from any one of the several subtypes of leukemia whereby malignant white cells infiltrate the gingiva in large numbers.

Predilections

Contrary to some popular thought, any white blood cell derived from bone marrow can produce a leukemic gingival infiltrate. However, it is worthy to note that acute lymphocytic leukemia (ALL) occurs mostly in pre-teenage children, acute myelogenous leukemia (AML) occurs mostly in teenagers and young adults, and both chronic lymphocytic leukemia (CLL) and chronic myelogenous leukemia (CML) occur mostly in adults over 40 years of age.

Clinical features

The gingiva will be enlarged and soft, often with a red/bluish color, and will easily bleed upon manipulation. This presentation is often referred to as "puffy gums." It is painless. Tooth mobility can occur due to alveolar bone resorption.

Radiographic presentation

The alveolar bone is usually of normal appearance. However, severe periodontal bone loss such as that seen in Langerhans cell histiocytosis and rapid progressive periodontitis may also be observed.

Differential diagnosis

The generalized friable nature of a leukemic gingival infiltrate is similar to that of advanced nonspecific gingivitis/periodontitis or rapid progressive periodontitis from a macrophage/neutrophil deficiency related to *Aggregatibacter actinomycetemcomitans* organisms or their related expression in Papillon-Lefèvre syndrome. Hereditary gingival fibromatosis and drug-induced gingival hyperplasia may also be considered but are clinically firm rather than friable.

Microscopic features

A dense infiltration of a monotony of identical-appearing lymphocytes are seen in the subepithelial layers of the gingiva.

Suggested course of action

Referral to a hematologic oncologist for workup and treatment.

Treatment

Each subtype of leukemia is treated with a separate and a specific chemotherapy protocol, sometimes supplemented with either a bone marrow or stem cell transplant.

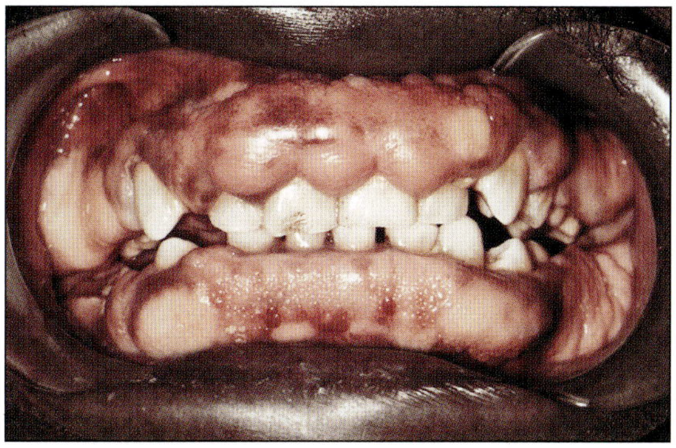

► Gingival fibromatosis caused by Dilantin (Pfizer) therapy for seizures.

Drug-Induced Gingival Fibromatosis

Nature of disease

A stimulation of gingival fibroblasts by certain drugs (ie, phenytoin, cyclosporine, calcium channel blockers) that results in the deposition of dense extracellular collagen, imparting a firm enlargement to the gingiva.

Predilections

No specific age, sex, or racial predilection is known. May occur in any person taking these drugs but does not occur in the majority of those receiving these drugs.

Clinical features

The gingiva will be firm and enlarged without ulceration or changes in the surface. The gingiva is painless and will not bleed upon probing unless secondary gingival inflammation has developed from pseudopocket formation.

Radiographic presentation

Usually none. However, some periodontal bone loss may be seen in cases where secondary gingival inflammation developed from pseudopocket formation.

Differential diagnosis

A firm gingival enlargement is also seen in hereditary gingival fibromatosis, hereditary neurofibromatosis, and in the rare variant of cherubism known as *Ramon syndrome*. A leukemic gingival infiltrate may be considered but will be soft and friable rather than firm and unresilient.

Microscopic features

The subepithelial connective tissue will appear as a poorly cellular, dense collagen composite with an intact epithelium and without inflammation.

Suggested course of action

Review the patient's history and confirm the use of medications known to produce gingival fibromatosis. Compose a letter to the prescribing physician about your findings and/or refer the patient to an oral and maxillofacial surgeon for diagnosis confirmation and workup.

Treatment

If feasible, discontinuation of the offending drug or prescription of an alternative drug for the same indication will result in a gradual, albeit incomplete reduction of the gingival enlargement. Gingivectomy is the treatment of choice. If the offending drug has been discontinued, the gingival enlargement will not recur. If the offending drug is required, the gingival enlargement will gradually recur, often requiring repeated surgeries.

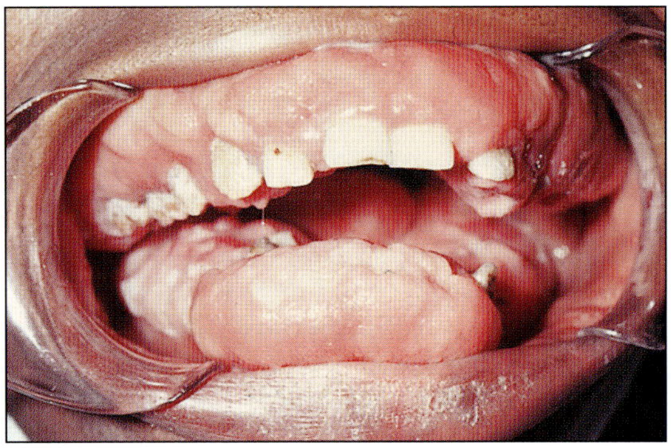

► Gingival enlargement from hereditary neurofibromatosis type 1.

Hereditary Neurofibromatosis Type 1

Nature of disease

An autosomal dominant inherited trait due to a mutation in the pericentromeric proximal gene locus on chromosome 17. However, only half of cases are caused by direct parental gene inheritance. The other half are caused by a spontaneous new mutation (sporadic occurrence), after which that individual transmits the new mutation to his or her offspring.

Predilections

Most cases are suspected before the age of 10 years with the emergence of café au lait spots and confirmed in the preteen/teen years with the development of neurofibromas. There is no known sex or racial predilection.

Clinical features

Café au lait spots are most noted in the axilla but are also frequently seen on the buttocks and chest. They are noted to have smooth, regular borders. Neurofibromas mostly occur on the skin of the face as raised nodules that gradually increase in size and number throughout the years. Other skin areas are also involved to varying degrees. Oral neurofibromas affect mostly the tongue, floor of the mouth, and palate. When they occur within the gingiva, the clinical presentation will mimic that of hereditary gingival fibromatosis. Brown pigmented spots on the iris (Lisch nodules) are also very common, and central bony lesions representing a neurofibroma can occur occasionally. Rare and more concerning are intra-abdominal neurofibromas, which have a greater propensity for malignant transformation. Such tumors may produce cramping, abdominal pain, nausea, or constipation.

Radiographic presentation

Neurofibromas in bone will be seen as a radiolucency with irregular borders. Intra-abdominal neurofibromas are best seen on a CT scan or MRI scan in which a high water content mass or masses will be noted within the peritoneum.

Differential diagnosis

Individual neurofibromas will be soft in texture mimicking a lipoma, lymphangioma, or a deep-seated hemangioma. Gingival lesions will suggest hereditary gingival fibromatosis, drug-induced gingival hyperplasia, and Ramon syndrome.

Microscopic features

Neurofibromas are unencapsulated. They will show spindle cells with wavy collagen and numerous small blood vessels and capillaries. →

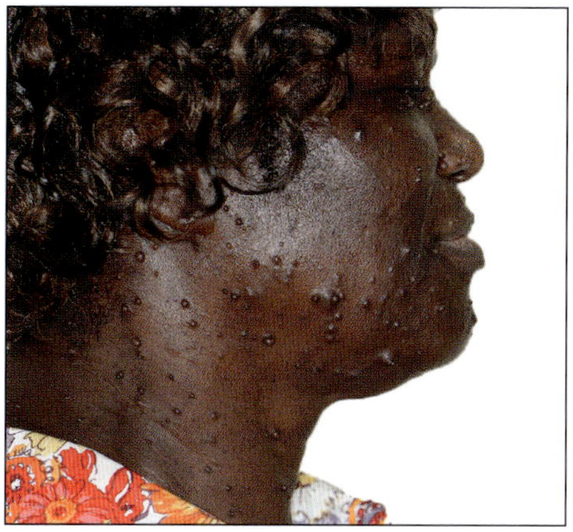

► Neurofibromas of skin in a beginning expression of hereditary neurofibromatosis type 1.

Suggested course of action

Take photographs of the face and oral cavity to document the number and size of any neurofibromas present. Look for café au lait spots and document their size and locations. Refer the patient to a major medical center for a comprehensive workup and genetic testing.

Treatment

There is no cure for hereditary neurofibromatosis type 1. Large lesions limiting function or causing pain may be excised. Note: Partial excision of a neurofibroma is often accomplished so as not to create excessive surgical morbidity. The partially excised neurofibroma will not grow back at a rate faster than the original growth rate when the lesion was removed.

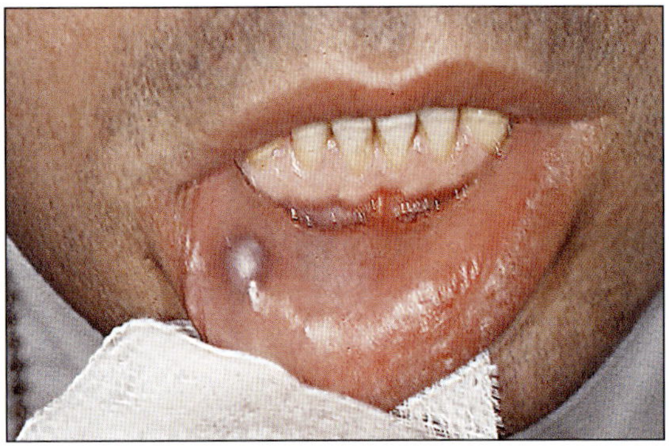

► Mucocele of the lower lip.

Mucoceles

Nature of disease

A disruption of a minor salivary gland duct resulting in extravasation of saliva into the surrounding area. Note: Mucoceles of the maxillary sinus are not true mucoceles but represent inflammatory hyperplasia of the mucus-secreting cells in the sinus membrane.

Predilections

Most occur in children, teenagers, and young adults. Slightly more common in females, with no known racial predilection. They are most common in the lower lip but also may occur in other mucosal surfaces.

Clinical features

Mucoceles will be seen as discrete, small (usually less than 1 cm) mucosal nodules with a thin surface. Most will imply a fluid content, and many will have a bluish color. Most are nonpainful. Contrary to popular assumption, a history of lip biting or trauma is not present. This is because mucoceles and even ranulas mostly arise from developmental defects in salivary ducts, which explains to some extent their predilection for children and young adults.

Radiographic presentation

None.

Differential diagnosis

Blue nodules in the lower lip may also represent low-grade mucoepidermoid carcinomas or even some other minor salivary gland tumors such as acinic cell carcinomas. One may also include pleomorphic adenomas if the blue quality is not as pronounced or absent altogether. Other considerations include scar accumulations from previous lip trauma or surgery and minor salivary gland sialoliths.

Microscopic features

Mucoceles will have a connective tissue–lined cavity filled with mucin in which scattered macrophages and other inflammatory cells are present. Adjacent normal mucous salivary glands are also often seen on excisional biopsy specimens.

Suggested course of action

Local excision observing 2.0-mm margins and obtaining primary closure, or referral to an oral and maxillofacial surgeon. Note: One must be sure to submit any suspected mucocele specimen for a pathologic assessment to rule out a salivary gland tumor or another unanticipated diagnosis.

Treatment

Excisional biopsy observing 2.0-mm margins.

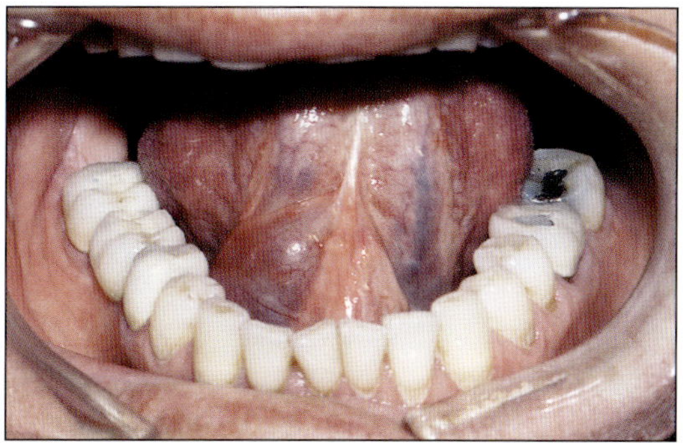

► Ranula in the floor of the mouth.

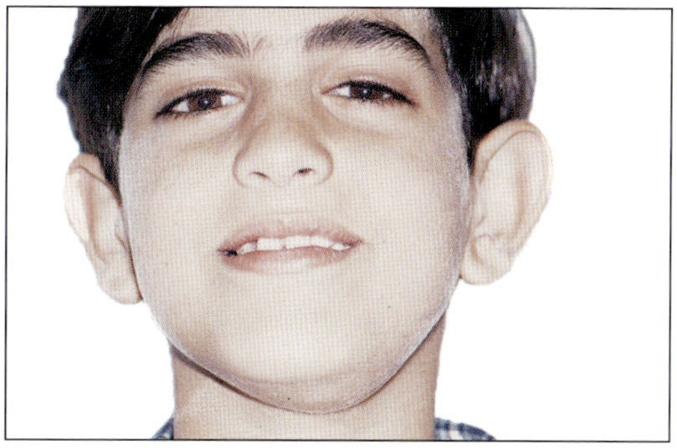

► Plunging ranula seen as a soft expansion in the submental area.

Ranulas

Nature of disease

A disruption of one of the many ducts arising from a sublingual salivary gland that results in the extravasation of saliva into the floor of mouth.

Predilections

Most occur in children, teenagers, and young adults. There is a slight female predilection, with no known racial predilection.

Clinical features

Most ranulas are confined to the floor of the mouth and will present as a dense, blue-colored expansion. The "plunging ranula" will also present as a fluid-filled compressible expansion in the submental triangle. In both areas, the mucosa and skin are intact, and the expansion is painless.

Radiographic presentation

Plain radiographs will not identify a ranula. However, CT scans will identify a hypodense area on the side of the affected sublingual gland. An MRI scan will identify the high water content of a ranula and will also imply the offending sublingual gland.

Differential diagnosis

Ranulas are somewhat distinctive. However, mucoepidermoid carcinomas and other salivary gland tumors should be considered as well. Additionally, the uncommon dermoid cyst, which is known to occur in the floor of the mouth or in the submental triangle, and an odontogenic abscess that has created a floor of the mouth space infection and/or a submental space infection may be considered.

Microscopic features

Like mucoceles, ranulas are soft tissue cavities lined by connective tissue that will contain mucin in which macrophages and inflammatory cells are scattered.

Suggested course of action

Refer to an oral and maxillofacial surgeon for workup and treatment.

Treatment

Some ranulas respond to unroofing procedures. However, for those that recur and for the most curative approach, excision including removal of the offending sublingual gland is preferred. Note: Plunging ranulas require an extraoral approach to remove the entire ranula and the offending sublingual gland.

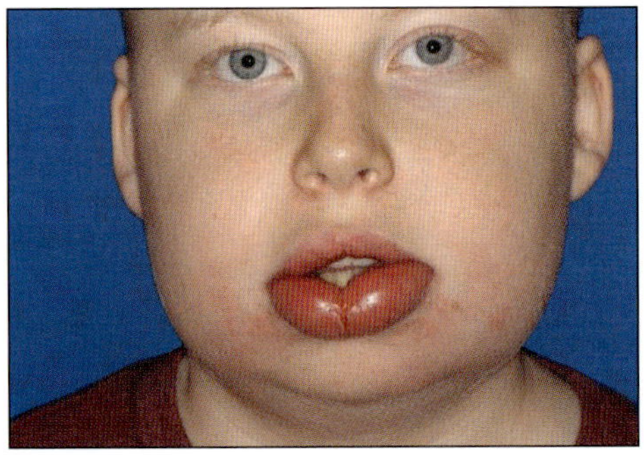

► Symmetric enlargement of the lips and cheeks in orofacial granulomatosis.

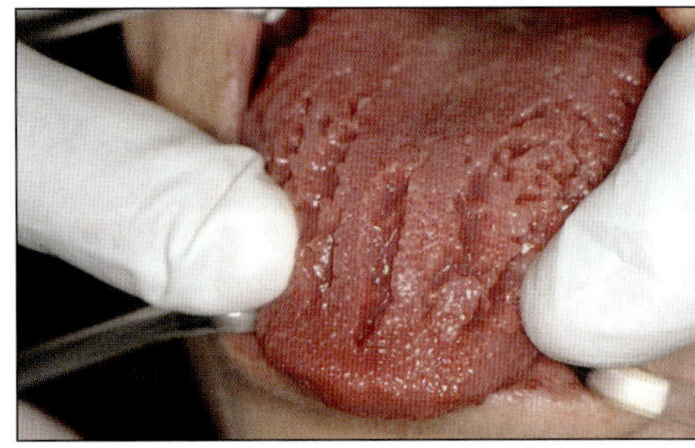

► Fissured tongue seen in the Melkersson-Rosenthal syndrome variant of orofacial granulomatosis.

Orofacial Granulomatosis

Nature of disease

A disease of unknown etiology in which true histologic discrete granulomas develop in the lips, cheeks, and/or gingiva, resulting in expansion that is sometimes extensive, causing disfigurement. This relatively new terminology encompasses the older terms of *cheilitis granulomatosis* and *Melkersson-Rosenthal syndrome*. Oral expressions of Crohn disease are also considered under this term, even though Crohn disease is more widespread in the gastrointestinal tract and is discussed separately in this text.

Predilections

A slight female predilection as well as a tendency for young adults. There is no known racial predilection.

Clinical features

The upper and lower lips are the main sites of occurrence, followed by the cheeks and gingiva. If or when the tongue becomes fissured or a transient facial muscle paralysis occurs, it may be called the *Melkersson-Rosenthal syndrome*. The enlargement of the lips and cheeks is not usually painful but can be disfiguring.

Radiographic presentation

None.

Differential diagnosis

Enlargement of the lips and/or cheeks may also be seen in cheilitis glandularis and angioneurotic edema. A diffuse cellulitis, surgery causing lymphedema, or trauma to the area may also result in a similar clinical picture.

Microscopic features

Noncaseating, organized granulomas composed of epithelioid histiocytes, lymphocytes, and an occasional Langhans giant cell are seen to infiltrate the submucosa and replace the minor salivary glands in the area.

Suggested course of action

Refer to an oral and maxillofacial surgeon or rheumatologist for workup and diagnosis.

Treatment

Intralesional steroid injections of triamcinolone 10 mg/mL once each month for 3 months is the mainstay treatment and usually resolves the enlargement in the long term. Recurrent cases may require retreatment. Multiple recurrences or cases refractory to intralesional steroids may require a systemic prednisone protocol or adalimumab (Humira, AbbVie).

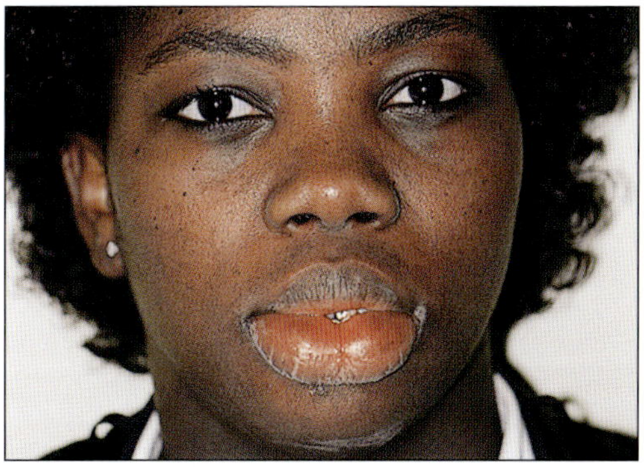

► Cheilitis glandularis.

Cheilitis Glandularis

Nature of disease

A nonspecific inflammatory enlargement of the lips involving the minor salivary glands and their ducts.

Predilections

Occurs more commonly in older adults, with a male predilection. No racial predilection is known. It targets the lower lip much more than the upper lip.

Clinical features

The lip is enlarged with a nodularity representing hypertrophied minor salivary glands. Pain is often present but is mild. The enlargement may cause a slight fissuring of the lower lip vermillion or a scaly appearance.

Radiographic presentation

None.

Differential diagnosis

Cheilitis granulomatosis and the cheilitis granulomatosis portion of Melkersson-Rosenthal syndrome should be considered along with angioneurotic edema, a diffuse cellulitis, or lymphedema from recent surgery or trauma to the area.

Microscopic features

The minor salivary glands will be hypertrophied, admixed with inflammatory cells (mostly neutrophils and lymphocytes).

Suggested course of action

Rule out a history of recent surgery or trauma. If surgery or trauma was the etiology, prescribe antibiotics to resist infection and observe for no more than 2 weeks. If there is no resolution or the etiology remains unknown, refer to an oral and maxillofacial surgeon for workup, diagnosis, and treatment.

Treatment

Persistent lip enlargement of such a nonspecific nature is usually treated with a reduction cheiloplasty.

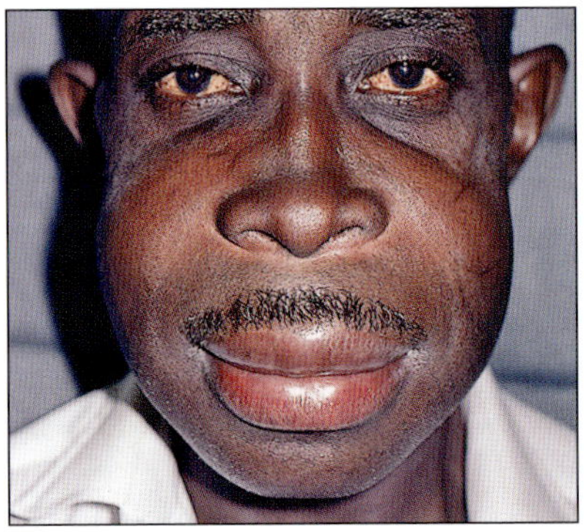

► Symmetric soft tissue expansion of angioedema.

Angioedema

Nature of disease

Acquired angioedema results when immunoglobulin E becomes fixed to mast cells by a previous sensitization and is then activated when a drug or other chemical containing the same or similar antigenic structure causes release of histamine and other coactive compounds. Hereditary angioedema results from an autosomal dominant trait whereby a deficiency of an inhibitor to the C1 esterase enzyme causes an overactive triggering of the complement cascade, resulting in excessive edema and in rare cases anaphylaxis.

Predilections

No age, sex, or racial predilection is known.

Clinical features

Both forms will be seen as a rapid symmetric and diffuse soft edema of the lips and face. Urticaria may accompany the edema but usually not pain.

Radiographic presentation

None.

Differential diagnosis

The history and clinical appearance of angioedema are distinctive. Nevertheless, a consideration of a diffuse cellulitis or a lymphedema from recent surgery, trauma, or radiotherapy is prudent.

Microscopic features

Specimens are usually not taken. However, the intercellular edema and a nonspecific inflammatory cell infiltrate with numerous mast cells (basophiles) would be expected.

Suggested course of action

If severe with airway compromise and/or hypotension suggesting anaphylaxis, call 911 for emergency help. If it is present in your emergency kit, administer epinephrine. If the pulse is lost, begin basic life support protocol and transport the patient to a local hospital emergency room. If nonprogressive with no symptoms, review the patient's history to rule out the hereditary form and pinpoint the allergen that may have triggered the response. If an allergen is noted, withdraw further contact with the allergen and refer to an allergist.

Treatment

The rare form of anaphylaxis is treated with airway support via endotracheal intubation or tracheostomy and blood pressure support usually with epinephrine in an intensive care unit. The less severe form is self-limiting in less than 1 week once the allergen is withdrawn, requiring only observation. The inherited form is treated with a C1 esterase blocker, icatibant, 30 mg/3 mL subcutaneously.

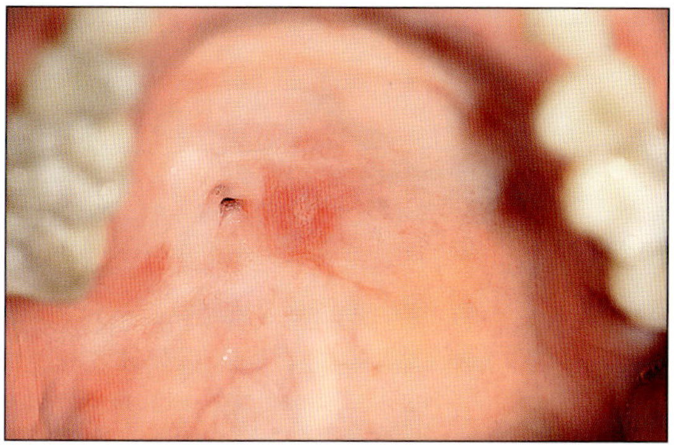

► Granuloma from an infected foreign body (a non-resorbable suture).

Foreign Body Granuloma

Nature of disease

A tissue reaction to either the physical surface characteristics or eluded chemical from a foreign body in tissues that provokes an inflammatory response containing macrophages and/or giant cells.

Predilections

No age, sex, or racial predilection is known.

Clinical features

The reaction causes a diffuse swelling in the area that is mild to moderately painful. The tissue may be boggy to palpation and at times will appear reddened.

Radiographic presentation

Some foreign bodies will appear on plain radiographs as dense metal objects, while others of less density will appear opaque, and yet others may be radiolucent. In some cases, bone erosion may also be present. CT scans will often reveal an increased soft tissue mass due to the edema and, in chronic cases, fibrosis. A MRI scan will show the increased water content of the edema.

Differential diagnosis

The diffuse edema and pain will suggest a cellulitis. If bone erosion is part of the radiographic picture, an osteomyelitis or a malignancy should be considered.

Microscopic features

A variable degree of inflammation will be present, frequently associated with macrophages and/or giant cells that are engulfing foreign particles. Interstitial edema fluid separating native cells is also seen.

Suggested course of action

Review the patient's history to ascertain the type of foreign body (ie, metal, silicone, cosmetic fillers, resorbable cribs or membranes, etc). If known, refer to an oral and maxillofacial surgeon for workup and treatment.

Treatment

Symptomatic foreign bodies require removal. Due to the scarring and fibrosis they create, reconstructive surgery is often required later.

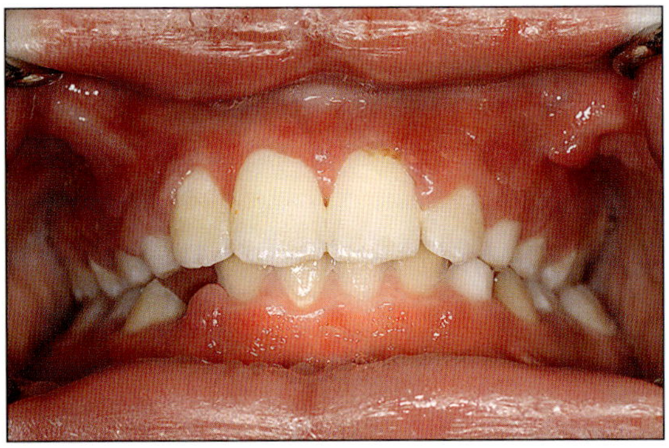

► Cobblestone appearance of the gingiva and oral mucosa in Crohn disease.

Crohn Disease

Nature of disease

A granulomatous transmucosal inflammatory condition of unknown etiology involving mostly the gastrointestinal tract, including but much less commonly the oral mucosa and/or lips.

Predilections

Mostly adults. No sex or racial predilection is known. Most commonly affects the colon.

Clinical features

In the oral cavity, Crohn disease will appear as submucosal nodules imparting a cobblestone appearance to the mucosa, small aphthous ulcers, or hyperplastic gingiva. The lesions in the oral cavity are mostly asymptomatic or mildly painful.

Radiographic presentation

None.

Differential diagnosis

Crohn disease lesions in the oral cavity may resemble aphthous stomatitis, particularly major aphthous stomatitis, as well as reactive arthritis (formerly termed *Reiter syndrome*) and Behçet syndrome.

Microscopic features

Noncaseating, organized, epithelioid granulomas with Langhans giant cells will be seen throughout the mucosa together with a dense inflammatory cell infiltrate of mostly lymphocytes and inflammatory cells.

Suggested course of action

Suspicious cases should be referred to a rheumatologist for evaluation and workup. At times, a biopsy of the oral lesions is necessary to confirm the diagnosis.

Treatment

Most cases of Crohn disease are treated with either the anti–tumor necrosis factor alpha (anti-TNF-α) drug infliximab (Remicade, Janssen), 5 mg/kg intravenously every 8 weeks, or with protocols of prednisone or azathioprine.

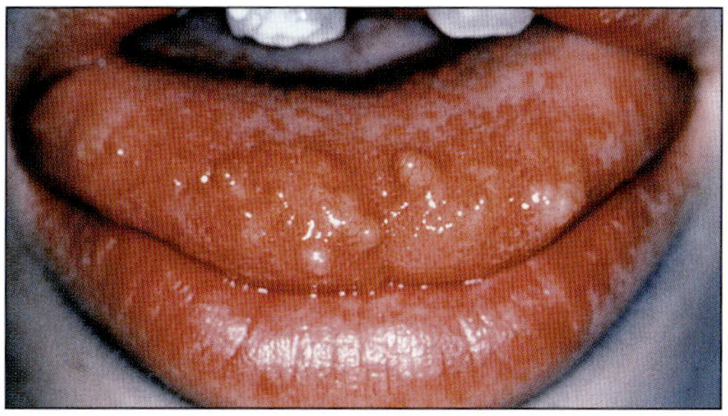

► Nonpainful neuromas in the tongue of an individual with multiple endocrine neoplasia type IIb.

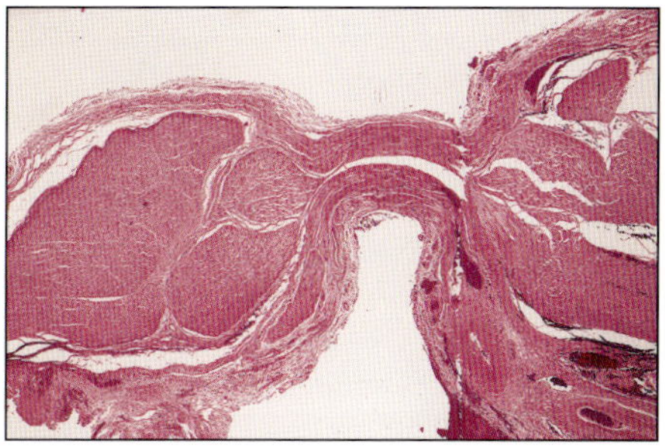

► Painful traumatic neuroma from selective C-fiber regeneration from a transected nerve.

Painful and Nonpainful Neuromas

Nature of disease

Painful neuromas are a selective regeneration of the unmyelinated C fibers from a damaged nerve. Because C fibers are the pain-conducting fibers to the brainstem's gating system and because unmyelinated fibers regenerate somewhat more completely than myelinated fibers, these nodules of neuroma will be painful. Nonpainful neuromas are a mixed fiber regeneration from a damaged nerve. This mixture of some pain fibers as well as larger myelinated touch and proprioceptive fibers send a mixed signal to the gating system that is not merely unbalanced pain-input fibers. This results in no recognition of pain by the individual. Note: All of these neuromas may be traumatic neuromas, but not all traumatic neuromas are painful.

Predilections

More common in adults. No sex or racial predilection is known.

Clinical features

Many neuromas will not have a clinical presence. Others will present as a small (less than 1 cm), freely movable nodule within the mucosa or as a bulge within a nerve known as an *incontinuity neuroma*. Painful neuromas will elicit a sharp painful response to palpation. Some painful neuromas will produce a constant burning pain. Most are seen together with paresthesia or anesthesia of the involved nerve distribution.

Radiographic presentation

Usually none. However, central neuromas may appear as a widened mandibular canal or a focal, small, round radiolucency.

Differential diagnosis

Painful nodules within the oral mucosa are often abscess cavities. Others are foreign bodies provoking inflammation. Nonpainful neuromas may be seen in young individuals as part of the multiple endocrine neoplasia type IIb (MEN IIb). Other nonpainful mucosal nodules may represent fibromas, minor salivary gland neoplasms, or Crohn disease.

Microscopic features

A discrete proliferation of nerve bundles surrounded by collagen is seen with an intact mucosal surface.

Suggested course of action

Referral to an oral and maxillofacial surgeon for evaluation and treatment.

Treatment

Nonpainful neuromas are removed for diagnosis and resolution. When identified as part of MEN IIb, a prophylactic thyroidectomy is recommended to prevent the inevitable development of thyroid cancer in this diagnosis. Painful neuromas are also removed with the offer for nerve grafting.

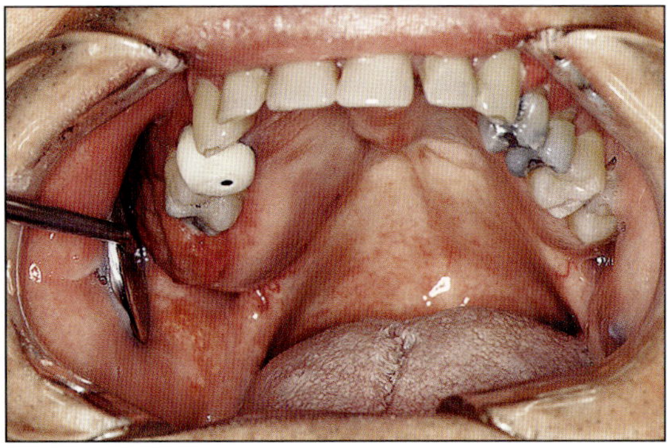

► Fibrosarcoma of the maxilla.

Sarcomas

Fibrosarcoma

Nature of disease

A malignant proliferation of mesenchymal stem cells and/or fibroblast precursors that partially differentiate into still-immature fibroblasts.

Predilections

A slight predilection for young adults. No sex or racial predilection is known.

Clinical features

Fibrosarcomas will present as fleshy to firm soft tissue masses adherent to and intertwined with adjacent tissues. If the tumor invades into bone or arises as a central fibrosarcoma, tooth mobility is likely. The mass is not painful unless biting trauma or secondary infection from ulcerations occurs.

Radiographic presentation

If the fibrosarcoma is limited to soft tissue, no radiographic features will be seen. If it invades into bone from the soft tissue or arises centrally from bone, an irregular osteolysis will be seen with a variable extent, up to a pathologic fracture in some cases.

Differential diagnosis

Aggressive fibromatosis and nodular fasciitis are considerations in children, teenagers, and young adults, as are osteosarcomas and Ewing sarcoma. In older adults, squamous cell carcinoma and a metastatic deposit to the jaws should also be considered.

Microscopic features

Fibrosarcomas are spindle cell neoplasms; depending on their grade, they may show a small amount of collagen production or none at all. Well-differentiated tumors will often show a herringbone pattern and will have only a few mitotic figures. Less-differentiated tumors have less collagen (and sometimes none) and a greater number of mitotic figures.

Suggested course of action

Referral to an oral and maxillofacial surgeon or a cancer center for biopsy, workup, and treatment.

Treatment

Fibrosarcomas are treated with soft tissue and bony resection if bone is involved, observing 2.0-cm margins controlled by frozen sections (for soft tissue). Neck dissection is not usually required. Chemotherapy may be considered but is not usually used.

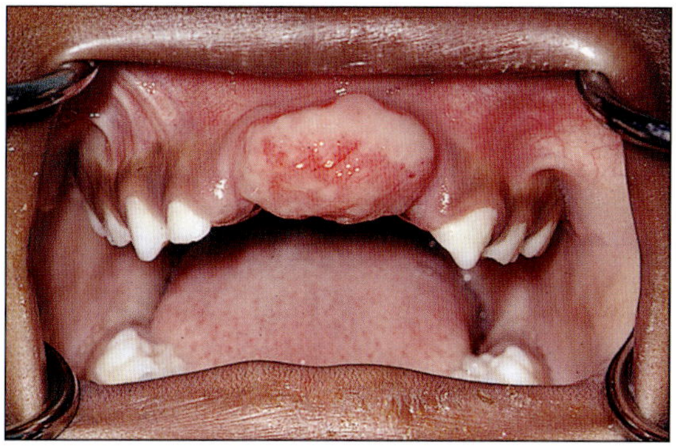

► Aggressive fibromatosis arising from the periosteum of the maxilla.

Aggressive Fibromatosis

Nature of disease

A benign fibrous proliferation that exhibits destructive infiltrative growth similar to a low-grade fibrosarcoma but without the ability to metastasize.

Predilections

Children and teenagers are most commonly affected. No sex or racial predilection is known.

Clinical features

Aggressive fibromatoses often arise from fascia at muscle insertion points or from periosteum to produce a painless, poorly circumscribed, firm mass. They may have a rapid onset of only 2 to 6 weeks and can reach a very large size. Paresthesias are very rare.

Radiographic presentation

Those limited to soft tissue will not have a radiographic presence on plain radiographs. On CT scans, a hyperdense homogenous soft tissue mass is seen. Those involving bone will show an irregular bony destruction form the cortex on into the marrow space.

Differential diagnosis

In these young individuals, fibrosarcomas and rhabdomyosarcomas should be considered. Smaller lesions on the gingiva may be similar to a peripheral ossifying fibroma or even a central ossifying fibroma.

Microscopic features

Fibroblasts and myofibroblasts will be seen as uniform, elongated spindle cells together with broad collagen bands. These cells will be seen to infiltrate adjacent muscle but will not show atypia or mitotic figures.

Suggested course of action

Referral to an oral and maxillofacial surgeon for biopsy, workup, and treatment.

Treatment

Aggressive fibromatoses are treated with a wide local excision, observing 1.0- to 1.5-cm margins that include the muscle fascia or periosteum into which they have arisen or infiltrated. If bone involvement is present, a resection of bone is also required.

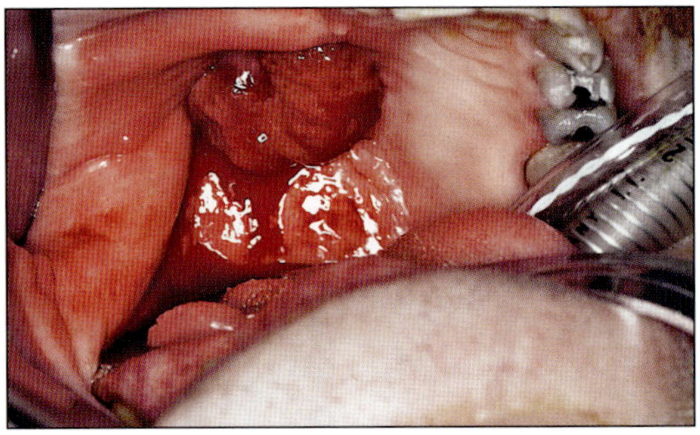

► Pleomorphic sarcoma (an aggressive malignancy).

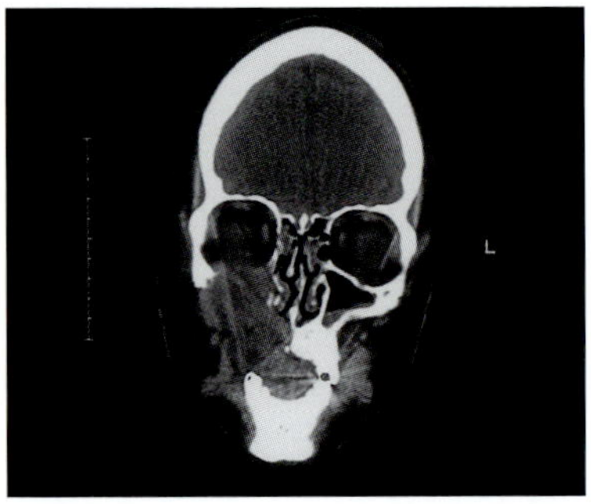

► Bony destruction and orbital invasion from a pleomorphic sarcoma.

Pleomorphic Sarcoma of the Jaws

Nature of disease

A highly aggressive proliferation of primordial stem cells that show a slight fibroblastic differentiation or histiocytic differentiation. Note: Previously known as *malignant fibrous histiocytoma*.

Predilections

Adults, with no known sex or racial predilection.

Clinical features

A very destructive soft tissue mass growing out of and resorbing bone. Paresthesia and overt anesthesia are common. Pain is sometimes present. Tooth mobility and displacement are common.

Radiographic presentation

A soft tissue mass is seen to replace bone via resorption. Tooth roots are often resorbed. Tooth displacement is common.

Differential diagnosis

Other high-grade malignancies such as some osteosarcomas, squamous cell carcinomas, fibrosarcomas, metastatic carcinoma, and even a suppurative osteomyelitis may be considered.

Microscopic features

A cellular proliferation of pleomorphic fibroblast-appearing cells with clear cytoplasm resembling a histiocyte often in a swirled pattern of darker-staining cells around a center of lighter-staining cells referred to as the *storiform pattern*.

Suggested course of action

Incisional biopsy and/or referral to an oral and maxillofacial surgeon.

Treatment

Resection of the tumor, observing 3.0-cm margins, followed by postoperative chemotherapy and radiation therapy.

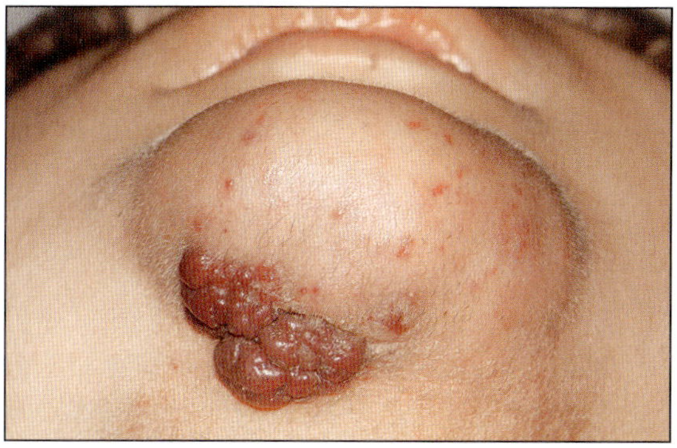

► Angiosarcomas are nodular and fleshy but do not bleed excessively.

Angiosarcoma

Nature of disease

A very rare malignant tumor that arises from the endothelial cells of either blood vessels or lymphatics.

Predilections

Male predilection (2:1) except after radical mastectomy in women due to lymphedema. Generally more common in areas of chronic lymphedema or radiation therapy. The scalp is the most common site in the head, neck, and oral cavity region. No age or racial predilection is known.

Clinical features

Angiosarcomas will appear as painless, lobulated, red fleshy masses. Induration is often present, and despite their name they do not usually blanch upon pressure or bleed.

Radiographic presentation

Those limited to soft tissue will not have a radiographic presentation. Those that erode into bone or arise within bone will show an irregular osteolysis.

Differential diagnosis

The red fleshy mass of an angiosarcoma may be indistinguishable from a rhabdomyosarcoma, osteosarcoma, Kaposi sarcoma, and some benign hemangiomas and lymphangiomas. When in the scalp, basal cell carcinomas, skin squamous cell carcinomas, and the cylindroma of the scalp may also be considered.

Microscopic features

Intercommunicating vascular channels lined by cytologically atypical cells with large nuclei and frequent mitotic figures is the most common histopathology.

Suggested course of action

Referral to a cancer center or to an oral and maxillofacial surgeon for workup and biopsy.

Treatment

As a highly aggressive malignancy, angiosarcomas are treated with radical excision, observing 4.0- to 5.0-cm margins, followed by radiotherapy of 7,000 cGy or greater.

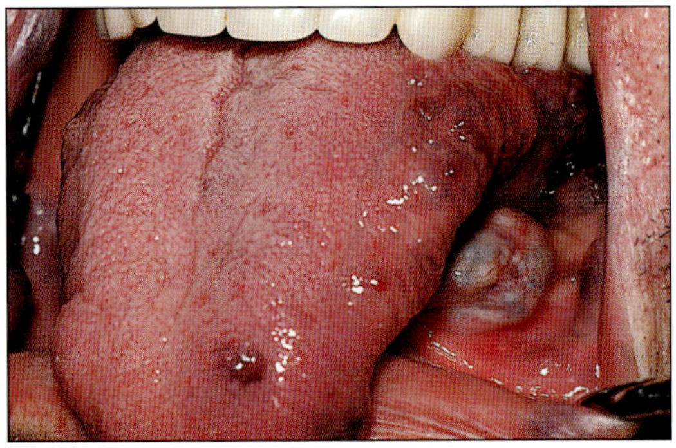

► Classic Kaposi sarcoma.

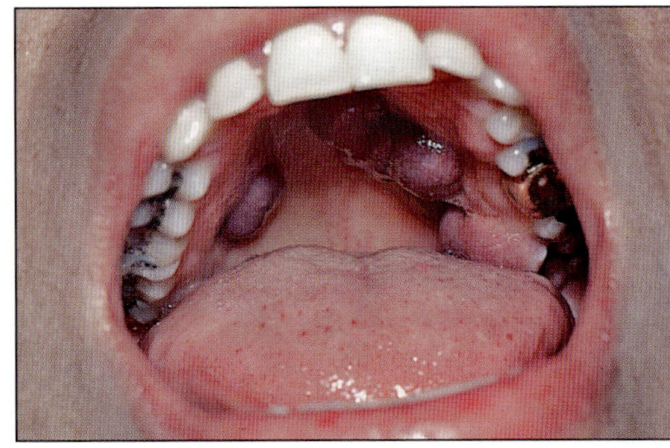

► AIDS-related Kaposi sarcoma.

Kaposi Sarcoma

Nature of disease

A low-grade multifocal vascular malignancy due to a viral infection in an individual with a genetic HLA-DR5 antigen predisposition.

Predilections

There are four types of Kaposi sarcoma:

1. Classic Kaposi sarcoma: This type affects mostly men over 60 years of age and has a strong predilection for those of Greek, Italian, or Jewish ethnicity.
2. African cutaneous Kaposi sarcoma: This type also occurs more commonly in men, specifically men 35 years or older, and is endemic in native black African men.
3. African lymphadenopathic Kaposi sarcoma: This type is endemic in black African children.
4. AIDS-related Kaposi sarcoma: This type is more common in adult men but also can occur in women and children.

Clinical features

The two most common types seen in the United States—classic Kaposi sarcoma and AIDS-related Kaposi sarcoma—appear as bluish-red submucosal or subdermal collections. Some will produce a soft tissue lobulated mass. The African cutaneous type is limited to the skin and is much more infiltrative, producing induration, and will spread rapidly in a proximal direction. The African lymphadenopathic type is a fulminant type involving lymph nodes, salivary glands, and internal organs, often leading to a rapid death.

Radiographic presentation

Usually none unless the mass invades bone; then it is usually only a superficial erosion.

Differential diagnosis

Many cases will mimic an area of ecchymosis from capillary fragility or platelet dysfunction. Those with a mass will suggest an angiosarcoma, rhabdomyosarcoma, hemangioma, lymphangioma, or a low-grade mucoepidermoid carcinoma.

Microscopic features

With some variability, there will be numerous blood-filled channels appearing like slits between spindle cells.

Suggested course of action

Refer to a cancer center or to a medical oncologist for workup.

Treatment

Isolated lesions are treated with intralesional injections of vinblastine 0.1 to 0.5 mg/mL or radiotherapy 1,800 to 2,400 cGy. Systemic treatment is via chemotherapy using vinblastine, etoposide, bleomycin, doxorubicin, and interferon alpha-2 as an adjunct.

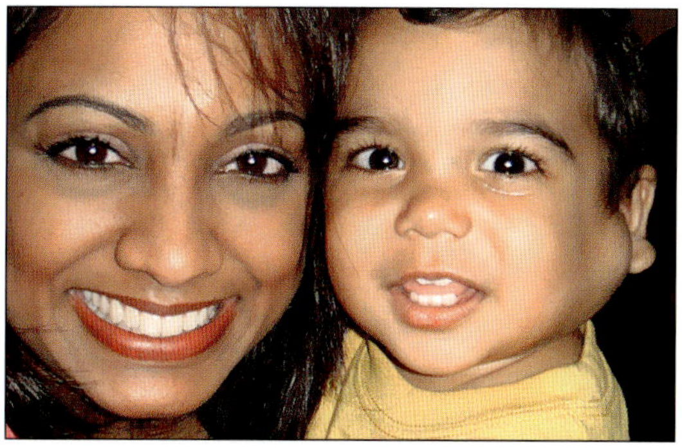

► Capillary hemangioma in a 1-year-old.

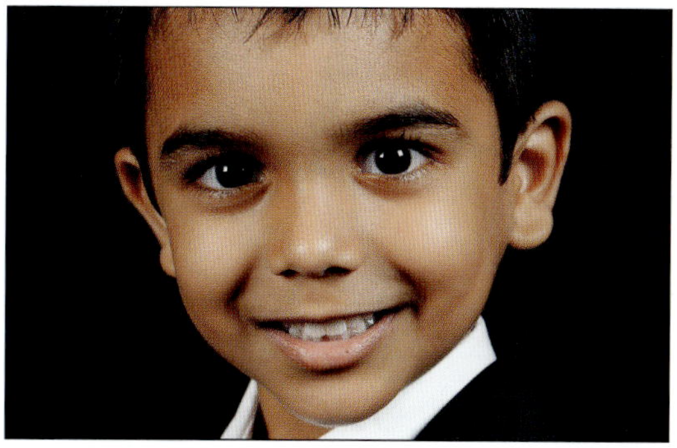

► Same child at 5 years old. The capillary hemangioma regressed.

Hemangiomas

Capillary Hemangioma

Nature of disease

An overproliferation of capillaries due to overexpression of basic fibroblast growth factor.

Predilections

Rare in bone. Most commonly seen in the soft tissues of a newborn or within the first 2 years of life. Some are congenital. These are often termed *juvenile capillary hemangiomas* (see page 72). Those in bone occur in older individuals.

Clinical features

Soft tissue lesions will be semifirm and nodular. A bluish or red coloration may appear but is uncommon. In bone, most are diagnosed radiographically as the clinical picture is normal. Some will produce a mild, painless expansion.

Radiographic presentation

When in bone, a multilocular radiolucency with thinned cortices and mild expansion is seen.

Differential diagnosis

Soft tissue lesions will suggest a fibroma, schwannoma, or minor salivary gland tumor. Due to its rarity in bone, lesions such as central giant cell tumors, ameloblastic fibromas, odontogenic myxomas, and odontogenic keratocysts are more realistic considerations.

Microscopic features

Very cellular lesions composed of endothelial cells forming tortuous but poorly canalized lumen.

Suggested course of action

Incisional biopsy and/or referral to an oral and maxillofacial surgeon. Note: Capillary hemangiomas will not return blood upon aspiration.

Treatment

Because capillary hemangiomas in bone are not true neoplasms with continuous growth, they are removed by enucleation and curettage. Those in soft tissue mostly regress over 5 to 10 years; otherwise, they are excised, observing 2.0-mm margins.

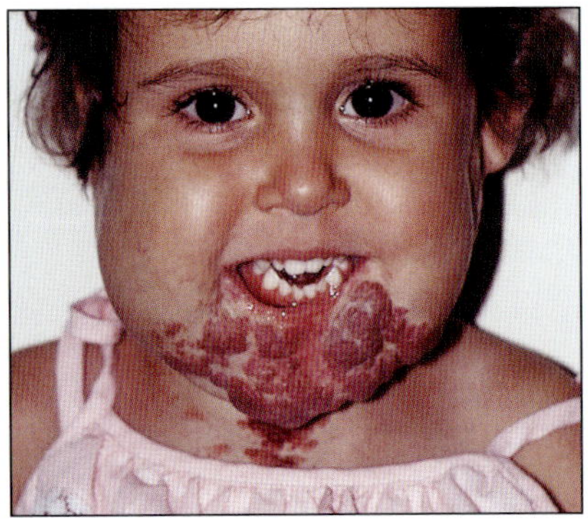

► Juvenile capillary hemangioma.

Juvenile Capillary Hemangioma

Nature of disease

A distinctive proliferation of endothelial cells around the chin, cheeks, and upper neck that begins shortly after birth. It is not a true neoplasm but a defect in the control of capillary regeneration within a developmental territory, often caused by the oversecretion of basic fibroblast growth factor (bFGF).

Predilections

Begins in children less than 1 year of age. There is a female predilection of 3:1. Mostly seen in white children.

Clinical features

They begin as a painless, red-blue, multinodular thickening of the skin that is mostly symmetric about the midline of the chin and neck. It will extend to just beyond the commissures of the mouth and taper down the midline toward the sternum. As the lesion regresses, it remains nodular but gradually becomes smaller, flatter, and more pale.

Radiographic presentation

None.

Differential diagnosis

Juvenile capillary hemangiomas are clinically distinctive with few similar-appearing lesions other than a lymphangioma, which is a related lesion.

Microscopic features

Juvenile capillary hemangiomas will begin as cellular proliferations of endothelial cells forming poorly canalized blood vessels containing a few erythrocytes. As they regress, fewer endothelial cells are seen, and a fibrotic stroma develops.

Suggested course of action

Refer to centers familiar with vascular lesions. Oftentimes these lesions are overtreated, resulting in deformity.

Treatment

These lesions will spontaneously regress but may take 10 to 12 years to do so. However, the skin will be scar filled and irregular. A more rapid regression can be obtained from oral prednisone 1 mg/kg per day at 2-week intervals interrupted by 2 weeks of a drug holiday for a 3-month period. For those cases in which a 24-hour urine collection identifies an increase in bFGF, interferon alpha-2a prescribed at a dose of 1 million to 4 million units per day has been shown to induce a regression.

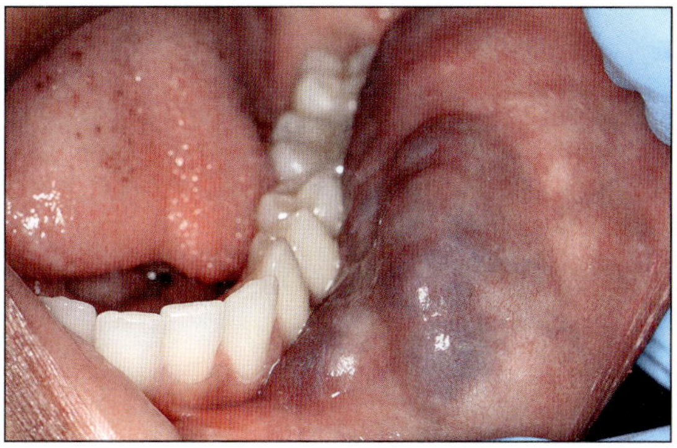

► Cavernous hemangioma.

Cavernous Hemangioma

Nature of disease

A dilation and proliferation of vascular channels presumably due to a dysregulation of vasculogenesis in a limited vascular territory.

Predilections

Unlike juvenile capillary hemangiomas, cavernous hemangiomas can occur in adults as well as children and will have less of a female predilection. White individuals are affected more than other races.

Clinical features

Most occur as a discrete bluish mass in soft tissue. Less commonly, they can occur in bone as a radiolucent-radiopaque mass. In some cases, cavernous hemangiomas will occur in the parotid gland as a soft bluish enlargement of the gland.

Radiographic presentation

Soft tissue cavernous hemangiomas will not usually appear radiographically but will show an outlined high water content on MRI scans. Intraosseous cavernous hemangiomas will have some radiolucency but surprisingly will be somewhat radiopaque as well due to the increased blood flow inducing reactive bone formation. Cavernous hemangiomas in the parotid gland will show a complete outline of the parotid gland with an increased water uptake. Note: As a cavernous hemangioma ages and involutes, phleboliths form due to trapped blood. These will appear on plain radiographs as discrete opacities.

Differential diagnosis

Cavernous hemangiomas must be differentiated from arteriovenous hemangiomas by either Doppler sounding or angiography. Similar-appearing lesions would include lymphangiomas, angiosarcomas, some low-grade mucoepidermoid carcinomas, as well as mucoceles and ranulas.

Microscopic features

Dilated vascular channels with flattened endothelial cells filled with erythrocytes. In older lesions, dystrophic calcifications forming phleboliths are often seen.

Suggested course of action

Refer to an oral and maxillofacial surgeon for workup and treatment.

Treatment

Despite the concerning term *cavernous hemangioma*, these lesions do not pose a serious bleeding threat during surgery because the dilated vascular channels are under low pressure. Parotid lesions in children are left to involute over the first 5 to 10 years of life. Intraosseous lesions are resected, observing 5.0-mm margins. Soft tissue lesions may be excised, observing 5.0-mm margins, or treated for resolution nonsurgically using sodium morrhuate 50 mg once or 60 mg/2 mL of sodium tetradecyl sulfate (Sotradecol 3%, Mylan).

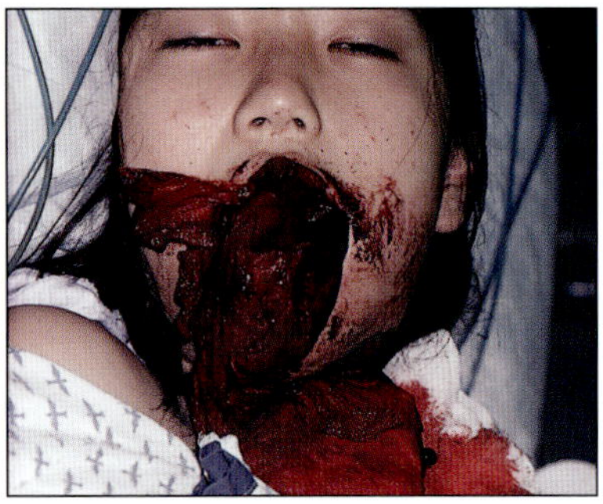

► Young girl in hypovolemic shock from an arteriovenous hemangioma bleed.

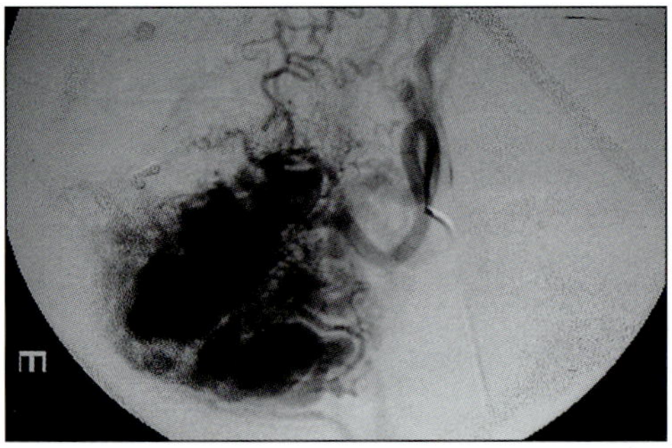

► Angiogram of an arteriovenous hemangioma showing large vascular networks.

Arteriovenous Hemangioma

Nature of disease

A developmental defect in the adventitia around arterioles and capillaries caused by the failure of endothelial cells to secret platelet-derived growth factor and transforming growth factor-beta 1 that recruit adventitial supporting cells. It occurs in a defined vascular developmental territory. The defective vessels enlarge as the cardiovascular system matures to develop dilated arteriovenous connections under arterial pressure.

Predilections

Clinical signs and symptoms emerge around age 10 years. Most are first noticed in the early teen years up to the early 20s. It is more common in females. No racial predilection is known.

Clinical features

Many are first discovered when an excessive high-pressure bleeding occurs when a primary tooth is exfoliated or a tooth is extracted. Others may be noticed as a pulsatile mobile tooth or a pulsatile oral mass. Others may be discovered due to a severe spontaneous bleeding episode.

Radiographic presentation

Those limited to soft tissues will not appear on plain radiographs but will appear on a CT scan as a hypodense area and on an MRI scan as an area of high water content. Those that develop within bone, which is the more common oral presentation, will appear as a radiolucency or a mixed radiolucent-radiopaque lesion similar to a fibro-osseous lesion.

Differential diagnosis

Clinically, arteriovenous hemangiomas will appear similar to a cavernous hemangioma or a lymphangioma. Venous varicosities in the sublingual area and ranulas may also appear in a similar fashion. Those that arise in bone will appear similar to an ameloblastoma, odontogenic myxoma, odontogenic keratocyst, or at times fibrous dysplasia or an ossifying fibroma.

Microscopic features

Large dilated vessels with a single layer of endothelial cells without adventitial supporting layers is characteristic of an arteriovenous hemangioma. →

Suggested course of action

Suspicious cases should be referred to an oral and maxillofacial surgeon. Avoid tooth removals and surgeries in the area of a suspected arteriovenous hemangioma. In the event of a rapid high-pressure bleed, place a gauze pad under handheld heavy pressure, place the patient's head in an upright position, and call 911 for immediate assistance and transport to an emergency room. Note: Replacing an extracted tooth back into a bleeding socket from an arteriovenous hemangioma is much less effective than a gauze packing.

Treatment

Arteriovenous hemangiomas are worked up with diagnostic angiography and treated with polyvinyl alcohol beads, alcohol, or cyanoacrylate embolizations or embolizations followed by surgery within 72 hours.

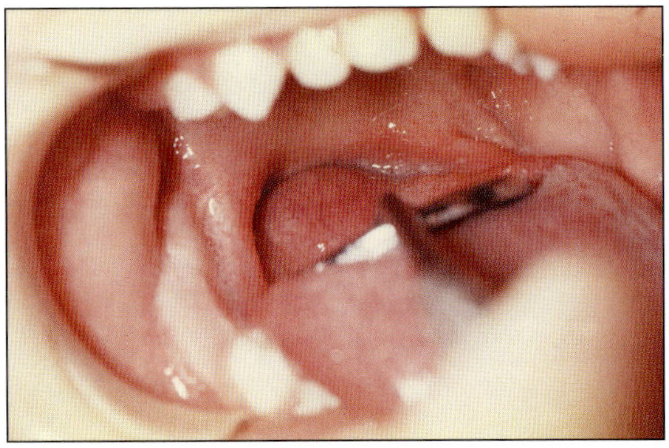

► Persistent lingual thyroid as the entire thyroid gland with no presence in the neck.

Persistent Lingual Thyroid

Nature of disease

Failure of the thyroid primordial cells to migrate from the junction of the anterior two-thirds of the tongue and posterior third down through the hyoid bone to develop a mature thyroid gland at the level of the larynx and trachea in the midline of the neck. The result is the development of a mature functional thyroid gland in the substance of the posterior third of the tongue.

Predilections

Persistent lingual thyroids are congenital but not usually noticed until the age of 4 years or older. It is too rare to have any known sex or racial predilection.

Clinical features

A persistent lingual thyroid is almost always a painless incidental finding. Occasionally, a large gland will cause gagging or bleeding. The gland will appear as a soft fleshy mass in the midline of the posterior tongue. At times it will be lobulated. It will generally have a thin overlying mucosa.

Radiographic presentation

A CT scan will show a discrete hyperdense mass in the posterior tongue. An MRI will identify an increased water content.

Differential diagnosis

A fleshy mass in the tongue of a child or young adult should suggest a rhabdomyosarcoma, hemangioma, or lymphangioma. More rarely, a mucocele or salivary gland tumor, particularly a mucoepidermoid carcinoma, will present in a similar fashion.

Microscopic features

Specimens are usually not available. In fact, biopsy of a suspected persistent lingual thyroid should be discouraged and avoided so as not to create an inadvertent hypothyroid state. The gland would be a normal thyroid with amorphous thyroid colloid admixed with the glandular cells and numerous small blood vessels. →

Suggested course of action

Avoid biopsy or referral to someone intent on a biopsy. Instead, order a radioactive iodine (I^{131}) scan, which will diagnose the thyroid tissue in the tongue as an uptake similar to the bilateral parotid glands, which concentrate halides like the thyroid gland with no uptake in the neck. Also order thyroid function tests to document a euthyroid state. Discuss with the family that the persistent lingual thyroid is functional and normal and to avoid biopsy or cautery if later bleeding develops. If the above cannot be accomplished, refer to an endocrinologist or an oral and maxillofacial surgeon to accomplish this workup, including a medical alert bracelet.

Treatment

No treatment is required. Biopsy should be discouraged. If symptoms of repeated gagging or bleeding develop, the gland is transplanted into the neck or into a muscle pouch, which will retain the gland in a functional state.

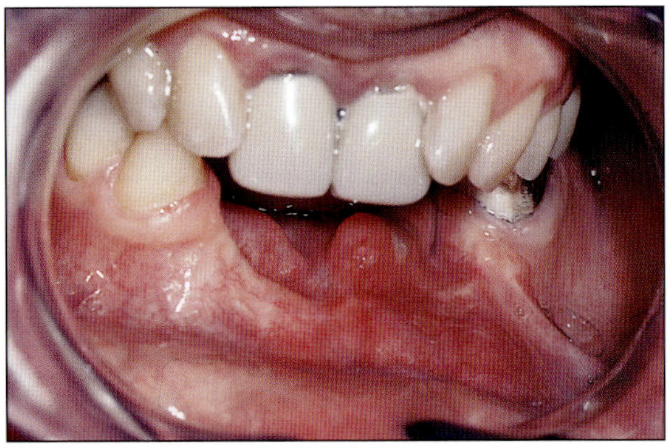

► Heterotopic gastrointestinal cyst in the floor of the mouth.

Heterotopic Gastrointestinal Cyst

Nature of disease

A rare, small developmental cyst that occurs along the gastrointestinal tract from the mouth to the anus. It arises from residual pluripotent stem cells from the development of the gastrointestinal lining.

Predilections

Almost all are found in boys from 4 months to 12 years. They occur very rarely in the mouth (0.3% in the tongue and an even smaller percentage in the floor of the mouth). Most occur in the small intestines. No racial predilection is known.

Clinical features

Heterotopic gastrointestinal cysts will be less than 1 cm and will present as a painless, submucosal, freely movable nodule or mass.

Radiographic presentation

None.

Differential diagnosis

A heterotopic gastrointestinal cyst is usually not on a differential list due to its rarity. Other similar lesions to consider are epidermoid and dermoid cysts, mucoceles, salivary gland tumors, and a granular cell tumor.

Microscopic features

The cyst will have a stratified squamous lining or at times a cuboidal lining with crypts and ductlike formations lined by glandular cells. A muscular layer around the cyst or glandular cysts may also be seen.

Suggested course of action

Referral to an oral and maxillofacial surgeon for an excisional biopsy.

Treatment

Heterotopic gastrointestinal cysts are diagnosed and resolved by a pericapsular excision.

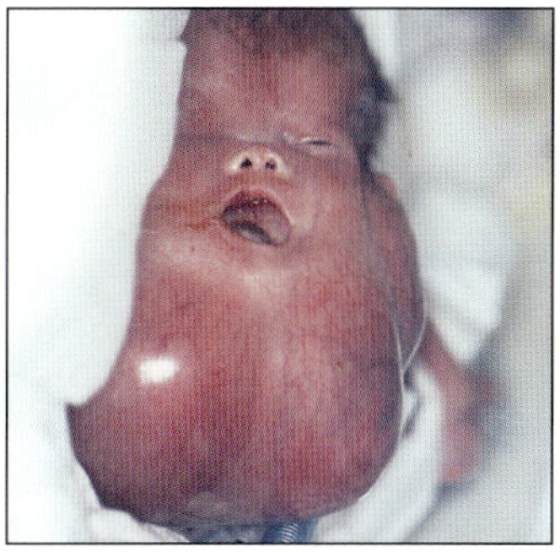

► Cervical cystic hygoma.

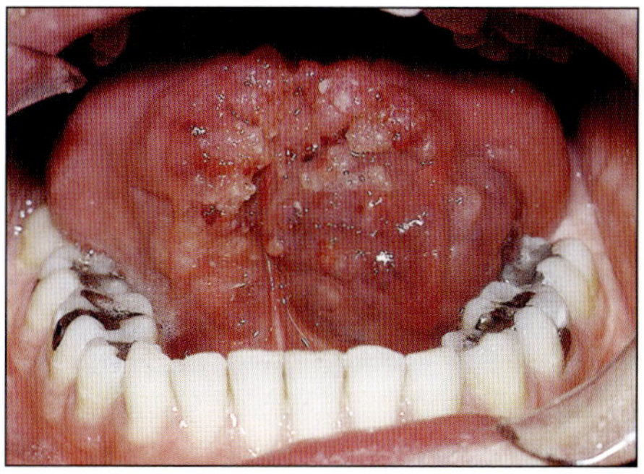

► Adult superficial type of lymphangioma.

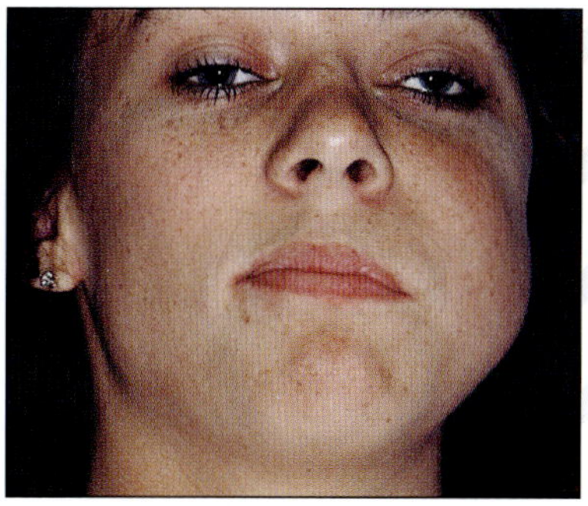

► Adult deep type of lymphangioma.

Lymphangioma

Nature of disease

A defect in the development of lymphatic channels within an embryologic field that can occur at any age and results in a dilation and a disorganized proliferation of endothelial-lined lymphatic channels.

Predilections

A strong predilection for females. White individuals are more commonly affected. One type is congenital or may develop within the first year (ie, cystic hygoma). Other types occur in adults (ie, superficial type and deep type).

Clinical features

- Cervical cystic hygoma: This type appears at birth or in early life as a large, seemingly painless, soft-textured and fluid-filled enlargement in the lateral neck. Most occur unilaterally, but some are bilateral.
- The adult superficial type: This type will appear as a mass of doughy to firm consistency with a red-brown pebbly surface that does not blanch upon pressure.
- The adult deep type: This type appears as a semisoft expansion with an intact and smooth surface.

Radiographic presentation

Lymphangiomas are not well seen on plain radiographs. They are best seen on MRI scans, which will usually identify a lobulated or irregular outline of a mass lesion with a high water content.

Differential diagnosis

The cystic hygoma type is clinically distinctive. However, it may resemble a mass from a rhabdomyosarcoma, neuroblastoma, or hemangioma in the child. The adult superficial type may resemble a verrucous hyperplasia, verrucous carcinoma, or squamous cell carcinoma. The adult deep type may present as several deeply located benign tumors such as schwannomas, neurofibromas, and salivary gland tumors.

Microscopic features

Lymphangiomas will appear as large, empty endothelial-lined spaces with sparse or absent adventitial cells.

Suggested course of action

Refer to an oral and maxillofacial surgeon or a major medical center for workup and treatment.

Treatment

Some cystic hygomas are incompatible with life and are left untreated. Others are partially removed because complete excision is not usually possible. Superficial and deep lymphangiomas do not require treatment unless they interfere with function. In such cases, they are debunked or incompletely excised.

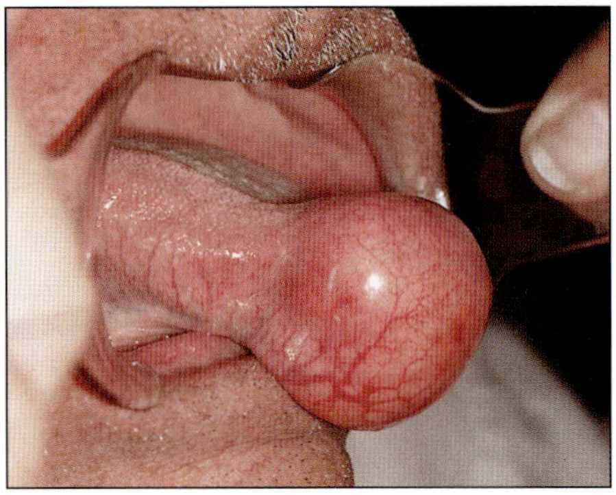

► Schwannoma of the tongue.

Schwannoma of Soft Tissue

Nature of disease

Schwannomas are benign proliferations of the Schwann cells covering nerves.

Predilections

Most are seen in adults. No sex or racial predilection is known. Although schwannomas can arise from any nerve, those in the neck tend to arise from more deeply located nerves.

Clinical features

Schwannomas will present as a painless, oval-shaped, freely movable mass. They are not associated with any paresthesia or paresis. The mass will be of a doughy to firm consistency.

Radiographic presentation

As soft tissue masses, schwannomas will not appear on plain radiographs. CT scans will show a well-encapsulated mass with a density similar to or slightly less than that of adjacent muscle. MRI scans will show an increased water content in the mass on a T2-weighted image.

Differential diagnosis

Oval-shaped soft tissue masses also suggest Hodgkin or non-Hodgkin lymphoma, cat-scratch disease, dermoid cysts, and, when around the parotid gland, benign parotid tumors.

Microscopic features

The mass will have a readily identifiable capsule of collagen. Within the capsule, a gray matrix is seen to be associated with darkly staining cell arrangements. One arrangement is a single-file alignment that may be noted to palisade. These cells are referred to as *Antoni A cells.* The matrix between two rows of Antoni A cells is referred to as a *Verocay body.* The second cell arrangement is a scattered cell arrangement without any organization. These cells are referred to as *Antoni B cells.* Throughout the mass, numerous blood vessels will also be noted.

Suggested course of action

Refer to an oral and maxillofacial surgeon for workup and treatment.

Treatment

Schwannomas are curable with a pericapsular excision. Those that arise from a nerve trunk can be removed from the nerve trunk without sacrificing the nerve. In those arising from small peripheral nerve fibers or nerve endings, the parent nerve is not seen and is removed with the tumor.

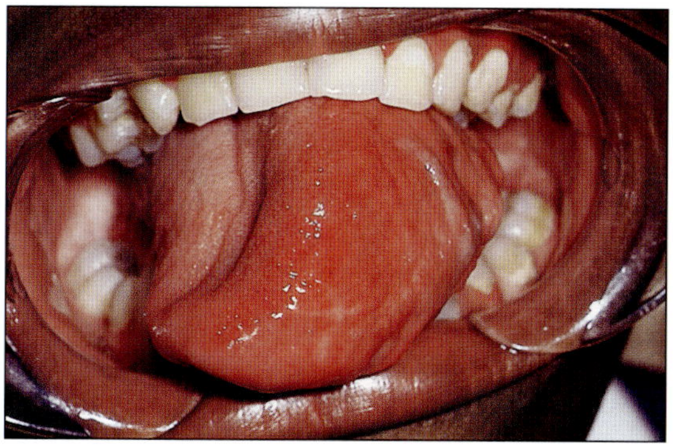

► Neurofibroma of the tongue.

Neurofibroma

Nature of disease

A benign but unencapsulated tumor of neurofibroblasts from peripheral nerve sheaths.

Predilections

Ninety percent of neurofibromas occur unassociated with hereditary neurofibromatosis type 1 or 2; these are termed *solitary neurofibromas*. They have no sex or racial predilection but do occur more frequently in young adults.

Clinical features

Patients will present with a diffuse, painless submucosal or subcutaneous mass. The mass will feel as if it has cords within it, often termed the "bag of worms" presentation. The mass will also infiltrate into surrounding tissues, making it somewhat immobile.

Radiographic presentation

Most neurofibromas are within soft tissue and have no plain radiograph projections. CT scans will outline the mass as a diffuse unencapsulated soft tissue density blending into adjacent tissues. MRI scans will identify a high water content indicative of the vascularity of a neurofibroma. The rarer central neurofibroma will appear as a diffuse radiolucency often seen as an expansion arising from the mandibular canal.

Differential diagnosis

In soft tissue, the "bag of worms" texture will suggest a deep-seated hemangioma, lymphangioma, lipoma, rhabdomyoma, or even a rhabdomyosarcoma.

Microscopic features

The mass will be unencapsulated with spindle-shaped fibroblasts in a serpentine arrangement amid a wavy pattern of collagen. Numerous small blood vessels will permeate throughout the specimen.

Suggested course of action

Refer to an oral and maxillofacial surgeon for workup and treatment.

Treatment

Because neurofibromas have slow and limited growth, many are incompletely excised to improve function and appearance. Complete excision observing 1.0-cm margins is recommended when possible.

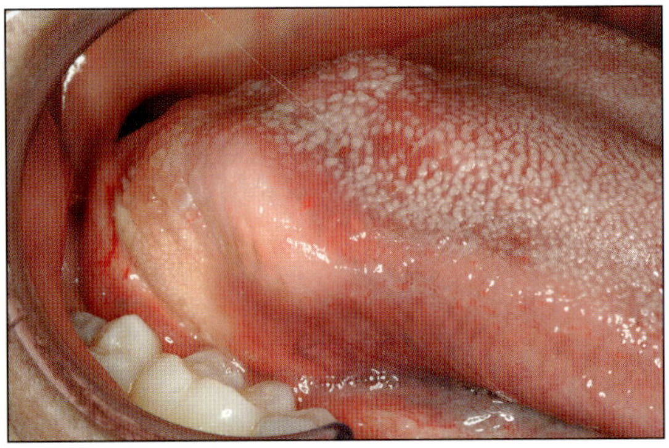

► Granular cell tumor of the tongue with characteristic pale surface.

Granular Cell Tumor

Nature of disease

A proliferation of altered neural cells that contain numerous cytoplasmic lysosomal vesicles imparting a granular appearance under light microscopy. The proliferation is the biology of a hamartoma and therefore of limited growth.

Predilections

There is a female predilection, and most occur in young adults within the tongue or more rarely in the lips or buccal mucosa. They are also well known to occur in the skin of the breast.

Clinical features

Oral lesions present as an indurated, firm fixed mass with an intact surface that is pale to white. Paresthesia or pain is not present.

Radiographic presentation

None on plain radiographs. CT scans will show a soft tissue density with indistinct and irregular borders.

Differential diagnosis

Because the surface is intact, squamous cell carcinoma does not hold a prominent place on a differential list. Instead, rhabdomyomas, rhabdomyosarcomas, schwannomas, neurofibromas, and salivary gland tumors are the more serious considerations.

Microscopic features

Pale and somewhat large granular cells will be seen interspersed among muscle fibers. Some of the muscle fibers may seem to be undergoing lysis. Most but not all will also show pseudoepitheliomatous hyperplasia extending into the granular cell layer but not the muscle fibers themselves. The pseudoepitheliomatous hyperplasia at times may show keratin pearls, creating a false suspicion for cancer.

Suggested course of action

Incisional biopsy or referral to an oral and maxillofacial surgeon for workup and treatment.

Treatment

Most require removal to rule out more serious diseases or to improve function to the affected area. However, complete removal is not necessary, because granular cell tumors are limited in their growth and some surgeries to remove this unencapsulated mass can be deforming or create functional deficit.

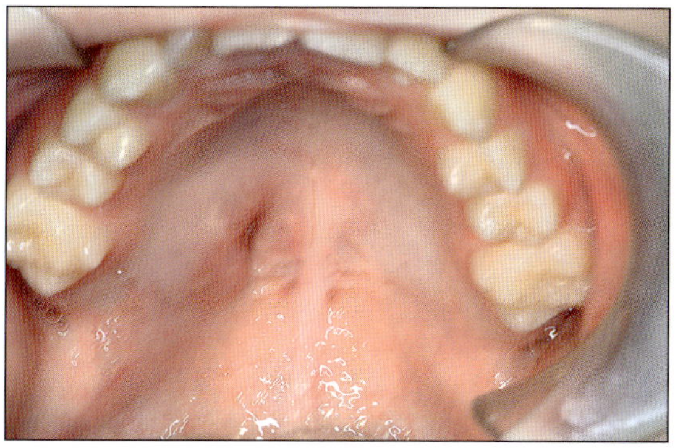

► Leiomyoma.

Leiomyoma

Nature of disease

A very rare, benign neoplasm of smooth muscle cells when it occurs in the oral and maxillofacial region. However, it is the most common benign tumor of the uterus, where it is often referred to as a *fibroid tumor*.

Predilections

There seems to be a young female predilection in the maxillofacial region. However, the rarity of this neoplasm in this area precludes confirmation. They may occur at any site throughout the maxillofacial region and arise from the smooth muscle precursors of capillaries and arterioles.

Clinical features

Leiomyomas will present as semifirm to firm masses within the submucosa at the site of occurrence. Paresthesia or pain is not present.

Radiographic presentation

Plain radiographs will not show a soft tissue leiomyoma. CT and MRI scans will identify a soft tissue density with indistinct borders.

Differential diagnosis

The rarity of leiomyomas in the maxillofacial region preclude its consideration on a differential list. Instead, the more likely schwannomas, granular cell tumors, neurofibromas, and salivary gland tumors should be considered.

Microscopic features

Leiomyomas will have numerous plump, elongated, or spindle-shaped cells with blunted tips. There is no discernible capsule, and mitotic figures are rarely seen or absent.

Suggested course of action

Incisional biopsy and/or referral to an oral and maxillofacial surgeon for workup and treatment.

Treatment

Leiomyomas are true neoplasms with continual growth potential, requiring excision with 0.5- to 1.0-cm margins.

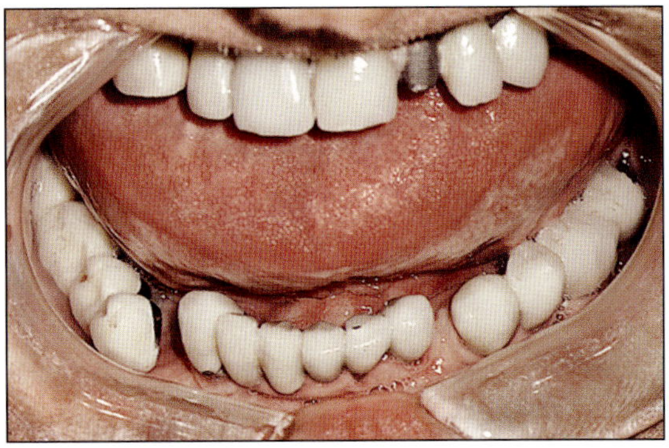

► Secondary amyloidosis causing a firm macroglossia that splayed the dentition and created diastemas.

Amyloidosis

Nature of disease

There are two types of amyloidosis, and both are rare. The rarer is primary amyloidosis, which is an inborn error in protein metabolism resulting in amyloid deposits through the soft tissues of the body. The less rare secondary amyloidosis results from aberrant proteins produced by diseases such as multiple myeloma and Waldenström macroglobulinemia, which result in amyloid deposits throughout the body, particularly in the tongue and to a lesser extent the gingiva.

Predilections

A predilection for adult males is noted in both types. The tongue is the primary site in the oral and maxillofacial region.

Clinical features

In both types, amyloid deposits will make the area firm and enlarged. The surface will be intact. Pain is rare, as is any paresthesia.

Radiographic presentation

Plain radiographs will not show amyloid deposition. CT and MRI scans will identify a diffuse increase in the soft tissue density of the involved area. The area of involvement will be enlarged but will maintain its general anatomical morphology.

Differential diagnosis

Differentiating between primary and secondary amyloidosis can only be accomplished by history. Other entities that can produce a diffuse enlargement of an anatomical area such as the tongue include neurofibromas, rhabdomyomas, hemangiomas, and lymphangiomas.

Microscopic features

The submucosal connective tissue will be seen to have a whorled area of amorphous eosinophilic-staining material. Congo red staining or fluorescence with thioflavin T will confirm this extracellular material to be amyloid.

Suggested course of action

Suspicious cases should be referred to the patient's primary care physician. If it is associated with an existing malignancy, the patient should be referred to his or her oncologist. In both cases, a report about the oral and maxillofacial findings should be sent to the appropriate physician. An incisional biopsy confirming the presence of amyloid may be considered as well.

Treatment

There is no known effective treatment for either type of amyloidosis. In the secondary type, control of the malignancy may reduce the size of the deposit slightly.

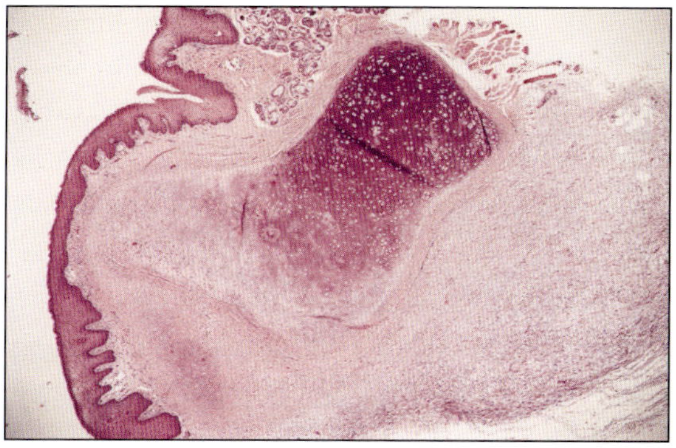

► Well-defined mass of normal cartilage and bone within the tongue representing an osteocartilaginous choristoma.

Osteocartilaginous Choristoma

Nature of disease

All choristomas are defined as a dysmorphic limited proliferation of non-native tissues. In the case of an osteocartilaginous choristoma, it is one that grows to a certain extent in a soft tissue space and then ceases growth. Therefore, it is not a neoplasia.

Predilections

Those that occur in the oral cavity mostly occur in the tongue or floor of the mouth. Some may also occur within the area of the invasive papilla. Their rarity precludes any accurate determination of a predilection for age, sex, or race.

Clinical features

An osteocartilaginous choristoma will present as a firm to hard painless mass with an intact overlying mucosa. Most will also be moveable within the soft tissue space.

Radiographic presentation

Plain radiographs and CT scans will show a round to oval mixed radiolucent-radiopaque mass within soft tissue. The degree of radiopacity will be a function of the bone content, which is radiopaque, and the cartilage content, which is radiolucent.

Differential diagnosis

Osteocartilaginous choristomas are very rare and may not be considered on a differential diagnosis unless they are clearly at a distance from native bone. Therefore, most differential considerations are such entities as a torus, ossifying fibroma, osteoblastomas, and even osteosarcomas. However, other somewhat radiopaque masses strictly within soft tissues include phleboliths, sialoliths, and sequestra from an infected bony area.

Microscopic features

A mixture of mature cartilage and bone within a normal soft tissue space. There is usually a fibrous capsule around the mass.

Suggested course of action

Obtain clear quality imaging. Refer to an oral and maxillofacial surgeon for an exploration and excisional biopsy.

Treatment

Osteocartilaginous choristomas are excised using a pericapsular dissection or with a 1.0- to 2.0-mm cuff of surrounding tissue.

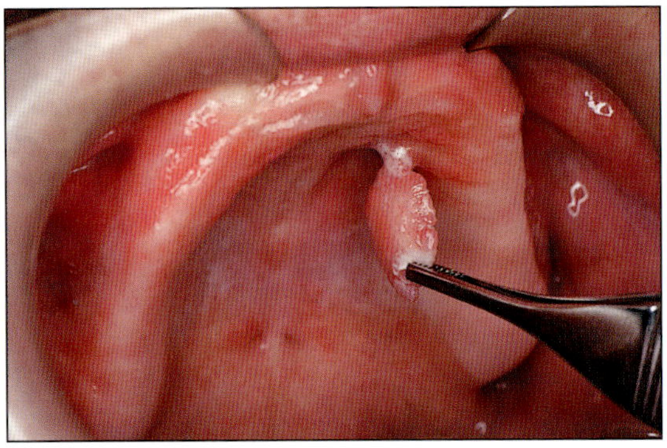

► Oral squamous papilloma.

Squamous Papilloma

Nature of disease

A benign proliferation of surface epithelial cells containing a fibrovascular core. Although an etiology for one of the many human papillomaviruses (HPV) has been suspected and shown in some cases, others have no proven link to HPV.

Predilections

There is a strong predilection for the hard and soft palate mucosa and lip vermilion. There is no known age, sex, or racial predilection.

Clinical features

Most will present with a sessile base, while others will have a thin stalk. The surface will be intact but may be verrucoid or have defined fingerlike or hairlike projections. They will be painless and will not readily bleed or blanch upon manipulation.

Radiographic presentation

None.

Differential diagnosis

The clinician must always consider the more concerning possibilities of a verrucous carcinoma or a papillary exophytic invasive squamous cell carcinoma. Other entities to consider are granulation tissue from an underlying wound or infection, verruciform xanthoma, and the viral venereal disease condyloma acuminatum.

Microscopic features

Squamous papillomas will show mature squamous epithelium growing out of a fibrovascular core in fingerlike projections.

Suggested course of action

Excise the mass, including the base, to cure and to rule out more concerning lesions, or refer to an oral and maxillofacial surgeon for evaluation and excisional biopsy.

Treatment

Squamous papillomas are excised at their base to a depth within the submucosa.

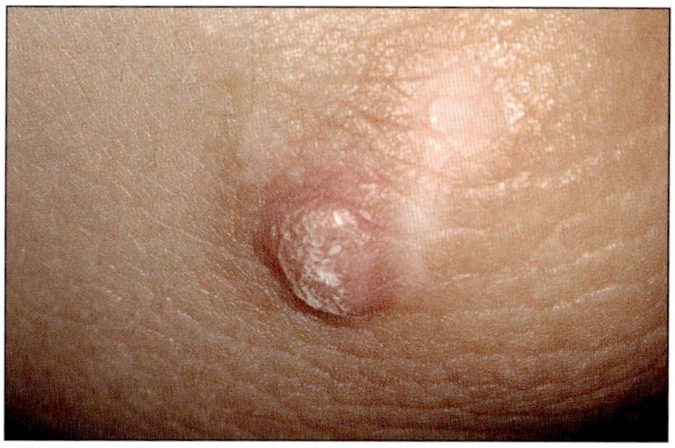

► Exophytic verruca vulgaris.

Verruca Vulgaris (Common Wart)

Nature of disease

A DNA human papillomavirus (HPV)-induced proliferation of skin epithelial cells.

Predilections

Mostly seen in children and young adults. Most lesions are seen on the skin, but some may also appear on the vermilion border. No sex or racial predilection is known.

Clinical features

Verruca vulgaris lesions are white with a sessile base. The lesion is elevated with a papillary surface. It is painless. Satellite lesions may be seen adjacent to a main lesion.

Radiographic presentation

None.

Differential diagnosis

On the vermillion border, one should consider a condyloma acuminatum (venereal wart) or a squamous papilloma. On skin, some may bear a resemblance to an early keratoacanthoma or skin basal cell or squamous cell carcinoma.

Microscopic features

Thin, pointed, exophytic epithelial proliferations arising from surface epithelium with no endophytic invaginations are the distinguishing features of verruca vulgaris. Thickened surface keratin as well as intranuclear viral inclusion bodies in the keratinocyte layer may also be seen.

Suggested course of action

Oral lesions often respond to a topical silver nitrate application or freezing. Skin lesions may be treated with numerous over-the-counter remedies or prescription podophyllum for unresponding cases. For refractory cases in the oral cavity or facial skin, refer to an oral and maxillofacial surgeon for excision. For skin lesions elsewhere, refer to a dermatologist.

Treatment

Topical therapy from silver nitrate and/or freezing to the numerous commercial topical applications available, such as 5% imiquimod cream or podophyllum. Refractory lesions are excised.

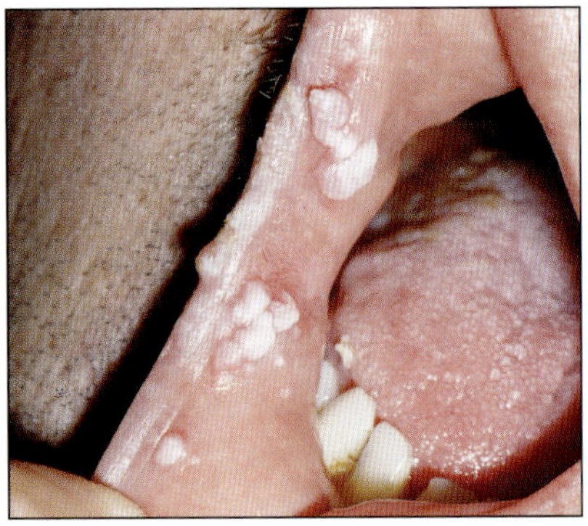

► Multiple warty lesions of condyloma acuminata.

Condyloma Acuminata (Venereal Warts)

Nature of disease

Condyloma acuminata are caused by DNA human papillomavirus (HPV) 6 and 11. It is highly transmissible by direct surface-to-surface contact.

Predilections

Ninety percent occur in men, with most occurring in men between 15 and 40 years of age. No racial predilection is known.

Clinical features

Oral lesions appear in clusters and are white with a sessile base. They will occur mostly around the commissures and lip vermillion. Less commonly, some may be seen in the floor of the mouth and tongue. These arise from either hand-to-mouth transmission from concomitant genital lesions or from oral sex. Skin lesions look similar but generally have a more red-white appearance and are found on the glans penis in men and the labia or vulva in women. Anal lesions also occur related to anal sex.

Radiographic presentation

None.

Differential diagnosis

Single or a few lesions may appear as the nonvenereal wart (verruca vulgaris) or squamous papillomas. Clusters of lesions will appear similar to a verrucous carcinoma or an exophytic squamous cell carcinoma.

Microscopic features

Lesions will have a marked acanthosis with broad, elongated rete ridges but without hyperparakeratosis or hyperkeratosis. Frequent mitoses are seen, and some nuclei will have a perinuclear halo suggestive of a viral involvement.

Suggested course of action

Suspicious lesions require protective barrier techniques for the dental provider, dental hygienist, and staff. The patient's history should be reviewed related to genital lesions and behavioral risks, and the patient should be referred to either an infectious disease specialist or a dermatologist.

Treatment

All areas with lesions require treatment. This can be accomplished with a CO_2 laser, cryotherapy, topical 25% podophyllum resin, topical 50% trichloroacetic acid, or imiquimod 5% cream. Refractory lesions may require excision.

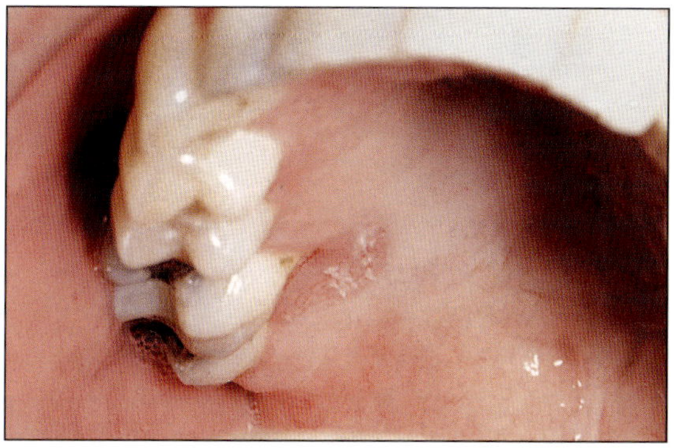

► Characteristic pebbly surface of a verruciform xanthoma.

Verruciform Xanthoma

Nature of disease

A rare but distinct proliferation of epithelial cells producing a warty surface from excess parakeratin and with numerous foamy macrophages in its connective tissue papilla. The etiology remains uncertain. No viral cause has been found.

Predilections

The attached gingiva, edentulous alveolar ridge, and palate are sites of predilection and underscore its focus on keratinized oral mucosa. Most occur in patients older than 45 years, with no sex or racial predilection.

Clinical features

Lesions are mostly singular painless lesions that are raised and of pale white to red color. The surface is pebbly. Most lesions are about 1 cm in size.

Radiographic presentation

None.

Differential diagnosis

The rarity of verruciform xanthomas preclude its inclusion on most differential lists. Instead, the more likely squamous papilloma, condyloma acuminatum, verrucous carcinoma, and exophytic squamous cell carcinoma should be considered as well as a soft tissue lesion of Langerhans cell histiocytosis.

Microscopic features

The unique histopathology of a verruciform xanthoma centers around the foamy macrophages within a connective tissue papilla beneath an acanthotic epithelial proliferation with abundant parakeratin and an equally elongated and widened endophytic epithelial proliferation. Note: The foamy macrophages have no association with hyperlipidemia or hypercholesterolemia.

Suggested course of action

Excisional biopsy or referral to an oral and maxillofacial surgeon.

Treatment

Local excision observing 1.0- to 3.0-mm margins.

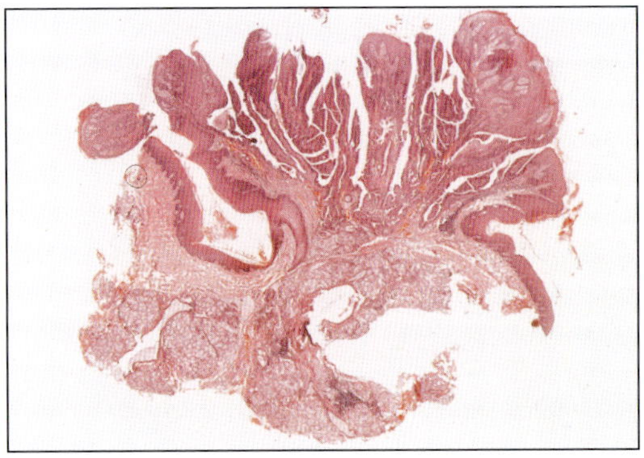

► Sialadenoma papilliferum with an exophytic papillary appearance.

Sialadenoma Papilliferum

Nature of disease

An exophytic, limited verrucous proliferation from the superficial portion of an excretory duct of a minor salivary gland.

Predilections

Occurs more in men over 50 years of age. There is no known racial predilection. Occurs more in areas of greater minor salivary gland density.

Clinical features

A sialadenoma papilliferum will present as a small (< 2 cm) verrucous-like proliferation at the opening of a minor salivary gland. The lesion will be painless and fixed to the oral mucosa.

Radiographic presentation

None.

Differential diagnosis

The rarity of a sialadenoma papilliferum will mostly leave it off a differential list that instead will include a squamous papilloma, verrucous carcinoma, and an exophytic squamous cell carcinoma. Additionally, the equally rare verruciform xanthoma may also be considered. On skin, the lesion will appear similar to a small keratoacanthoma, a folliculitis, or a small epidermoid inclusion cyst.

Microscopic features

An exophytic/endophytic squamous proliferation occurs above ductal and glandular elements from minor salivary gland structures.

Suggested course of action

Excisional biopsy or referral to an oral and maxillofacial surgeon.

Treatment

Excisional biopsy observing 2.0- to 3.0-mm margins and into the submucosa is curative.

Warty Dyskeratoma

Nature of disease

A rare, benign focal disturbance in the maturation and shedding of epithelial cells.

Predilections

Mostly a skin lesion but does occur on the palate, alveolar ridge, and lateral border of the tongue on occasion. Adults are affected, with no known sex or racial predilection.

Clinical features

Warty dyskeratomas will appear as a small ($\leq$ 1 cm) papule or verrucous lesion with a central pit resembling and sometimes incorrectly reported as an oral keratoacanthoma. The lesion will be painless and will seem thick and immobile upon palpation.

Radiographic presentation

None.

Differential diagnosis

Orally, the lesion will be similar to a plugged minor salivary gland duct, a stone in the duct, or even a small salivary gland tumor. Additionally, a traumatic lesion may appear similar. On skin, the lesion will appear similar to a small keratoacanthoma, a folliculitis, or a small epidermoid inclusion cyst.

Microscopic features

An acanthosis is seen with a central invagination and cells undergoing individual keratinization. Additionally, a projection of rete ridges will be seen with disruption and necrosis of epithelial cells (acantholysis).

Suggested course of action

Excisional biopsy or referral to an oral and maxillofacial surgeon.

Treatment

Excisional biopsy observing 2.0- to 3.0-mm margins and into the submucosa is curative.

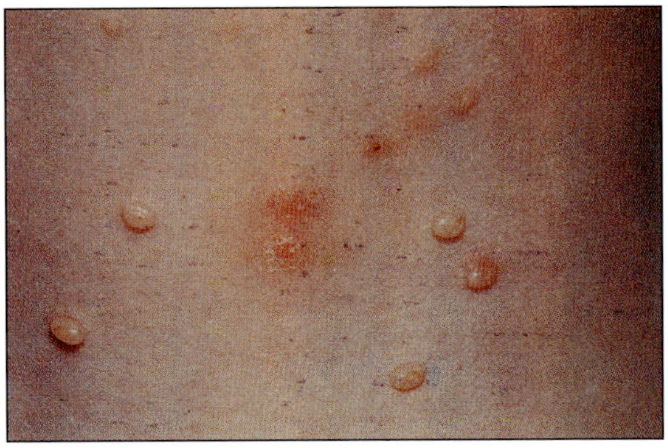

► Circular rings and a central caseous plug are typical features of molluscum contagiosum.

Molluscum Contagiosum

Nature of disease

A skin disease caused by an unclassified pox virus that produces single or multiple small, dome-shaped papules.

Predilections

Mostly affects immune-competent children and young adults but has occurred at all ages. Occurs with a more prolonged course in immune-compromised individuals. There is no sex or racial predilection.

Clinical features

Early lesions will be firm and flesh colored. Most begin on the hands, face, abdomen, and/or genital area. Mature lesions are gray in color and develop a caseous center. Transmission is by direct surface-to-surface contact.

Radiographic presentation

None.

Differential diagnosis

Molluscum contagiosum will appear similar to cystic acne or a folliculitis. Individual lesions may appear similar to a solitary keratoacanthoma. The more common presentation of multiple lesions will mimic syndromes in which multiple keratoacanthomas occur (ie, Muir-Torre syndrome, Ferguson-Smith syndrome in children, and Grzybowski syndrome in adults).

Microscopic features

A crateriform appearance of acanthotic epithelium in which a central component of enlarged, ballooned epithelial cells with large viral inclusions compressing the nucleus will be seen.

Suggested course of action

Suspicious cases should be referred to a dermatologist or infectious disease specialist.

Treatment

Molluscum contagiosum is self-healing and requires no specific treatment unless a quickened healing time is required or the patient is immune compromised. In those instances, topical 25% podophyllum or topical 5% imiquimod cream applied three to five times weekly for 4 to 8 weeks is effective.

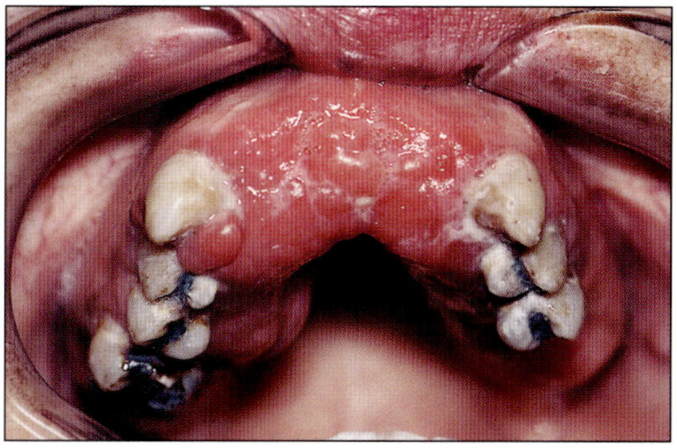

► Inflammatory papillary hyperplasia, like peri-implantitis and epulis fissuratum, is an example of chronic inflammatory response to a continuous stimulus.

Inflammatory Papillary Hyperplasia, Peri-implantitis, and Epulis Fissuratum

Nature of disease

A combined epithelial and fibrous proliferation of oral mucosa in response to one of the many inflammatory stimuli that the oral mucosa endures (ie, *Candida* infection, ill-filling dentures, repetitive trauma, etc).

Predilections

Adults are affected more frequently than children. No sex or racial predilection is known.

Clinical features

The most common presentation is that of a papillary reddened area of slightly edematous oral mucosa beneath an ill-fitting removable denture. Today, peri-implantitis represents a focal area of a similar pathogenesis where either microorganisms and/or repetitive trauma create the inflammatory response. Additionally, the term *epulis fissuratum* has been applied to an inflammatory proliferation around the flange of a denture.

Radiographic presentation

Vertical bone loss with thread exposure is commonly seen around an implant with peri-implantitis; otherwise, there are no radiographic changes noted.

Differential diagnosis

The red-white nature of all three clinical presentations is suspicious for epithelial dysplasia, verrucous carcinoma, or squamous cell carcinoma. Additionally, lichen planus may present with a similar appearance. Candidiasis should be considered as well and is often a co-etiology of inflammatory papillary hyperplasia.

Microscopic features

All three presentations will be seen to have an inflammatory cell infiltrate mostly of lymphocytes and plasma cells within the connective tissue below the basement membrane. Inflammatory papillary hyperplasia will show a multinodular response of fibrous tissue with an intact surface and multiple rete ridges. *Candida* organisms can frequently be seen on the surface and in the internodular cervices. Epulis fissuratums will have a fibrous proliferation with nodularity but also with an intact surface. ⟶

Inflammatory Papillary Hyperplasia, Peri-implantitis, and Epulis Fissuratum *(cont)*

Suggested course of action

Remove the ill-fitting denture and reduce any overextended flanges. Reline the denture with a tissue conditioner or rebase the denture if feasible. Treat the *Candida* initially with nystatin oral suspension 100,000 units/mL, 5 mL three times daily swish and spit. For refractory cases, add fluconazole (Diflucan, Pfizer) 100 mg once daily for 5 days. If lesions persist despite treatment and patient compliance, refer to an oral and maxillofacial surgeon for excision.

Treatment

Denture rebase or remake along with anti-*Candida* medications as noted above. Excision into the sub-basement membrane without grafting or grafting with palatal mucosa or skin may be required in persistent cases.

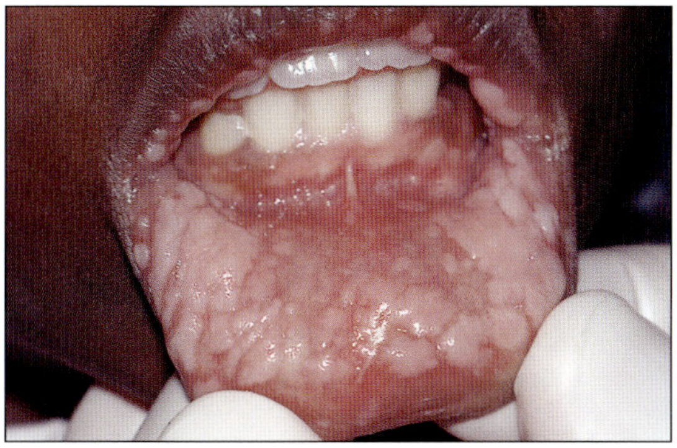

► Slightly raised, asymptomatic white mucosal patches of focal epithelial hyperplasia.

Focal Epithelial Hyperplasia (Heck Disease)

Nature of disease

An epithelial hyperplasia caused by DNA human papillomavirus (HPV) 13 and 32.

Predilections

Once thought to be limited to Native Americans, Eskimos, and Brazilian ethnicities, it is now recognized to occur in all races and ethnicities. It is seen mostly in preteens and teenagers but can occur at any age. There is no known sex predilection. It involves mostly the labial and buccal mucosa and to a lesser degree the tongue.

Clinical features

Multiple painless, white raised areas of the oral mucosa measuring 1.0 to 1.5 cm will be seen. The lesions are part of the oral mucosa and therefore are not movable and will not blanch.

Radiographic presentation

None.

Differential diagnosis

Multiple painless white thickenings of the oral mucosa may resemble condyloma acuminata, the multiple neuromas seen in multiple endocrine neoplasia type IIb, orofacial granulomatosis, or Crohn disease.

Microscopic features

There will be a focal, raised dome-shaped acanthosis without subepithelial inflammation or ulceration. Viral particles and perinuclear halos in the epithelial cells are often seen.

Suggested course of action

No action is required if the clinical diagnosis is evident. This is because the lesions will spontaneously involute over 3 to 5 years. If uncertain, obtain an incisional biopsy to rule out other considerations or refer to an oral and maxillofacial surgeon for evaluation, opinion, and biopsy.

Treatment

None required. Observational follow-up is recommended every 6 months.

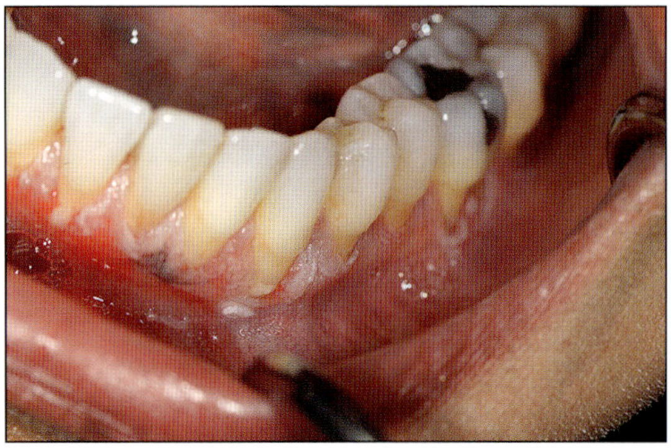

► Pyostomatitis vegetans.

Pyostomatitis Vegetans

Nature of disease

An intense, necrotizing focal inflammatory response forming pustules and exudates related to inflammatory bowel disease and ulcerative colitis.

Predilections

Mostly occurs in adults over 40 years of age, with a slight female predilection. No racial predilection is known.

Clinical features

An intense oral exudative and polypoid response seen on the labial mucosa, gingiva, and tongue. Pain is less severe than the clinical picture will suggest.

Radiographic presentation

None.

Differential diagnosis

Lesions may be similar to verrucous carcinoma or squamous cell carcinoma but also may appear similar to secondarily infected pemphigus, often referred to as *pemphigus vegetans*, or to paraneoplastic pemphigus. Severe erosive lichen planus may also appear similar.

Microscopic features

A polypoid proliferation of the epithelium sometimes with ulceration is seen over a connective tissue with microabscesses filled will a collection of eosinophils and some neutrophils.

Suggested course of action

Consult with a gastroenterologist to coordinate treatment. Inform him or her that oral lesions frequently become infected with anaerobic bacteria and that penicillin-metronidazole or doxycycline-metronidazole may be of benefit.

Treatment

Treatment is coordinated with a gastroenterologist, who may treat the patient with prednisone and/or infliximab (Remicade, Janssen), which is an anti–tumor necrosis factor alpha drug. Oral antibiotics as recommended above will complement the effectiveness of the ulcerative colitis/enteritis treatment on the oral mucosa.

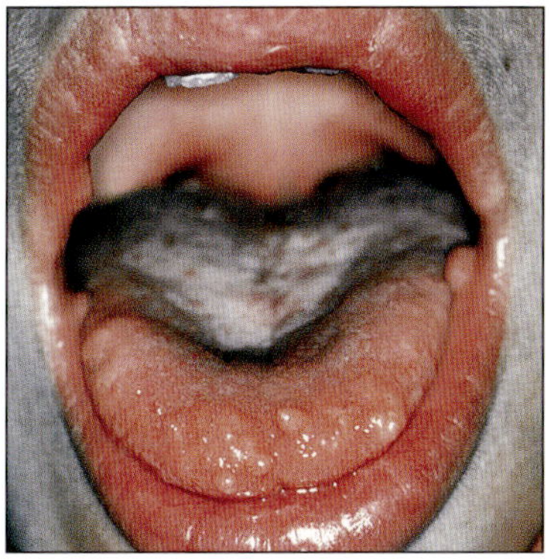

► Oral neuromas seen in MEN IIb.

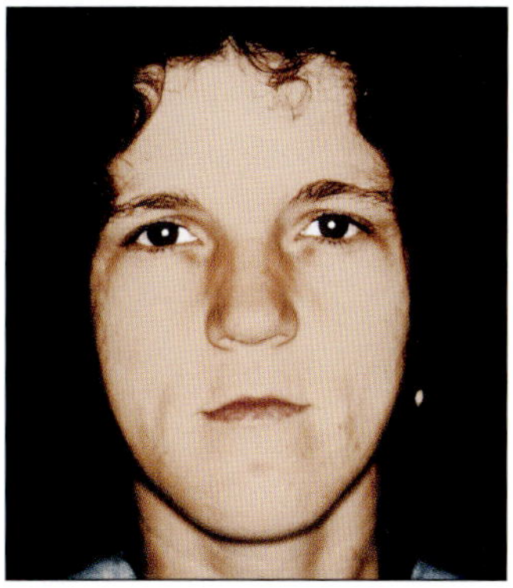

► Vertical maxillary excess (long face syndrome) may be a subtle clue focusing on MEN IIb if oral neuromas are also present.

Multiple Endocrine Neoplasia Type IIb (MEN IIb)

Nature of disease

A composite of clinical signs and symptoms arising from a mutation in the *RET* proto-oncogene located on chromosome 10q, 11.2. The syndrome comprises mucosal neuromas, pheochromocytoma, and early aggressive thyroid carcinoma. MEN type IIa (Sipple syndrome) also results from a mutation in the same proto-oncogene. This different mutation does not include mucosal neuromas, and the thyroid cancers are somewhat less aggressive, but it also includes primary hyperparathyroidism and Hirschsprung megacolon.

Predilections

Mucosal neuromas usually appear first and are usually seen in children and/or teenagers. No sex or racial predilection is known.

Clinical features

The oral mucosal neuromas are small, painless nodules with an intact surface and are mostly seen on the borders of the tongue or lips. Similar neuromas may also be seen arising from the conjunctiva of the eyes. The pheochromocytoma may not be recognized but may be indicated by tachycardia and hypertension. The medullary thyroid cancer may appear as a mass in the neck but not usually. Most patients also have a long face appearance and some element of vertical maxillary excess and temporal wasting.

Radiographic presentation

None except that a total body PET scan will identify a hypermetabolic focus in the thyroid if thyroid cancer is present or any area of its metastasis. It will also identify any pheochromocytoma.

Differential diagnosis

Because the multiple mucosal neuromas appear first, early cases may resemble focal epithelial hyperplasia (Heck disease), condyloma acuminata, or merely plugged or inflamed taste buds on the tongue or oral minor salivary glands. In the eyes, such neuromas may be similar to plugged meibomian glands (styes).

Microscopic features

Oral mucosal neuromas will show Schwann cells and identifiable nerve fascicles surrounded by perineurium within normal connective tissue lacking fibrosis and inflammation. →

Multiple Endocrine Neoplasia Type IIb (MEN IIb) *(cont)*

Suggested course of action

For the dental provider, it is important to know that early identification of this syndrome by recognizing the multiple oral neuromas can be life-saving. Suspicious cases need to be immediately referred to an endocrinologist for evaluation.

Treatment

The oral mucosal neuromas are painless and do not require excision unless they represent a functional impairment. The thyroid is treated with a prophylactic thyroidectomy; if cancer is already present, a thyroidectomy and a bilateral cervical lymphadenectomy usually followed by radiotherapy is accomplished. Pheochromocytomas usually develop later and, if mild, are treated medically. If significant symptoms occur, an adrenalectomy is performed.

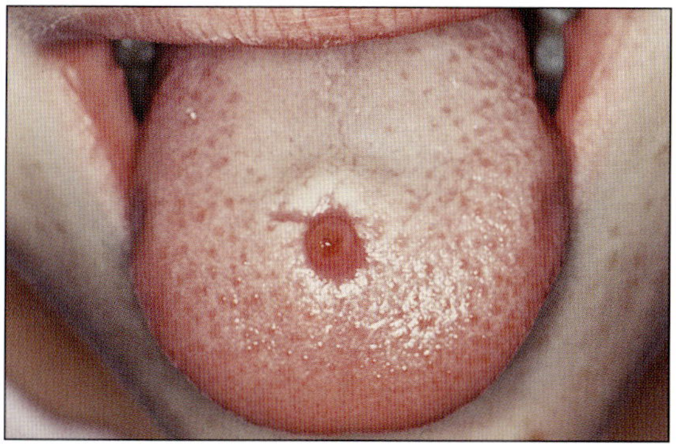

► Small dermoid cyst in the midline of the tongue.

Dermoid Cyst

Nature of disease

May arise from entrapped epithelia in the midline from fusion of the lateral tongue and floor of the mouth anlages or in facial skin from hair follicle epithelium.

Predilections

Mostly seen in children and young adults aged 1 to 35 years. There is no sex or racial predilection.

Clinical features

A slow-growing, round to oval, painless mass. Developmental dermoid cysts are found as a midline mass or paramidline mass in either the floor of the mouth, tongue, or anterior neck. Those that arise from hair follicle epithelium can be found on any hair-bearing skin.

Radiographic presentation

CT scans or MRI scans will show a round to oval homogenous soft tissue density well demarcated from surrounding tissues.

Differential diagnosis

In the midline area of the tongue, one must consider an epidermoid cyst and a granular cell tumor. In the midline of the floor of the mouth area, a ranula and salivary gland tumors are also strong considerations. In the midline of the neck, a plunging ranula, lipoma, and lymphoma are considerations. When these cysts occur from hair follicle epithelium, an epidermoid cyst and adnexal skin tumors such as a syringocystadenoma are considerations.

Microscopic features

An epithelial-lined lumen with adnexal structures (ie, hair follicle epithelium, sebaceous glands, and sweat gland structures) is characteristically seen in the wall of the cyst.

Suggested course of action

Refer to an oral and maxillofacial surgeon for definitive workup and treatment.

Treatment

All dermoid cysts are removed with a pericapsular excision. In those that arise from facial skin, the skin is later treated with retinoic acid compounds (ie, isotretinoin), antibiotics (eg, doxycycline), or commercial skin cleansers for prevention.

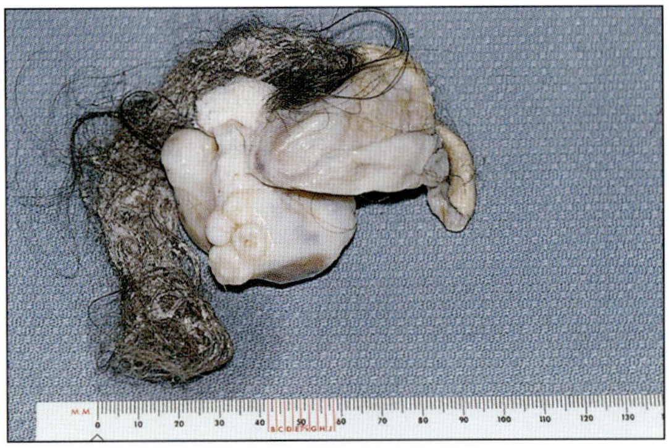

► Teratoid cyst/teratoma from the ovary seen with all three germ layer structures developed.

Teratoid Cyst

Nature of disease

A developmental disturbance in all three germ layers (ectoderm, endoderm, and mesoderm) resulting in a cyst in which structures from each of the three germ layers are present.

Predilections

Oral teratoid cysts are extremely rare. Most occur in the female ovary. In the oral region, they occur in the floor of the mouth, anterior mandible, or submental triangle. Oral lesions are mostly congenital but may first be found in children or young adults, with no sex or racial predilection. Ovarian teratoid cysts occur mostly after menarche.

Clinical features

Teratoid cysts in the oral cavity will present as an asymptomatic but firm expansion with an intact overlying mucosa. Those in the ovary are often found as an incidental radiographic or scan finding but may also be discovered after the patient complains of abdominal pain and/or dysmenorrhea.

Radiographic presentation

Detailed images will show bone with some morphologic resemblance to a recognizable bone (ie, maxilla or mandible). Many will also identify teeth.

Differential diagnosis

Those found around the floor of the mouth in young individuals will present similar to a dermoid cyst, a hemangioma, a lymphangioma, or a rhabdomyosarcoma.

Microscopic and gross specimen features

The gross specimen will be more revealing than the histopathology. Representatives from each germ layer will be microscopically normal. Gross specimens will show hair (ectoderm), intestinal lining (endoderm), cartilage or bone (mesoderm), and teeth with a periodontal ligament (ectoderm and mesoderm).

Suggested course of action

Large, firm oral expansions in a child require a referral to a pediatrician or an oral and maxillofacial surgeon.

Treatment

Teratoid cysts require enucleation or excision from whatever location they arise.

4

Oral Mucosal, Facial, and Neck Masses

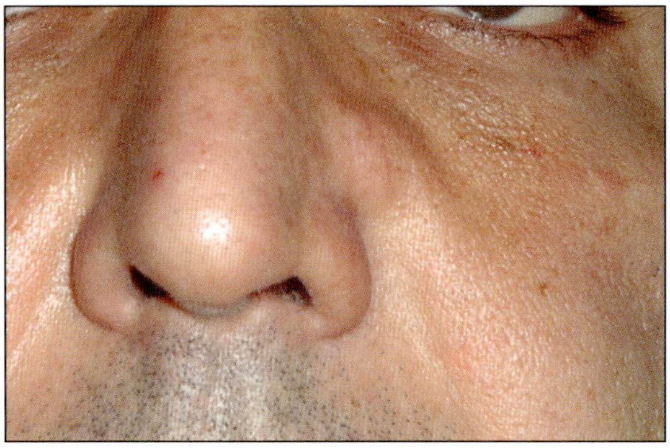

► Nasolabial cyst deep to the muscles of facial expression.

Nasolabial Cyst

Nature of disease

A rare cyst arising from epithelial remnants from the development of the nasolacrimal duct.

Predilections

There is no age, sex, or racial predilection.

Clinical features

Slow development of a painless mass appearing deep within the soft tissues in the paranasal area between the ala of the nose and the lacrimal sac.

Radiographic presentation

A true nasolabial cyst will not appear on plain radiographs. A medical CT scan will show an oval area of hypodensity as compared with the density of normal muscle.

Differential diagnosis

Epidermoid and dermoid cysts can occur in the same area and will strongly mimic the presentation of a nasolabial cyst. Additionally, tumors such as syringomas and trichilemmomas may be considered.

Microscopic features

The cyst is lined by pseudostratified ciliated columnar epithelium. The connective tissue wall is thin or of medium thickness.

Suggested course of action

Palpate the lesion intranasally and externally to determine if the mass is superficial or deep to the muscles of facial expression. Nasolabial cysts are deep to the muscles of facial expression, whereas skin cysts and tumors are superficial. Obtain a medical CT scan with contrast. Refer to an oral and maxillofacial surgeon for definitive treatment.

Treatment

Where possible, a transnasal pericapsular excision is preferred. Otherwise, a transcutaneous pericapsular excision is performed, separating and retracting the muscles of facial expression for access.

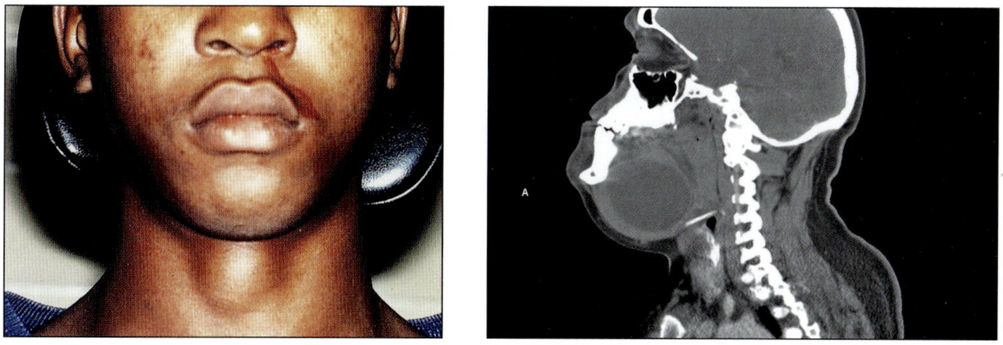

► Thyroglossal tract cyst.

Thyroglossal Tract Cyst

Nature of disease

Arises from residual epithelia that invaginated from the tuberculum impar of the tongue as a second brachial arch derivative and migrated to develop the thyroid gland over the larynx and upper trachea.

Predilections

Mostly seen in teenagers and young adults between 15 and 35 years old. There is no sex or racial predilection.

Clinical features

The thyroglossal tract cyst will usually have a rapid development of a painless or mildly painful, round to oval soft tissue mass in the midline of the neck over the larynx. Rarely, thyroglossal tract cysts will be paramidline; even more rarely, they may develop in the root of the tongue deep to the hyoid bone. Many are preceded by an upper respiratory tract cold or flu. Because the thyroglossal tract (note that it is a tract and not a duct) goes through the body of the hyoid bone, the cyst will characteristically move upon swallowing.

Radiographic presentation

CT scans and MRI scans will show a homogenous round soft tissue density in the tissues over the larynx or within the root of the tongue.

Differential diagnosis

Lipomas, dermoid cysts, and plunging ranulas may also present as a midline mass. Less commonly, a thyroid goiter or thyroid carcinoma may mimic its clinical presentation.

Microscopic features

Thin (one to three cell layers) epithelial-lined lumen. The wall of the cyst will contain thyroid colloid and sparse thyroid glandular cells.

Suggested course of action

Confirm movement of the cyst upon swallowing. Refer to an oral and maxillofacial surgeon for definitive treatment.

Treatment

Pericapsular soft tissue excision with either transection of the tract at the body of the hyoid bone or resection of the body of the hyoid bone.

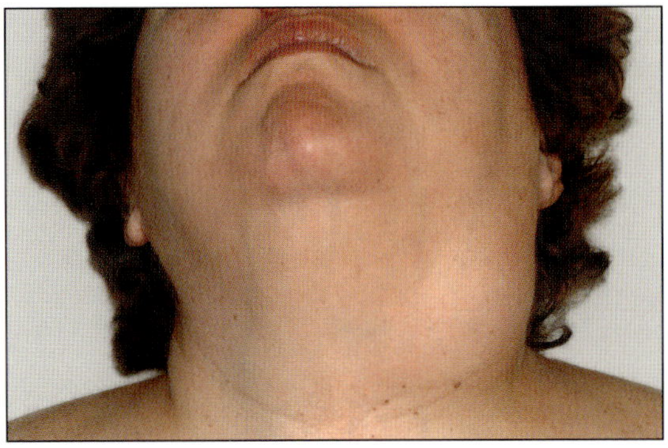

► Branchial cyst.

Branchial Cyst

Nature of disease

Arises from entrapped epithelia from the third branchial arch within a cervical lymph node.

Predilections

Mostly seen in teenagers and younger adults between 15 and 40 years old. There is no sex or racial predilection.

Clinical features

The rapid development of a painless or only mildly painful mass. Ninety percent develop in the lateral neck deep to the sternocleidomastoid muscle at its anterior border. The remaining 10% occur in either the preauricular area or the supraclavicular area. It is often preceded by an upper respiratory tract infection such as a cold or flu.

Radiographic presentation

CT scans or MRI scans will show a round soft tissue mass that will often reveal a hyperdensity representing a thickened cyst wall and a hypodense center representing fluid in the lumen. Others will be hypodense throughout compared with the density of adjacent muscle.

Differential diagnosis

Hodgkin lymphoma or less commonly non-Hodgkin lymphoma, metastatic squamous cell carcinoma from a cancer at the base of the tongue, a carotid body tumor, and cat-scratch disease should be considered.

Microscopic features

An epithelial-lined lumen with germinal centers and diffuse white blood cell collections in the cyst wall are characteristically seen.

Suggested course of action

Refer to an oral and maxillofacial surgeon for definitive treatment.

Treatment

Pericapsular soft tissue excision with transection of the tract superficial to the bifurcation of the carotid. Fifteen percent will not have a tract that would otherwise course through the carotid bifurcation to the pharyngeal wall.

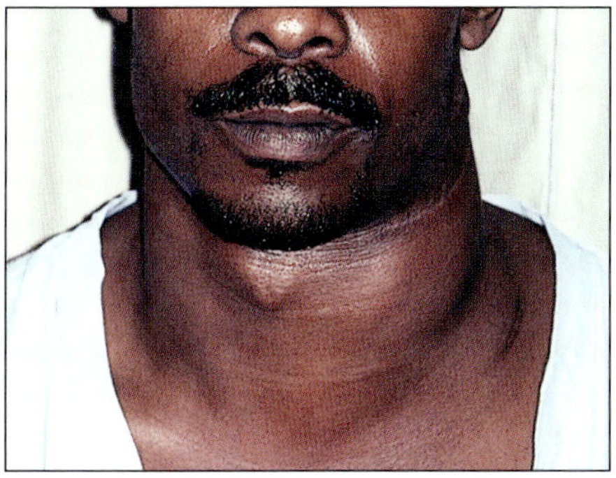

► Hodgkin lymphoma "bull neck" appearance.

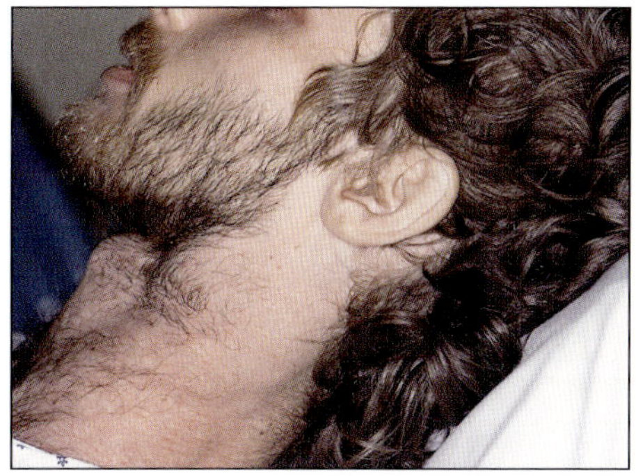

► Hodgkin lymphoma cachectic appearance.

Hodgkin Lymphoma

Nature of disease

A malignant disease of lymphoid cells, mostly B lymphocytes, that produces a peculiar cell termed the *Reed-Sternberg cell* and variations of that cell termed *lacunar cells* and *popcorn cells.*

Predilections

In general, Hodgkin lymphomas have a bimodal peak of incidence, most occurring between 15 and 35 years of age, with another smaller increase in incidence over 50 years of age. There is no racial predilection, but there is a male predilection of 1.5 to 1. The cervical lymph node chain is the most common one to be involved.

Clinical features

Hodgkin lymphomas present as one of two clinical pictures. The first is a healthy-appearing individual with large, bulky masses in the neck that give the impression of a "bull neck." The other is a thin, cachectic individual with smaller but obvious masses. If the weight loss is 10% of the person's normal body weight, it is referred to as a *B symptom.*

Radiographic presentation

CT scans, MRI scans, or PET scans are used to identify lymph node enlargements anywhere throughout the body.

Differential diagnosis

Lymph node enlargements in the cervical chain may also result from non-Hodgkin lymphoma, cat-scratch disease, sarcoidosis, tuberculous lymphadenitis, HIV infection, or infectious mononucleosis.

Microscopic features

There are five types of Hodgkin lymphoma, each with a somewhat different appearance but all with the identification of the malignant Reed-Sternberg cells or one of its variants: *(1)* Nodular lymphocyte-predominant Hodgkin lymphoma (NLPHL) has sheets of lymphocytes as a background with a scattering of Reed-Sternberg cells or its variants. *(2)* Nodular sclerosis Hodgkin lymphoma (NSHL) has sheets of lymphocytes and scattered eosinophils surrounded by thick collagen bands. *(3)* Mixed cellularity Hodgkin lymphoma (MCHL) has a mixture of lymphocytes, plasma cells, neutrophils, and eosinophils together with numerous Reed-Sternberg cells and no collagen bands. *(4)* Lymphocyte-depleted Hodgkin lymphoma (LDHL) has only sparse lymphocytes, eosinophils, and other normal cells replaced by numerous Reed-Sternberg cells or its variants, many with multinucleated bizarre forms resembling a poorly differentiated sarcoma. *(5)* Lymphocyte-rich Hodgkin lymphoma (LRHL) has mostly lymphocytes with some plasma cells and eosinophils but with only sparse Reed-Sternberg cells or its variants.

⟶

Hodgkin Lymphoma *(cont)*

Suggested course of action

Previously undiagnosed patients suspicious for Hodgkin lymphoma should be referred to a hematologist-oncologist. Already diagnosed patients should receive supportive dental care and required oral surgical care in consultation with the hematologist-oncologist. Note: Many Hodgkin lymphoma patients receive radiation therapy to the cervical, axillary, and mediastinal lymph node chains referred to as *mantle field radiation*. This field includes the mandible, but its dose is only 4,000 to 5,000 cGy, which is below the risk dose from osteoradionecrosis or the threshold for hyperbaric oxygen to improve the healing potential in the field.

Staging

Prior to treatment, Hodgkin lymphoma patients are staged according to the Ann Arbor staging system:

- Stage I is involvement of one lymph node chain (Stage I) or one extranodal site (Stage IE)
- Stage II is involvement of two or more lymph node chains on one side of the diaphragm (Stage II). If one site is an extranodal site, it is classified Stage IIE.
- Stage III identifies involvement on both sides of the diaphragm (Stage III). If one site is extranodal, an E is added (Stage IIIE). If the spleen is enlarged, an S is added for either Stage IIIS or Stage IIIES.
- Stage IV is disseminated multiorgan involvement with or without lymph node chain involvement.

Note: The letter B is added for weight loss or fever.

Treatment

- For cervical chain involvement Stages I and II, patients are treated with mantle field radiation alone.
- For cervical chain involvement Stages IB and IIB, mantle field radiation therapy is combined with multidrug chemotherapy.
- For Stages III and IV, multidrug chemotherapy is used with the addition of mantle field radiation therapy for the cervical chains in selected cases.

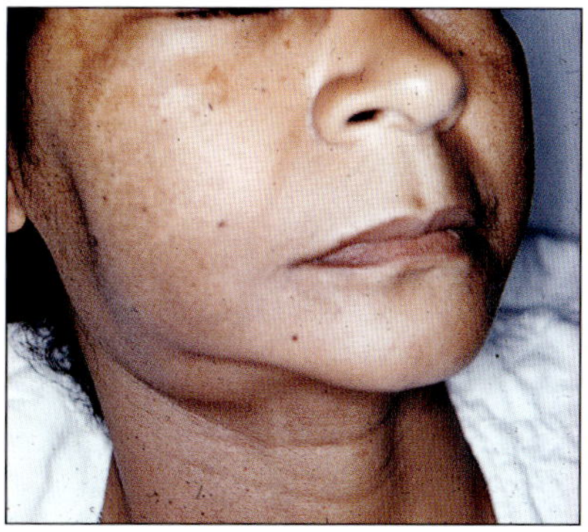

► Non-Hodgkin lymphoma.

Non-Hodgkin Lymphoma

Nature of disease

A proliferation of any one of several types of malignant lymphocyte precursors of the B-cell type or T-cell type.

Predilections

The risk for non-Hodgkin lymphoma increases with age. Extranodal sites, particularly in the palate, pharynx, and buccal mucosa, are more common than in Hodgkin lymphomas. There is no known sex or racial predilection.

Clinical features

In the oral cavity a diffuse, soft, fleshy expansion of the palatal and maxillary mucosa is a common presentation. Others include submucosal masses that may occur with or without cervical lymph node enlargement. Some patients will present with only large, painless neck masses. Many will be seen to have suffered weight loss or will report fatigue.

Radiographic presentation

CT, MRI, and PET scans will identify locations of either nodal or extranodal sites.

Differential diagnosis

Extranodal sites in the palate may be confused with a squamous cell carcinoma or an underlying bone necrosis, such as drug-induced osteonecrosis, osteoradionecrosis, or even an osteomyelitis. Masses within the submucosa will most closely resemble salivary gland tumors and benign schwannomas. Cervical chain lymph node masses may represent a Hodgkin lymphoma, cat-scratch disease, sarcoidosis, or HIV infection. →

Non-Hodgkin Lymphoma *(cont)*

Microscopic features

There are too many types of non-Hodgkin lymphoma to describe each variant. However, the central theme is a sheet of altered lymphocytes that resemble plasma cells instead of lymphocytes in a monotonous pattern where all cells look alike. The distinction for the specific type of non-Hodgkin lymphoma is based on cell size and whether it is a B-cell or T-cell lymphoma. The most recognized types of non-Hodgkin lymphoma are the following:

- Small, lymphocytic B-cell lymphoma
- Extranodal marginal B-cell lymphoma (MALT lymphoma)
- Follicular B-cell lymphoma
- Mantle cell lymphoma
- Diffuse large B-cell lymphoma
- Burkitt lymphoma (small noncleaved cell lymphoma), African type or American type
- Anaplastic large cell lymphoma
- Extranodal natural killer T-cell lymphoma nasal type (previously known as *midline lethal granuloma of the palate*)
- Mycosis fungoides (a peripheral lymphatic lymphoma of the T-cell type)

Note: Large-cell lymphomas generally have a poorer prognosis than small-cell lymphomas.

Suggested course of action

Previously undiagnosed patients suspicious for non-Hodgkin lymphoma should be referred to a hematologist-oncologist. Already diagnosed patients should receive supportive dental and oral care throughout their treatment course.

Treatment

Each type of lymphoma is treated with a different type of specific chemotherapy protocol, with the addition of radiation therapy in selected cases and for selected sites.

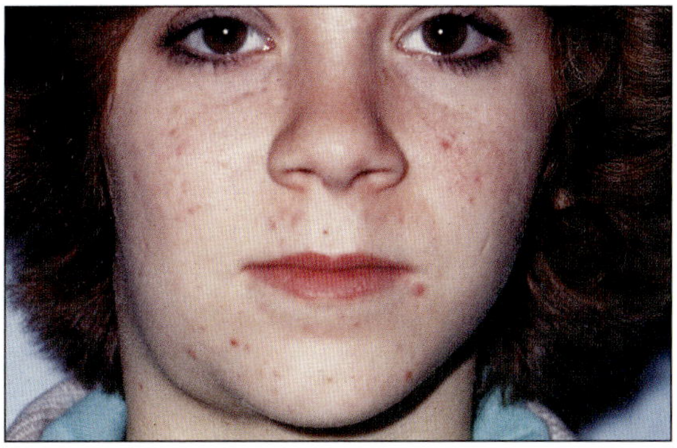

► Lymphadenopathy from cat-scratch disease.

Cat-Scratch Disease

Nature of disease

A necrotizing lymphadenitis caused by an infection from the microorganism *Bartonella henselae.*

Predilections

Can occur at any age but seen mostly in children and young adults. No sex or racial predilection is known. There is a strong association with kittens and cats younger than 1 year.

Clinical features

The involved lymph nodes will present as a firm, painless, lobulated mass of lymph nodes adhered together. Only 50% of patients are actually scratched by a cat, but nearly all have been around young cats. Additionally, if the patient has been scratched, the location of the lymphadenitis is usually not in the drainage field of the scratch. In late-stage cases, the lymph nodes may undergo liquefactive necrosis, presenting as a mildly painful abscess that may also drain pus.

Radiographic presentation

Cat-scratch disease will not be seen on plain radiographs. A medical CT scan will identify a hyperdense mass that may have a central area of hypodensity if liquefactive necrosis is present.

Differential diagnosis

Adherent, painless cat-scratch lymph nodes will appear identical to those of squamous cell carcinoma and tuberculous lymphadenitis. Other considerations are Hodgkin and non-Hodgkin lymphoma and infectious mononucleosis.

Microscopic features

A dense inflammatory infiltrate is seen between germinal centers that often have a central area of breakdown.

Suggested course of action

Obtain a serum cat-scratch antigen test for *Bartonella henselae*. (Note: Cat-scratch cases usually do not show a lymphocytosis.) A positive cat-scratch antigen value in a dilution equal to or greater than 1:320 is diagnostic. Refer to an infectious disease specialist or an oral and maxillofacial surgeon for definitive treatment.

Treatment

Although many cases resolve without treatment, most are treated with erythromycin or doxycycline to prevent liquefaction, necrosis, and drainage. In cases of necrosis and clinical abscess, incision and drainage is not recommended. Instead, complete removal of the necrotic lymph node is preferred.

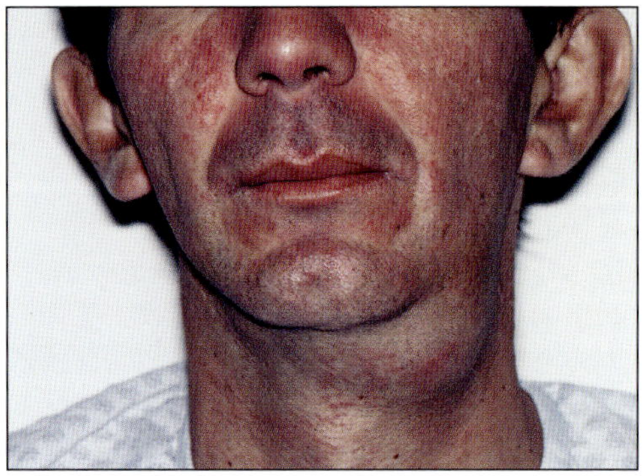

► Tuberculous lymphadenitis.

Tuberculous Lymphadenitis

Nature of disease

A lymph node infection caused mostly by *Mycobacterium scrofulaceum*. Other cases may be caused by *Mycobacterium tuberculosis* or, rarely, atypical *Mycobacterium* species.

Predilections

Today more common in HIV-infected patients. Seen mostly in adults. There is no sex or racial predilection.

Clinical features

Presents as either multiple small (< 3 cm) painless lymph node enlargements or as a single large (> 3 cm) mass that is mild to moderately painful. The node or nodes are usually freely movable and doughy in consistency.

Radiographic presentation

Tuberculous lymphadenitis does not appear on plain radiographs. A medical CT scan will identify a soft tissue mass or masses. If caseation is present within the lymph node, it will appear as a hypodense center.

Differential diagnosis

Hodgkin and non-Hodgkin lymphomas are the most serious considerations, followed by cat-scratch disease and infectious mononucleosis.

Microscopic features

The lymph node architecture will be replaced by epithelioid granulomas, which are seen as a central area of histiocytes (macrophages) surrounded by a ring of lymphocytes. This organization also contains Langhans giant cells (large cells that have a series of nuclei at the periphery and a pale central cytoplasm). This organization of cells is the description of a true granuloma. If caseation necrosis is present, there will be an area devoid of cells and filled with an amorphous eosinophilic substance.

Suggested course of action

Request patient consent for HIV testing. Refer to an infectious disease specialist.

Treatment

Cultures are obtained to ascertain drug sensitivities. Treatment consists of multiple antimycobacterial drugs that may include isoniazid, ethambutol, streptomycin, and rifampin, among others.

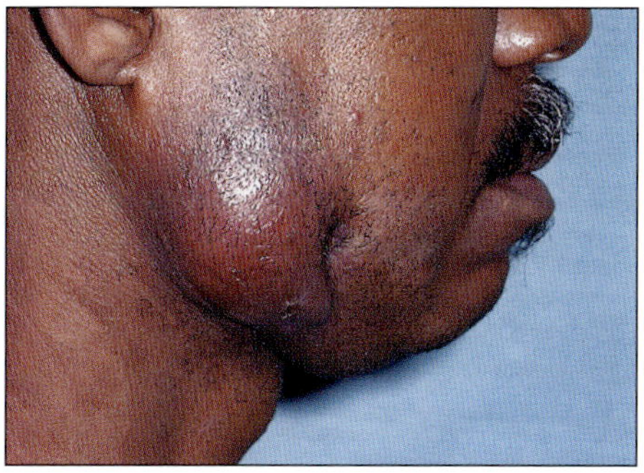

► Cervicofacial actinomycosis.

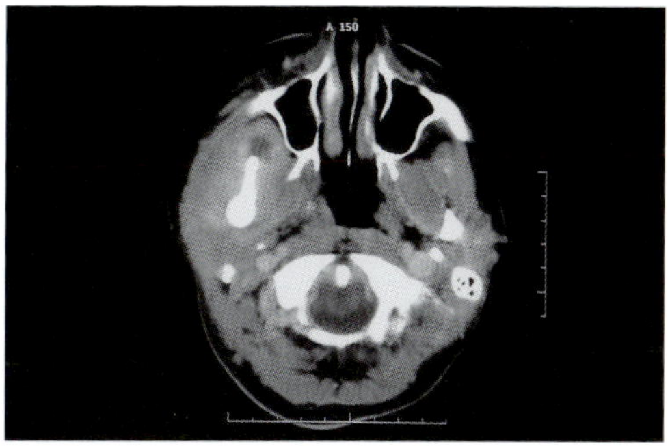

► Fibrosis in the muscles of mastication causing trismus in a patient with actinomycosis.

Cervicofacial Actinomycosis

Nature of disease

A soft tissue infection caused by one of the several species of *Actinomyces*, of which *Actinomyces israeli* is the most common. It is characterized by chronicity and fibrosis, giving it its historical name of "lumpy jaw." Note: *Actinomyces* is a common pathogen directly responsible (or as a co-pathogen) for most cases of osteomyelitis of the jaw, and it is well known to cause secondary bone infections in the exposed bone from osteoradionecrosis and drug-induced osteonecrosis. These infections are not referred to specifically as *cervicofacial actinomycosis.*

Predilections

There is no age, sex, or racial predilection.

Clinical features

The patient will present with firm fibrotic masses within the fascia and lymph nodes of the neck. The masseter and medial pterygoid muscles are often fibrotic as well, producing trismus. The masses are usually only mildly painful or painless and are fixed to the surrounding tissue. A source of infection, usually odontogenic, is generally found. Most commonly a cracked tooth, pulpal pathology, or a failing root canal treatment is found to be the focus of infection or, more rarely, cryptic tonsils, as *Actinomyces* is well known to reside in tonsillar crypts.

Radiographic presentation

Plain radiographs may show the portal of entry of the *Actinomyces*. However, CT scans and MRI scans will show the soft tissue hyperdensity indicative of fibrosis as well as any abscess cavity within the soft tissues. Frequently, the masseter and medial pterygoid muscles are noted to be enlarged and hyperdense, indicative of a diffuse fibrosis.

Differential diagnosis

On initial presentation, the patient's trismus and fibrosis will suggest radiation fibrosis and traumatic myositis ossificans. Trismus should also suggest a possible carcinoma within the pterygomandibular space.

Microscopic features

The fibrosis will be represented by dense acellular collagen. Scattered inflammatory cells may be noted. However, the pathognomonic feature is that of a basophilic-staining colony of *Actinomyces* organisms surrounded by neutrophils. This is known as a *sulfur granule.* Note: Today sulfur granules are very rarely seen clinically. In the past, more advanced and long-term cases produced macroscopic yellow flecks during drainage and debridement procedures, leading to the term *sulfur granules.* Today *sulfur granules* usually refer to this microscopic finding.

→

Cervicofacial Actinomycosis *(cont)*

Suggested course of action

Accomplish a thorough oral examination with radiographs, looking for a definitive focus of infection. Refer to an oral and maxillofacial surgeon for further workup and treatment.

Treatment

Removal of the focus of infection and debridement is crucial. Antibiotics of the penicillin type via a PICC line for 3 months is recommended. If the infection advances or persists, a more extensive debridement is required to remove fibrotic tissue, and intravenous antibiotics should be continued. Note: *Actinomyces* is incapable of penicillin resistance and should be used in all cases except in patients allergic to penicillin. Alternative antibiotic choices for the penicillin-allergic patient are doxycycline, cefoxitin, and vancomycin.

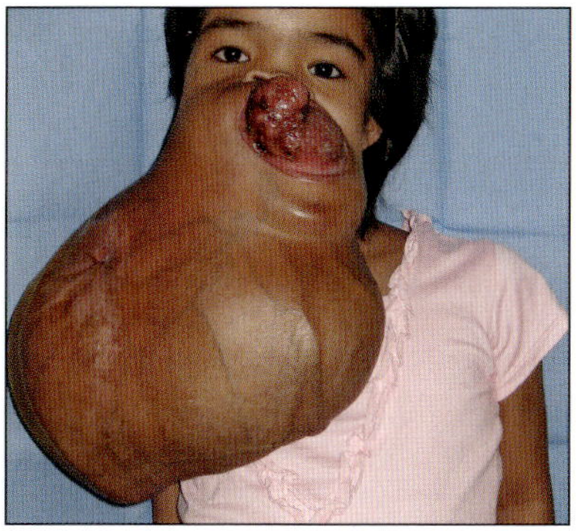

► Extreme-sized schwannoma.

Schwannoma of Soft Tissue

Nature of disease

Schwannomas are benign proliferations of the Schwann cells covering nerves.

Predilections

Most are seen in adults. No sex or racial predilection is known. Although schwannomas can arise from any nerve, those in the neck tend to arise from more deeply located nerves.

Clinical features

Schwannomas will present as a painless, oval-shaped, freely movable mass. They are not associated with any paresthesia or paresis. The mass will be of a doughy to firm consistency.

Radiographic presentation

As soft tissue masses, schwannomas will not appear on plain radiographs. CT scans will show a well-encapsulated mass with a density similar to or slightly less than that of adjacent muscle. MRI scans will show an increased water content in the mass on a T2-weighted image.

Differential diagnosis

Oval-shaped soft tissue masses also suggest Hodgkin or non-Hodgkin lymphoma, cat-scratch disease, dermoid cysts, and, when around the parotid gland, benign parotid tumors.

Microscopic features

The mass will have a readily identifiable capsule of collagen. Within the capsule, a gray matrix is seen to be associated with darkly staining cell arrangements. One arrangement is a single-file alignment that may be noted to palisade. These cells are referred to as *Antoni A cells*. The matrix between two rows of Antoni A cells is referred to as a *Verocay body*. The second cell arrangement is a scattered cell arrangement without any organization. These cells are referred to as *Antoni B cells*. Throughout the mass, numerous blood vessels will also be noted.

Suggested course of action

Refer to an oral and maxillofacial surgeon for workup and treatment.

Treatment

Schwannomas are curable with a pericapsular excision. Those that arise from a nerve trunk can be removed from the nerve trunk without sacrificing the nerve. In those arising from small peripheral nerve fibers or nerve endings, the parent nerve is not seen and is removed with the tumor.

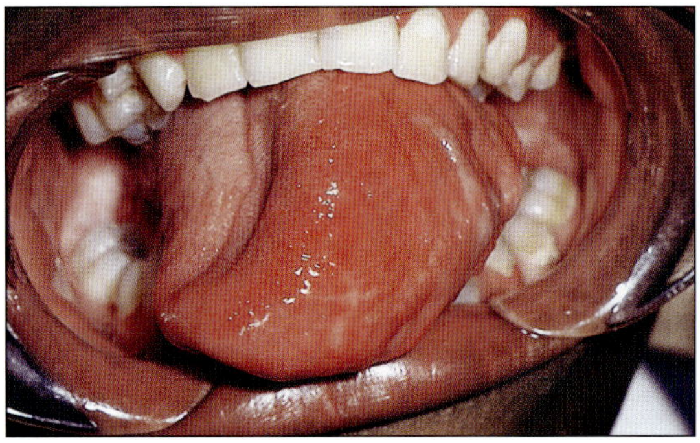

► Neurofibroma of the tongue.

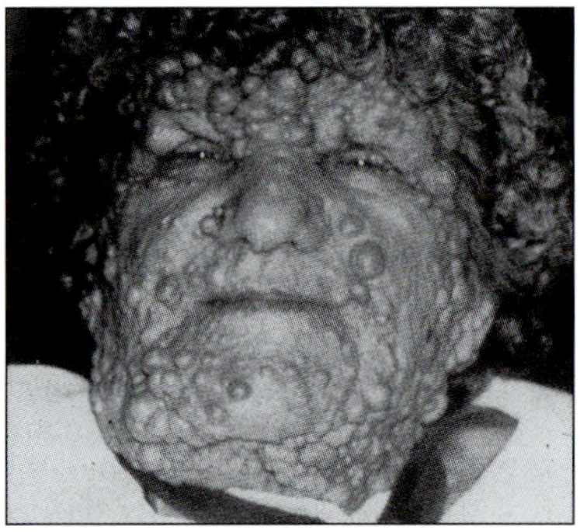

► Multiple neurofibromas from hereditary neurofibromatosis type 1.

Neurofibroma

Nature of disease

A benign but unencapsulated tumor of neurofibroblasts from peripheral nerve sheaths.

Predilections

Ninety percent of neurofibromas occur unassociated with hereditary neurofibromatosis type 1 or 2; these are termed *solitary neurofibromas*. They have no sex or racial predilection but do occur more frequently in young adults.

Clinical features

Patients will present with a diffuse, painless submucosal or subcutaneous mass. The mass will feel as if it has cords within it, often termed the "bag of worms" presentation. The mass will also infiltrate into surrounding tissues, making it somewhat immobile.

Radiographic presentation

Most neurofibromas are within soft tissue and have no plain radiograph projections. CT scans will outline the mass as a diffuse unencapsulated soft tissue density blending into adjacent tissues. MRI scans will identify a high water content indicative of the vascularity of a neurofibroma. The rarer central neurofibroma will appear as a diffuse radiolucency often seen as an expansion arising from the mandibular canal.

Differential diagnosis

In soft tissue, the "bag of worms" texture will suggest a deep-seated hemangioma, lymphangioma, lipoma, rhabdomyoma, or even a rhabdomyosarcoma.

Microscopic features

The mass will be unencapsulated with spindle-shaped fibroblasts in a serpentine arrangement amid a wavy pattern of collagen. Numerous small blood vessels will permeate throughout the specimen.

Suggested course of action

Refer to an oral and maxillofacial surgeon for workup and treatment.

Treatment

Because neurofibromas have slow and limited growth, many are incompletely excised to improve function and appearance. Complete excision observing 1.0-cm margins is recommended when possible.

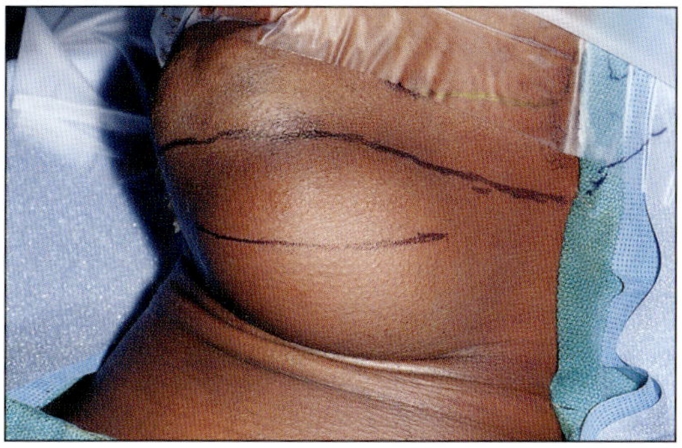

► Pulsatile mass from a carotid body tumor.

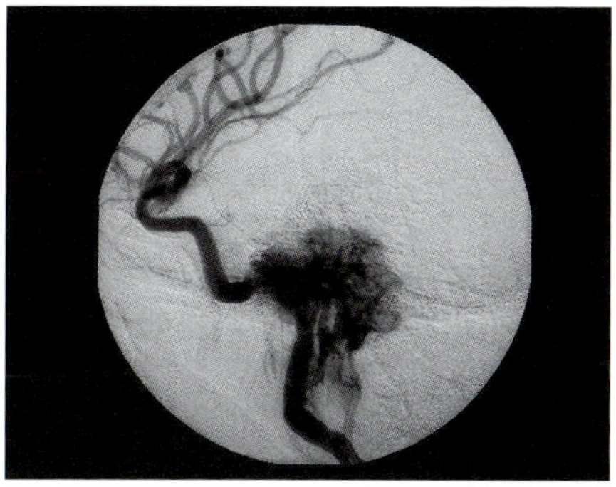

► Multiple blood vessels comprise a carotid body tumor as seen on this angiogram.

Carotid Body Tumor

Nature of disease

A rare, highly vascular tumor that arises out of specialized neural crest cells that develop into autonomic ganglia. The carotid body tumor, along with other paraganglioma tumors in the aorta, abdomen, thorax, etc, are known as *extra-adrenal paragangliomas.*

Predilections

Most cases occur between the ages of 40 and 60 years. It is more common in areas of high altitude (eg, Peru, Colorado, Mexico City), where it affects women more than men. Those that occur in areas of lower altitude are seen more commonly in men. There is no racial predilection.

Clinical features

The carotid body tumor will present as a painless, pulsatile mass in the area of the carotid bifurcation. Pulsation can often be readily seen from a distance of 5 feet. The mass will be movable in the anteroposterior direction but not in the superior-inferior direction. A bruit will be heard by stethoscope, auscultation, or by Doppler. A palpable pulsation "thrill" can also be felt.

Radiographic presentation

CT scans will identify a mass of increased soft tissue density. However, an angiogram will show numerous blood vessels circled around the carotid bifurcation.

Differential diagnosis

Other masses at the level of the carotid bifurcation may pulsate due to their proximity to the normal carotid artery. Therefore, regional lymph node metastasis from an oropharyngeal squamous cell carcinoma should be considered along with a branchial cyst, cat-scratch disease, Hodgkin and non-Hodgkin lymphomas, and sarcoidosis.

Microscopic features

Nests and balls of large, polygonal eosinophilic cells that have a somewhat granular cytoplasm will be seen and will be separated by a thin fibrovascular connective tissue. Nuclear pleomorphism is common, but mitotic figures are rare.

Suggested course of action

The finding of a pulsatile mass in the area of the carotid bifurcation requires a referral to a vascular surgeon.

Treatment

Carotid body tumors require a wide-access, slow, and delicate surgery to remove the lesion from its adherence to the carotid artery.

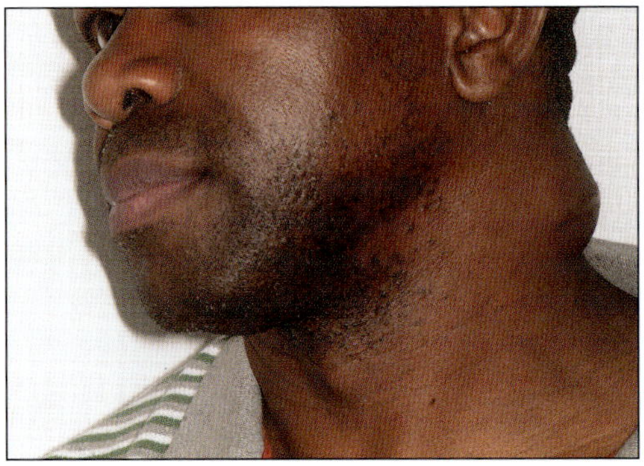

► Lipoma in the posterior triangle of the neck.

Lipoma

Nature of disease

Lipomas are benign neoplasms that arise from adipocyte precursors that slowly proliferate to produce an encapsulated mass of mature fat cells.

Predilections

Mostly seen in adults, with a slight female predilection. No racial predilection is known.

Clinical features

Lipomas can occur in any region of the neck. In the oral mucosa, most are seen around the mental foramen area. They are slow-growing, painless masses that will register a soft consistency when palpated. Most are freely movable.

Radiographic presentation

Lipomas will not appear on plain radiographs other than as a slight soft tissue density. On CT scans, they will be noted to appear as a well-delineated soft tissue mass with a density much less than that of adjacent muscle. On an MRI scan T2-weighted image, they appear as a well-delineated soft tissue mass with a high water content.

Differential diagnosis

Depending on its location in the neck, a lipoma may resemble a Hodgkin or non-Hodgkin lymphoma, a plunging ranula, or a dermoid cyst.

Microscopic features

Mature fat cells with collagen septa containing small blood vessels are seen encased within a thin capsule of collagen.

Suggested course of action

Refer to an oral and maxillofacial surgeon for workup and treatment.

Treatment

Lipomas are curable with a pericapsular dissection. Note: The capsule is extremely thin, so many will seem to have no capsule.

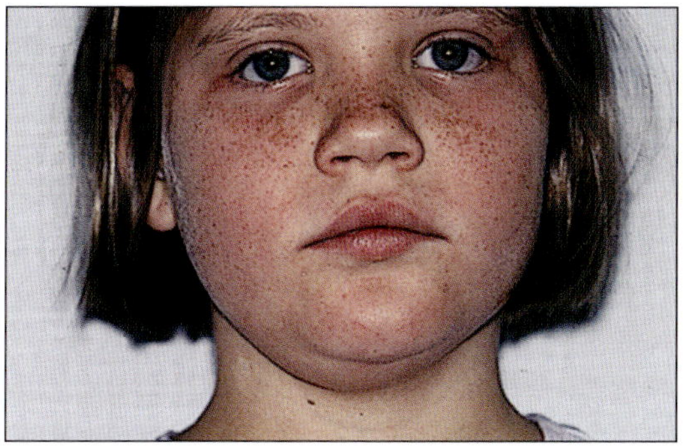

► Plunging ranula.

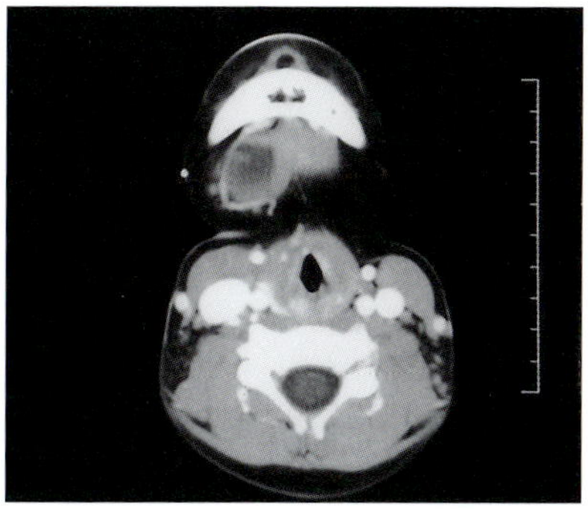

► Hypodense area of a plunging ranula seen on a CT scan.

Plunging Ranula

Nature of disease

A fibrous encapsulation of extravasated saliva from a ruptured sublingual gland duct in which the expanding backpressure against the floor of the mouth mucosa causes it to project into the submental triangle of the neck.

Predilections

Children and young adults mostly. No sex or racial predilection is known.

Clinical features

The component of the ranula in the floor of the mouth will appear as a bluish expansion causing thinning of the mucosa, giving it the appearance of a frog's belly, hence the name *ranula* after the Latin for *little frog.* The component in the submental triangle of the neck may also appear blue, but it is usually seen as a normal-colored, expanded skin mass. Both components will imply a fluid content upon palpation.

Radiographic presentation

Plain radiographs will not identify a ranula. CT scans will show a hypodense mass arising from one of the two sublingual glands. An MRI scan T2-weighted image will show a very high water content of a mass arising from one of the two sublingual glands.

Differential diagnosis

The bluish coloration and the soft texture will suggest a hemangioma or lymphangioma. Other considerations in this location include a low-grade mucoepidermoid carcinoma, a dermoid cyst, or a lipoma.

Microscopic features

A compressed fibrous capsule will be seen to contain remnants of mucin along with scattered inflammatory cells.

Suggested course of action

Refer to an oral and maxillofacial surgeon for workup and treatment.

Treatment

After aspiration of the lesion to test for a high level of amylase, which will confirm the diagnosis, the plunging ranula and the associated sublingual gland are removed with a pericapsular excision via an external approach.

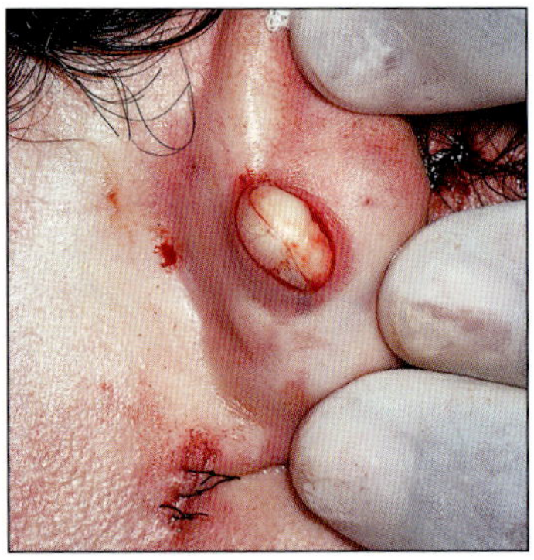

► Epidermoid inclusion cyst being removed from skin of the ear.

Epidermoid Inclusion Cyst

Nature of disease

Most arise from hair follicle epithelium or epithelium entrapped in the dermis.

Predilections

More common in teenagers and young adults and specifically those with acne. There is no sex or racial predilection. Note: Multiple epidermoid cysts can be part of Gardner syndrome.

Clinical features

A slow-growing dermal/subcutaneous mass that is sometimes painful if secondarily infected. It is usually fixed to the skin and dermis.

Radiographic presentation

None on plain radiographs. However, a CT scan or MRI will show a round or oval-shaped soft tissue mass in the dermis.

Differential diagnosis

Skin appendage tumors such as syringomas or other skin lesions such as trichofolliculomas and dermoid cysts should be considered. Additionally, a dermal metastasis from an oral squamous cell carcinoma or a metastasis from a distant malignancy should be considered.

Microscopic features

Squamous epithelial-lined lumen with a cyst wall of connective tissue devoid of adnexal structures.

Suggested course of action

Observe for other skin masses and acne. Palpate the mass in an attempt to elicit pain indicative of secondary infection. Refer to a dermatologist for evaluation or an oral and maxillofacial surgeon for excision.

Treatment

Pericapsular excision.

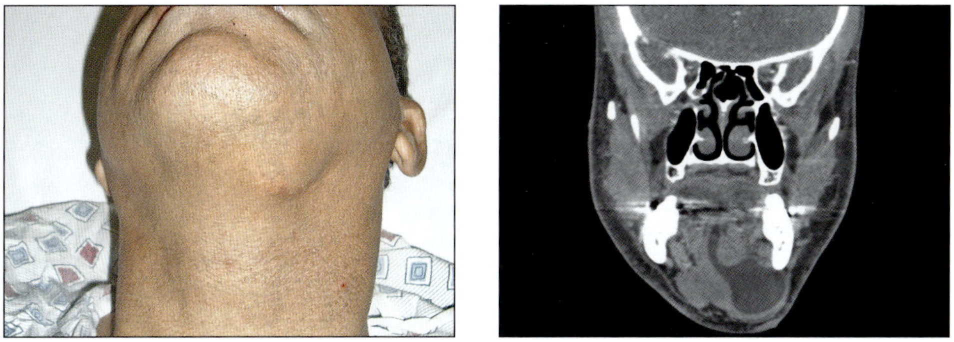

► Dermoid cyst that began in the midline of the tongue and presented off the midline in the neck.

Dermoid Cyst

Nature of disease

May arise from entrapped epithelia in the midline from fusion of the lateral tongue and floor of the mouth anlages or in facial skin from hair follicle epithelium.

Predilections

Mostly seen in children and young adults aged 1 to 35 years. There is no sex or racial predilection.

Clinical features

A slow-growing, round to oval, painless mass. Most are found as a midline mass or paramidline mass in either the floor of the mouth, tongue, or anterior neck.

Radiographic presentation

CT scans or MRI scans will show a round to oval homogenous soft tissue density well demarcated from surrounding tissues.

Differential diagnosis

In the midline area of the tongue, one must consider an epidermoid cyst and a granular cell tumor. In the midline of the floor of the mouth area, a ranula and salivary gland tumors are also strong considerations. In the midline of the neck, a plunging ranula, lipoma, and lymphoma are considerations. When these cysts occur from hair follicle epithelium, an epidermoid inclusion cyst and adnexal skin tumors such as a syringocystadenoma are considerations.

Microscopic features

Epithelial-lined lumen with adnexal structures (ie, hair follicle epithelium, sebaceous glands, and sweat gland structures) located in the wall of the cyst.

Suggested course of action

Refer to an oral and maxillofacial surgeon for definitive workup and treatment.

Treatment

All dermoid cysts are removed with a pericapsular excision. In those that arise from facial skin, the skin is later treated with retinoic acid compounds (ie, isotretinoin), antibiotics (eg, doxycycline), or commercial skin cleansers for prevention of future cysts.

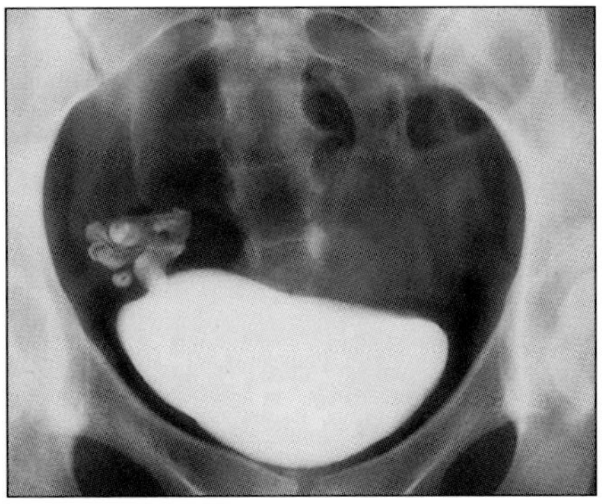

► Bone and teeth are apparent in this teratoid cyst from the ovary.

Teratoid Cyst

Nature of disease

A developmental disturbance involving all three germ layers (ectoderm, endoderm, and mesoderm) resulting in a cystic lumen in which structures from each of the three germ layers are present.

Predilections

Oral teratoid cysts are extremely rare. Most occur in the female ovary. In the oral region, they occur in the floor of the mouth, anterior mandible, or submental triangle. Oral lesions are mostly congenital but may first be found in children or young adults, with no sex or racial predilection. Ovarian teratoid cysts occur mostly after menarche.

Clinical features

Teratoid cysts in the oral cavity will present as an asymptomatic but firm expansion with an intact overlying mucosa. Those in the ovary are often found as an incidental radiographic or scan finding but may also be discovered after the patient complains of abdominal pain and dysmenorrhea.

Radiographic presentation

Detailed images will show bone with some morphologic resemblance to a recognizable bone (ie, maxilla or mandible). Many will also identify teeth.

Differential diagnosis

Those found around the floor of the mouth in young individuals will present similar to a dermoid cyst, a cystic hygoma-lymphangioma, or a rhabdomyosarcoma.

Microscopic and gross specimen features

The gross specimen will be more revealing than the histopathology. Representatives from each germ layer will be microscopically normal. Gross specimens will show hair (ectoderm), intestinal lining (endoderm), bone (mesoderm), and teeth with a periodontal ligament (ectoderm and mesoderm).

Suggested course of action

Large, firm oral expansions in a child require a referral to a pediatrician or an oral and maxillofacial surgeon.

Treatment

Teratoid cysts require enucleation or excision from whatever location they arise.

Thyroid Goiter

Nature of disease

A nonspecific term referring to an increased size of the thyroid gland. It may herald a nonfunctioning hyperplasia resulting in hypothyroidism or an overfunctioning hyperplasia resulting in hyperthyroidism, also known as *Graves disease*.

Predilections

Women are more commonly affected than men, and most are in their middle adult years. There is no known racial predilection.

Clinical features

A goiter will be seen as an almost symmetric mass just inferior to the larynx. The mass is usually painless and movable. Some will be multinodular.

Radiographic presentation

A CT scan will show a soft tissue density over the laryngotracheal area. A radioactive iodine (I^{131}) scan will identify a hyperthyroid gland by an increased uptake and imply a hypothyroid gland by a decreased uptake. However, serum thyroid function tests are the standard to identify a hypothyroid state, a euthyroid state, or a hyperthyroid state.

Differential diagnosis

A mass in the area of the thyroid gland should be considered to be a possible thyroid carcinoma. A thyroglossal tract cyst, lipomas, and lymphomas should also be considered.

Microscopic features

In the hypothyroid goiter ("cold goiter"), the follicular cells are replaced by or have differentiated to an adenomatous appearance. Thyroglobulin is seen in abundance within the thyroid follicles in the hyperthyroid gland ("hot goiter"). The follicles are more neuromatous, and the follicular cells are hyperplastic.

Suggested course of action

Examine the patient for signs of hypothyroidism (ie, lethargy, slow mentation, sparse hair, dry skin) and hyperthyroidism (ie, exophthalmos, thin body habitus, tachycardia, tense excitable affect). Note your findings and refer to an endocrinologist.

Treatment

If hypothyroidism is diagnosed, synthetic thyroid replacement is prescribed. If hyperthyroidism is diagnosed, radioactive iodine by mouth will atrophy the gland. Alternatively, the antithyroid drugs propylthiouracil and methimazole also cause thyroid atrophy and may be prescribed. At times, a subtotal thyroidectomy is used.

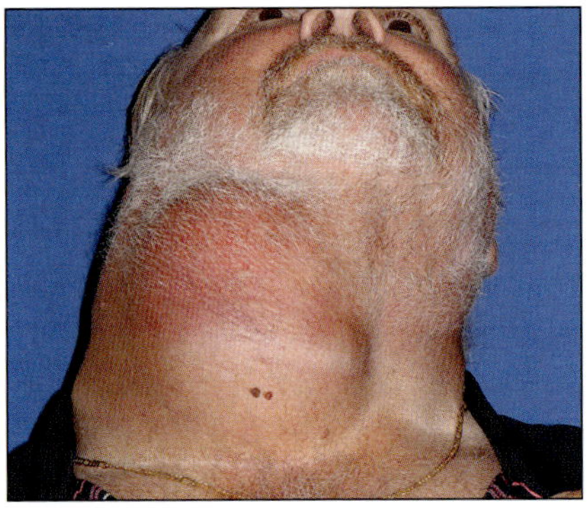

► Thyroid neoplasia.

Thyroid Neoplasias

Nature of disease

Benign or malignant proliferations of thyroid follicular cells.

Predilections

Both are more common in women. Most are seen in mature adults over 40 years of age. No racial predilection is known.

Clinical features

Some benign and some malignant tumors will be clinically unnoticed due to a small size. A benign tumor will be a soft movable nodule in one of the lateral poles of the gland. A malignant tumor will likely be firm and fixed in one of the lateral poles of the glands.

Radiographic presentation

CT scans and MRI scans will identify soft tissue with an increased density outlining the tumor.

Differential diagnosis

A nodule in the substance of the thyroid gland may represent a thyroid cyst or the early nodularity of a benign hyperplasia (goiter). Other entities that can appear as a nodule around the laryngotracheal area are lipomas, lymphomas, sarcoidosis, and cat-scratch disease.

Microscopic features

Benign tumors are varied, with most appearing as adenomatous proliferations amid a background of normal thyroid follicles and thyroglobulin. Malignant tumors show a proliferation of pleomorphic follicular cells, often with amyloid and some calcifications.

Suggested course of action

Nodules and masses in the area of the thyroid gland should be referred to an endocrinologist or a general surgeon for workup and treatment planning.

Treatment

Benign thyroid tumors are treated with a lobectomy of the involved area of the thyroid. Thyroid cancers are treated with a total thyroidectomy and a consideration for a bilateral neck dissection.

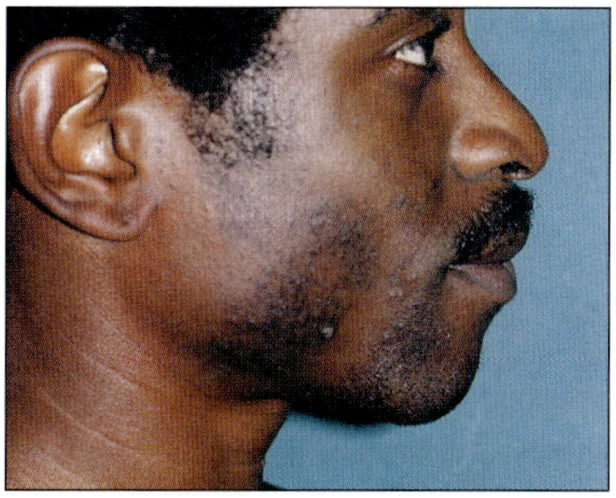

► Benign masseteric hypertrophy.

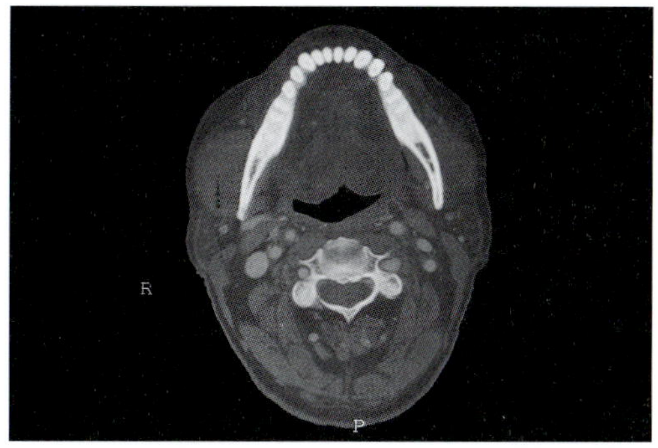

► Unilateral enlargement of the right masseter muscle readily seen on a CT scan.

Masseteric Hypertrophy

Nature of disease

Cellular hypertrophy resulting in clinical enlargement of one or both masseter muscles due to the isometric exercising of the muscle from either a teeth-clenching habit or an excessive gum-chewing habit.

Predilections

No age, sex, or racial predilection is known.

Clinical features

Usually a painless enlargement of one masseter muscle due to a patient preference of one side related to clenching or gum chewing. Occasionally, both masseter muscles are enlarged, but most often one side is somewhat larger than the other. The dentition is usually absent of wear facets and has deep intercuspation. The mandibular plane angle is usually less than 110 degrees.

Radiographic presentation

Panoramic views usually appear normal. Some cases may show an elongation of the coronoid process. Anteroposterior views often show a bony ridge at the insertion of the masseter at the inferior border of the ramus. CT or MRI scans will usually show a uniform enlargement of the involved masseter muscle or muscles. Rarely, and mostly seen in the excessive gum chewer, the temporalis muscle will be seen to be enlarged as well.

Differential diagnosis

Clinically, masseteric hypertrophy is often confused with parotid enlargement, thus suggesting such entities as parotid tumors, Sjögren syndrome, sarcoidosis, parotitis, and other entities that may cause a diffuse enlargement of the parotid gland. Other considerations may include an osteomyelitis or benign tumor of the ramus or a tumor within the masseter such as a rhabdomyosarcoma.

Microscopic features

If biopsied or removed to reduce the size of the muscle, normal striated muscle is seen without inflammation.

Suggested course of action

Ask the patient to clench his or her teeth while you palpate the involved masseter. If the mass tenses, it confirms that it is indeed the masseter. Examine the occlusion carefully for premature contacts, because they are often the trigger for a clenching habit. Accomplish an occlusal adjustment, if indicated, and evaluate for a night guard. Order a CT or MRI scan to rule out other conditions.

Treatment

Occlusal adjustment and splint therapy. In some cases, Botox injections (Allergan) are required, and in refractory cases, a partial myectomy and surgical contouring of the masseter is required.

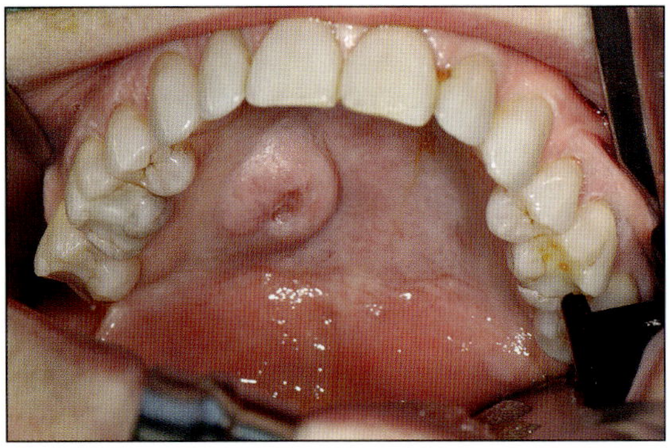

► Pleomorphic adenoma of the palate.

Pleomorphic Adenoma of the Oral Mucosa

Nature of disease

Benign neoplasms that arise from reserve cells within the ductal system of minor salivary glands.

Predilections

Adults. There is no sex or racial predilection. They occur most commonly within the posterior aspect of the palatal submucosa but may also occur in all places where minor salivary glands exist (ie, lips, buccal mucosa, floor of the mouth, etc).

Clinical features

Pleomorphic adenomas of the oral mucosa will present as a firm, movable mass within the submucosa. In its most common location in the palatal submucosa, it may not be mobile due to the restriction of the palatal mucosa itself. The mass is painless and will not be ulcerated unless trauma or a previous biopsy has taken place.

Radiographic presentation

Occasionally, a larger-sized tumor will create a concave, cupped-out thinning of the bony palate due to backpressure from the unyielding palatal soft tissues. Otherwise, no radiographic features are seen.

Differential diagnosis

In the palate, malignant salivary gland tumors such as adenoid cystic carcinomas, mucoepidermoid carcinomas, and polymorphous low-grade adenocarcinomas are the main considerations. In the upper lip, the canalicular adenoma, which is the more common tumor in this location, together with mucous cysts and the same three malignant salivary gland tumors should be considered.

Microscopic features

A diverse array of features may be present from a proliferation of ductal epithelium and myoepithelium. A chondromyxoid matrix is usually seen, foci of hyalinization or keratinization are occasionally seen, and even calcifications may be rarely seen. A collagenous capsule may be present, but it is not a true capsule that encases the tumor. Tumor cells are usually seen within the capsule.

Suggested course of action

Refer to an oral and maxillofacial surgeon.

Treatment

Pleomorphic adenomas cannot be removed for cure by enucleation because of the presence of tumor cells in the capsule. Instead, they require an excision with 1.0-cm margins controlled by frozen sections. In the palate, the palatal periosteum serves as an anatomical barrier. Excision of bone in any location of a pleomorphic adenoma is unnecessary.

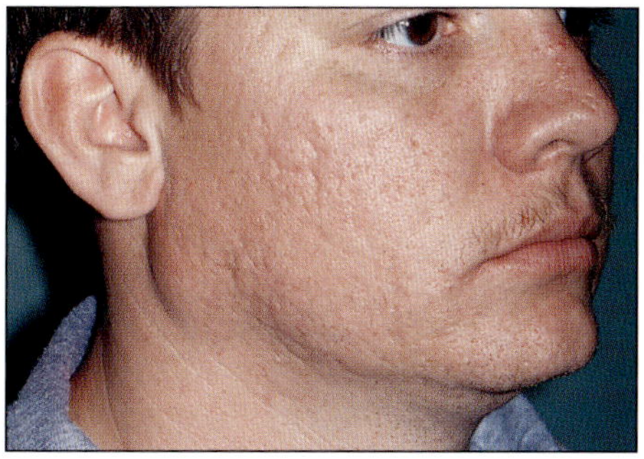

► Papillary cystadenoma lymphomatosum (Warthin tumor).

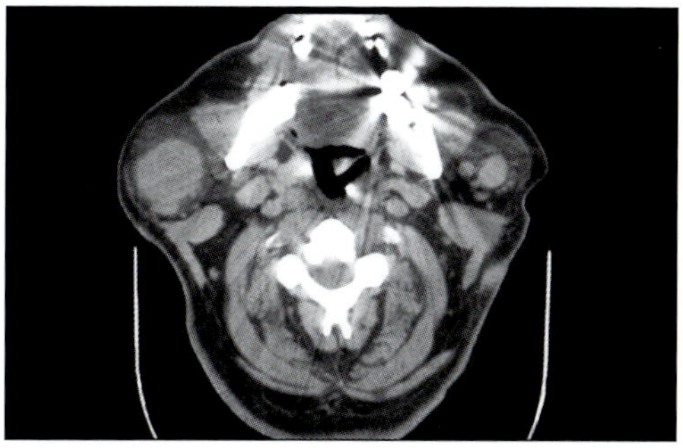

► This CT scan identified bilateral Warthin tumors.

Papillary Cystadenoma Lymphomatosum (Warthin Tumor)

Nature of disease

Warthin tumors are treated as unique true neoplasms but more likely represent entrapped embryologic foregut or primitive parotid ductal epithelium within parotid lymph nodes.

Predilections

Warthin tumors occur almost exclusively in the superficial lobe of the parotid gland. In about 10% of cases, they are known to occur bilaterally, most at the same time but occasionally several years apart.

Clinical features

The masses are painless and somewhat movable within the substance of the parotid gland. Facial nerve paresis does not occur, and there is no alteration in the flow of saliva.

Radiographic presentation

A CT scan or MRI scan will show the tumor mass in the superficial lobe of the parotid gland. Such scans will also reveal the presence of any multiple or contralateral Warthin tumors.

Differential diagnosis

The most common tumor in the parotid gland is the pleomorphic adenoma (75%), not the Warthin tumor (5%), so this should be a prime consideration. Mucoepidermoid carcinoma, adenocystic carcinoma, lipoma, and hemangioma should also be considered.

Microscopic features

A Warthin tumor has a unique and characteristic histopathology. Cystic spaces with papillary projections of highly eosinophilic epithelial cells known as *Warthin epithelium* are visible in double rows. Lymphocytic aggregates and even defined germinal centers are also seen.

Suggested course of action

Order a CT scan or MRI scan to confirm the presence of the tumor mass in the parotid gland rather than the dermis, which would imply a skin tumor or cyst. Refer to an oral and maxillofacial surgeon for definitive workup and treatment.

Treatment

Warthin tumors are treated with a nerve-sparing superficial parotidectomy, which is expected to be curative. Rare recurrences result from incomplete removal of the entire superficial lobe. Such rare recurrences are mostly new tumors that develop in the lymph nodes with the remaining superficial lobe.

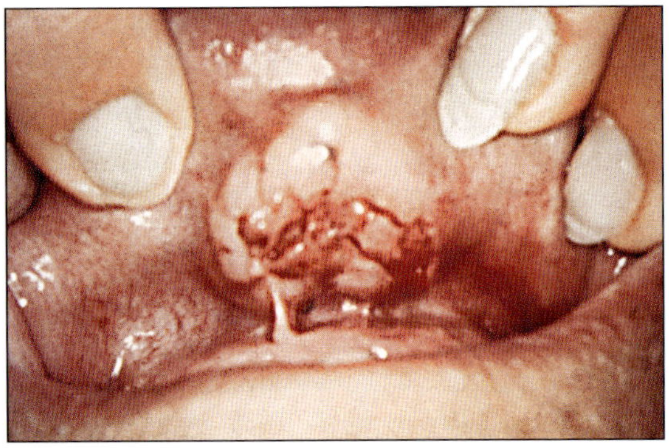

► Adenoid cystic carcinoma of the upper lip.

Adenoid Cystic Carcinoma of the Oral Mucosa

Nature of disease

A malignant salivary gland tumor that arises from reserve cells in the ductal system of minor salivary glands. It is well known to undergo perineural and intraneural invasion as well as to spread proximally along the involved nerve. It is also well known to grow slowly but metastasize readily, giving it a favorable 5-year prognosis but an unfavorable 10-year prognosis.

Predilections

Adults. There is no sex or racial predilection. In the oral mucosa, the most common site is the palate, but it has also been reported to occur in the tongue, lips, and buccal mucosa.

Clinical features

Most present as a painless submucosal mass. The surface may be intact but can also be ulcerated. Paresthesia is variably present, depending on the location of the mass, and may require objective testing to detect early subtle changes. Larger lesions may be painful and can cause facial asymmetry.

Radiographic presentation

In some early cases, no radiographic changes are evident. In more advanced cases, bone erosion and osteolysis are seen with a soft tissue density replacing the bone.

Differential diagnosis

Adenoid cystic carcinomas will present similar to other minor salivary malignancies such as mucoepidermoid carcinomas and polymorphous low-grade adenocarcinomas. If the overlying mucosa is intact, a pleomorphic adenoma should also be considered.

Microscopic features

Small, cuboidal, highly basophilic cells with little if any pleomorphism or mitotic figures are present in all cases. There will also be a mixture of three well-known patterns: cribriform, tubular, and solid. Most tumors contain two or more patterns, with one pattern predominating.

Suggested course of action

Suspected cases should be referred to an oral and maxillofacial surgeon for biopsy and workup.

Treatment

Aggressive surgery is required. In the palate, a hemimaxillectomy up to the skull base is followed by radiotherapy with or without adjunctive chemotherapy. In other soft tissue sites, a wide excision observing 3.0-cm margins and tracing any nerve trunk proximally to clear margins or to the base of the skull is performed, followed by radiotherapy. Note: Neutron or proton beam radiotherapy is more effective than other forms of radiotherapy for adenoid cystic carcinomas.

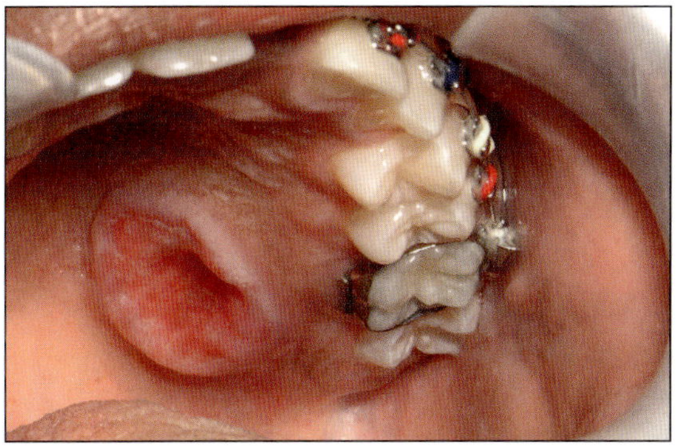

► Mucoepidermoid carcinoma of the palate.

Mucoepidermoid Carcinoma of the Oral Mucosa

Nature of disease

A malignant tumor that arises from reserve cells in the ducts of minor salivary glands and partially differentiates into mucus-secreting cells and epidermoid cells.

Predilections

In comparison with other mucosal salivary gland tumors, mucoepidermoid carcinomas have been known to occur more frequently in children and teenagers. However, the majority still develop in adults, with no sex or racial predilection. Most occur in the posterior palatal mucosa, but they also may occur in the lip, tongue, floor of the mouth, or buccal mucosa.

Clinical features

The tissue mass will appear firm or semifirm within the substance of the submucosa. It may be lobulated or noted as having a smooth surface. Ulceration may be present but often is not. In some low-grade mucoepidermoid carcinomas, the mucus production is significant enough to impart a translucent blue color to the mass. Pain or paresthesia is usually not noted.

Radiographic presentation

Most oral mucosal mucoepidermoid carcinomas are low grade and do not invade into bone. Intermediate- and high-grade mucoepidermoid carcinomas will often present with obvious osteolysis in an irregular invasive pattern.

Differential diagnosis

Mucoepidermoid carcinomas of the oral mucosa will appear similar to the other two prominent malignant salivary gland tumors: adenoid cystic carcinoma and polymorphous low-grade adenocarcinoma. If the mucosa is not ulcerated, pleomorphic adenoma should also be considered. If located within the substance of the upper lip, a canalicular adenoma should be considered.

Microscopic features

1. Low-grade mucoepidermoid carcinomas will have well-formed cysts containing mucin. Mucus-secreting cells will be numerous, but intermediate cells and epidermoid cells will be present as well. However, all cell types are mature and will not show atypia or mitotic figures.
2. Intermediate-grade mucoepidermoid carcinomas will have few if any mucus cysts and will be more solid. Intermediate and epidermoid cells are more numerous, and mucus-secreting cells are more sparse than with low-grade tumors. Some nuclear pleomorphism is usually seen but not mitotic figures.
3. High- grade mucoepidermoid carcinomas are solid without cystic spaces and consist only of intermediate cells and epidermoid cells. Cells will show considerable atypia and some mitotic figures. The absence of any mucus-secreting cells frequently requires the identification of intracellular mucin via a mucicarmine stain for diagnosis.

⟶

Mucoepidermoid Carcinoma of the Oral Mucosa *(cont)*

Suggested course of action

Refer to an oral and maxillofacial surgeon for excisional biopsy and workup.

Treatment

1. Low-grade tumors: Wide local excision observing 1.5-cm margins controlled with frozen sections.
2. Intermediate-grade tumors: Wide local excision observing 2.0-cm margins controlled with frozen sections. Excision of bone is required if imaging identifies bone involvement.
3. High-grade tumor: Very wide excision observing 3.0-cm margins controlled with frozen sections, likely resection of adjacent bone, and an ipsilateral or bilateral neck dissection as per the examination and imaging findings, followed by postoperative radiotherapy.

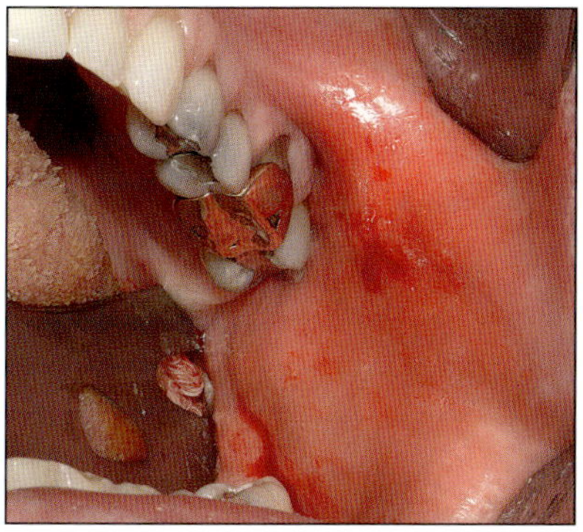

► Basal cell adenoma in the left buccal mucosa.

Basal Cell Adenoma of the Oral Mucosa

Nature of disease

A benign neoplasm arising from the reserve cells in the ductal epithelium of minor salivary glands.

Predilections

Adults over 50 years of age, with a male predilection. Most occur in the parotid gland (70%). However, when they occur in the oral mucosa, the upper lip is the most common site.

Clinical features

Similar to the canalicular adenoma, basal bell adenomas present as small (< 3 cm), round, painless, freely movable masses within the submucosa.

Radiographic presentation

None.

Differential diagnosis

When located on the upper lip, a canalicular adenoma, a mucous cyst, and a pleomorphic adenoma are strong considerations. Malignant salivary gland tumors such as a mucoepidermoid carcinoma and adenoid cystic carcinoma should also be considered.

Microscopic features

A collagen capsule encasing uniform eosinophilic cells with oval nuclei without pleomorphism or atypia may be seen in either a solid, trabecular, or tubular pattern. The background is a poorly collagenized but hyalinized stroma similar to that seen in canalicular adenomas.

Suggested course of action

Refer to an oral and maxillofacial surgeon for excisional biopsy.

Treatment

For basal cell adenomas occurring within the oral mucosa, a pericapsular excision is curative.

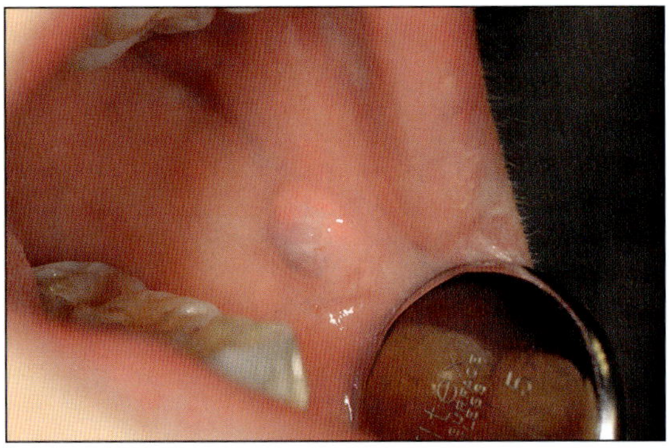

► Acinic cell carcinoma of the oral mucosa.

Acinic Cell Carcinoma of the Oral Mucosa

Nature of disease

A low-grade malignancy arising from the reserve cells of minor salivary gland ductal epithelium.

Predilections

Most occur in the parotid gland, but they can also be located in oral sites, especially the palatal and buccal mucosa. Most occur in adults, but rare cases have been reported in children. There is a slight female predilection, with no racial predilection known.

Clinical features

In the oral mucosa, they will appear as a small, lobulated, freely movable mass usually with an intact surface. Like the mucoepidermoid carcinoma, they may have a slight bluish appearance. There is no paresthesia noted with this tumor.

Radiographic presentation

Most have no radiographic presentation due to their usual low-grade biology. However, the rare high-grade counterpart will show extensive irregular bone resorption.

Differential diagnosis

If the mass has a slight bluish coloration, low-grade mucoepidermoid carcinoma would be the most serious consideration. Otherwise, pleomorphic adenomas, polymorphous low-grade adenocarcinomas, and adenoid cystic carcinomas should be considered.

Microscopic features

Oral mucosal acinic cell carcinomas are often encapsulated at least partially. A solid, papillary, or cystic pattern is created by rounded or polygonal cells with an eosinophilic cytoplasm but a deeply basophilic-staining eccentric nucleus. The cystic spaces are eosinophilic. The tumor cells frequently have coarse, dark-staining granules reminiscent of the zymogen granules seen in the normal parotid acini.

Suggested course of action

Refer to an oral and maxillofacial surgeon for workup and treatment.

Treatment

Excision with 1.5-cm margins controlled with frozen sections is curative. In the rare high-grade acinic cell carcinoma, a resection observing 3.0-cm margins as well as any involved bone followed by radiotherapy is the preferred treatment.

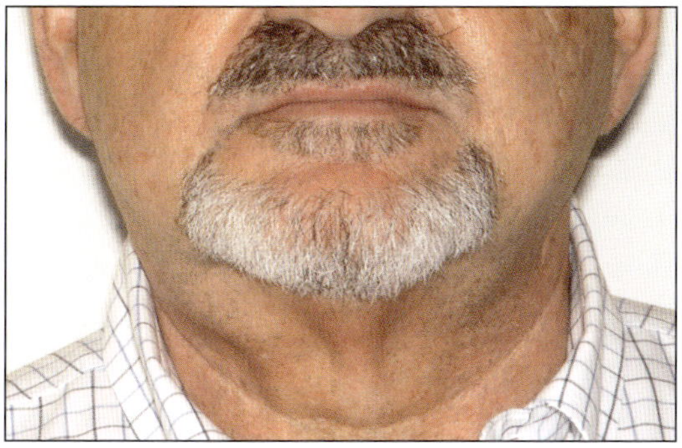

► Pleomorphic adenoma of the submandibular gland.

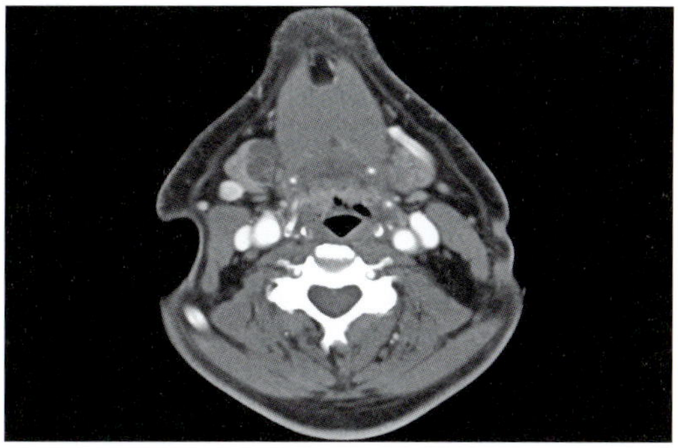

► Hypodense area in the right submandibular gland suspicious for a neoplasm.

Submandibular Gland Tumors

Nature of disease

Benign or malignant proliferations of the ductal reserve cells within the submandibular gland.

Predilections

Mostly adults, with no sex or racial predilection. Sixty percent of submandibular gland tumors are malignant, which is a much higher percentage than those in the parotid gland and slightly higher than those in minor salivary glands.

Clinical features

Both benign and malignant submandibular gland tumors will generally present as a firm mass within the submandibular triangle. The mass is usually painless. Paresthesia is uncommon and mostly involves the lingual nerve and is mostly caused by either adenoid cystic carcinoma or a high-grade mucoepidermoid carcinoma. Benign tumors and most malignant tumors are freely moveable, but some malignant tumors become fixed to the mandible or adjacent tissues.

Radiographic presentation

CT scans and MRI scans will show an increased soft tissue density within the gland and, in some malignant tumors, a spread outside the capsule of the gland. Note: On occasion a submandibular gland tumor will cause stasis with the duct, resulting in a sialolith and thus misleading the practitioner into pursuing a sialolith and sialadenitis instead of a tumor.

Differential diagnosis

Other pathologies that can result in a mass within the submandibular triangle are Hodgkin and non-Hodgkin lymphomas, cat-scratch disease, HIV infections, sarcoidosis, and infectious mononucleosis.

Microscopic features

The specific histopathology of the many benign and malignant tumors that can occur in the submandibular gland is beyond the scope of this text. However, the dental practitioner should know the following general rules:

- The most common benign tumor in this gland is the pleomorphic adenoma.
- The most common malignant tumor is the mucoepidermoid carcinoma, followed closely by the adenoid cystic carcinoma.
- Warthin tumors do not occur in the submandibular gland.
- Polymorphous low-grade adenocarcinomas do not occur in the submandibular gland. →

Submandibular Gland Tumors *(cont)*

Suggested course of action

Identification of a mass in the submandibular triangle is a concern for a significant pathology. Refer to an oral and maxillofacial surgeon; before doing so, inquire about any association with cats (particularly young cats), risk factors for HIV infection, and any recent fatigue, weight loss, or fever.

Treatment

Benign tumors are treated with removal of the entire gland. Some malignant tumors (eg, low-grade mucoepidermoid carcinoma) may also be treated with removal of the entire gland. Other malignant tumors will require a wider field of excision that may include a lymphadenectomy neck dissection, excision of the lingual nerve, or a continuity resection of the mandible depending on the type, size, and growth history of the malignancy.

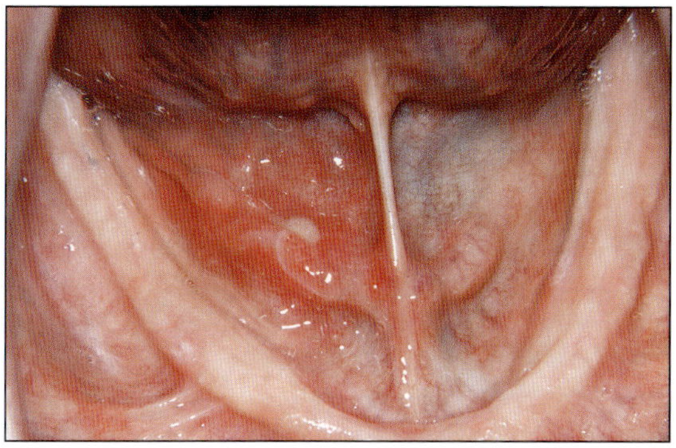

► Pus emanating from the submandibular duct due to sialadenitis.

Submandibular Gland Sialadenitis

Nature of disease

An inflammatory process within the gland that is usually infectious and caused by retrograde bacterial entry into the gland through the submandibular duct.

Predilections

There is no sex or racial predilection. Most cases occur in mature adults. Many are associated with a sialolith in the gland or ductal system.

Clinical features

Most will present with a tender fullness or mass in the submandibular triangle. The overlying skin may be red and warm if it is an acute infection. Pus is often noted emanating out of the ductal opening. The gland will be painful to palpation. Fever may be present as well.

Radiographic presentation

A panoramic radiograph will imply an increased soft tissue density in the submandibular triangle better seen with a CT scan. Sialoliths may be noted within the gland or within the duct.

Differential diagnosis

A painful mass in the submandibular triangle may result from a submandibular space abscess from a pulpal infection in a molar tooth, cat-scratch disease, cervical facial actinomycosis, infectious mononucleosis, or other infections causing inflamed or infected lymph nodes.

Microscopic features

An intense mixed infiltration of inflammatory cells is seen within the gland. In acute infections, neutrophils predominate, and areas of gland parenchymal necrosis may be seen. In chronic sialadenitis, lymphocytes and plasma cells predominate, and varying degrees of fibrosis will be seen.

Suggested course of action

Begin hydration and antibiotic therapy covering staphylococcal organisms (ie, doxycycline, cephalosporins) and anaerobes (ie, metronidazole, clindamycin). Refer to an oral and maxillofacial surgeon for workup and treatment.

Treatment

Excision of the infected gland is the most common treatment and is recommended. This is due to the possibility of a subtle tumor in the gland initiating the infection via stasis and the risk of relapse and reinfection after a nonsurgical course of antibiotics.

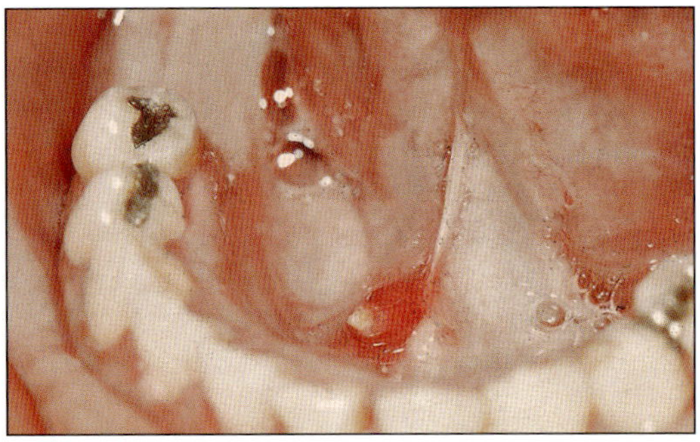

► Sialolith emerging from the opening of the submandibular duct.

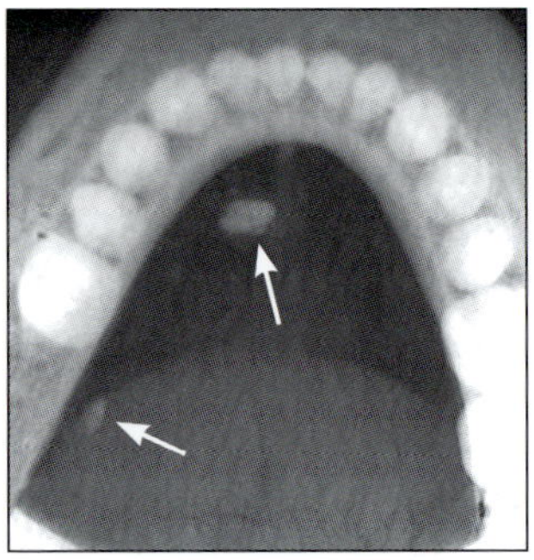

► Sialoliths appear on an occlusal radiograph.

Submandibular Gland Sialolithiasis

Nature of disease

The formation of calcium carbonate or, less commonly, calcium oxalate stones (sialoliths) within the substance of the gland or its duct. The stone forms around a nidus of either a bacterial colony or the thick glycoprotein content of submandibular gland saliva.

Predilections

Mostly adults. There is no sex or racial predilection.

Clinical features

Such sialoliths cause an obstructive sialadenitis and secondary infection. Therefore, the submandibular gland will be firm and at times even hard if the stone is within the gland and large. When a single stone or two or more stones are in the duct in the floor of the mouth, it will be swollen and tender. On occasion the stone(s) will be visible at the opening of the duct or will have partially eroded through the duct and oral mucosa to be visible in the floor of the mouth.

Radiographic presentation

A panoramic radiograph with identify a sialolith within the gland as an opaque structure just beneath the inferior border in the molar region. Sialoliths in the floor of the mouth are more subtle and may be unnoticed or superimposed over teeth or the mandible, suggesting some type of an intrabony calcification. Therefore, an occlusal radiograph is suggested and will identify sialoliths within the duct.

Differential diagnosis

Other radiopacities may be confused with a sialolith in the submandibular gland. These include calcified lymph nodes such as may be seen in resolved tuberculosis or fungal infections, phleboliths from long-standing hemangiomas, calcifications of the carotid bifurcation, and some tonsilloliths.

Microscopic and gross specimen features

Sialoliths will not have a true microscopic presentation because the required decalcification process dissolves the entire stone. However, the gross specimen will be chalky and flake off into several pieces. One can often discern concentric rings like that seen in a cross section of a tree trunk, indicating a layering around a central nidus. →

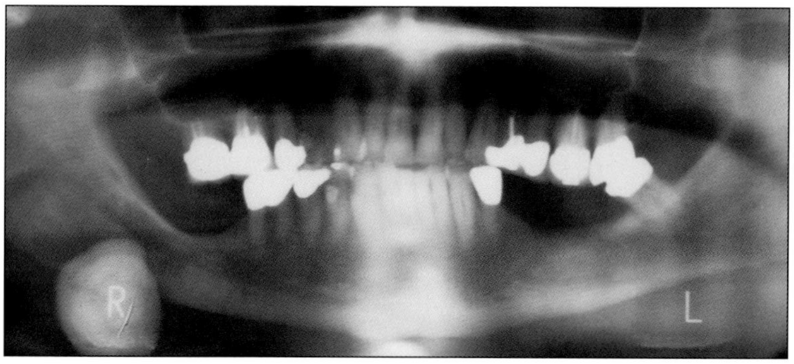

► Large sialolith as seen on a panoramic radiograph.

Suggested course of action

Obtain quality images such as occlusal and panoramic radiographs to document the presence and location of a sialolith. Refer the patient to an oral and maxillofacial surgeon for further workup and treatment.

Treatment

For sialoliths within the duct, removal of the stone (sialolithotomy) and suturing of the ductal lumen to the oral mucosa for salivary drainage (sialodochoplasty) usually resolves the secondary infection and maintains normal salivary flow. For cases in which the gland continues with pain and recurrent infection after transoral sialolithotomy, and for stones within the gland substance, complete excision of the gland via an extraoral approach is performed. Note: Sialoliths are not related to hypercalcemic states or to renal stones.

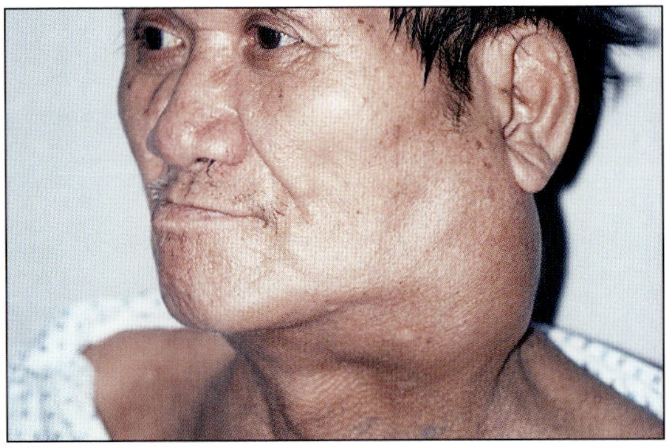

► Metastatic squamous cell carcinoma from an unknown primary at the base of the tongue.

Metastatic Deposits in the Neck

Nature of disease

Known as the "unknown primary" phenomenon, a large lymph node enlargement develops in the cervical lymphatic chain suspicious for a local regional metastasis without identification of the primary cancer.

Predilections

Adults, with a predilection for men. Occurs more in smokers, but some occur in nonsmokers positive for human papillomavirus. No racial predilection is known.

Clinical features

Usually an otherwise asymptomatic person develops a firm fixed mass in the cervical lymphatic chain on one side of the neck. The mass is often fixed to the sternocleidomastoid muscle or resides in the posterior triangle of the neck.

Radiographic presentation

CT scans and MRI scans will identify a round to oval mass of increased soft tissue density representing the lesion. In some cases, the mass will have a central area of hypodensity indicating tumor necrosis. A PET scan will show an increased uptake in the lesion indicating a hypermetabolic focus and may also point toward a subtle primary tumor, usually located at the base of the tongue or less commonly in the nasopharynx.

Differential diagnosis

Asymptomatic masses in the cervical lymphatic chain will suggest either a Hodgkin or non-Hodgkin lymphoma, a branchial cyst, cat-scratch disease, tuberculous lymphadenitis, or sarcoidosis.

Microscopic features

Most are from squamous cell carcinomas from the base of the tongue and will show the typical features of poorly differentiated pleomorphic epithelial cells with mitotic figures and rarely keratin pearls. The lymph node capsule will be seen as a band of eosinophilic collagen with lymphocytes condensed against its inner surface. The lymph node center will contain tumor cells and/or keratin or necrosis.

Suggested course of action

Refer to a cancer center for evaluation, workup, and treatment.

Treatment

Prior to treatment, an attempt to locate the often very small primary cancer site by PET scans and/or by direct laryngoscopy with directed or blind biopsies is undertaken. Specific treatment is accomplished with a modified neck dissection followed by a chemoradiation protocol.

5

Infectious Diseases of the Jaws and Oral Cavity

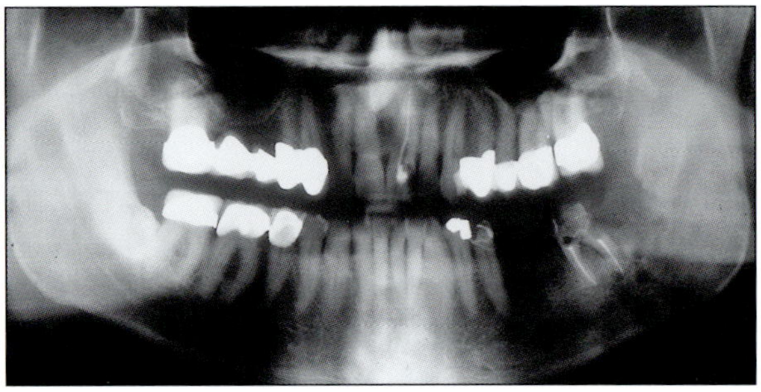

► Suppurative osteomyelitis from a failing root canal treatment.

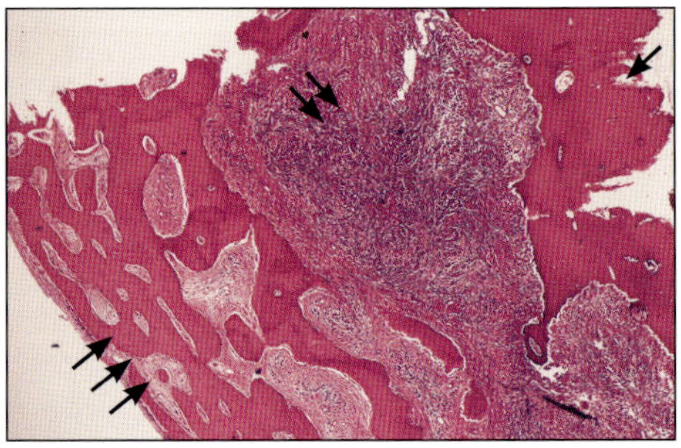

► Inflammation *(double arrow)* in the marrow space defines an osteomyelitis, here with necrotic bone *(single arrow)* and periosteal new bone formation *(triple arrow)*.

Bacterial Diseases

Primary Suppurative Osteomyelitis

Nature of disease

A primary bacterial infection of the marrow space usually involving a mixed group of microorganisms, especially anaerobic organisms that maintain a low–oxygen tension environment by small vessel thrombosis. Note: Secondary infections of the mandible or maxilla as seen in osteoradionecrosis or drug-induced osteonecrosis are infections of already necrotic bone. They represent a different pathogenesis and are treated differently.

Predilections

Occurs mostly in adults over 30 years of age and is very rare in the maxilla unless a significant medical compromise coexists (eg, HIV, drug immunosuppression, type 1 diabetes, etc). There is no sex or racial predilection. It is known to occur more frequently in patients with failing root canal treatments, in patients with a penicillin allergy, after trauma, and in association with foreign bodies.

Clinical features

Pain is usually mild. The overlying mucosa will be edematous, and an oral mucosal or orocutaneous fistula may be present. Skin erythema may also be noted. A suppurative drainage may be noted through the fistula or around teeth. Teeth may be mobile, and some teeth may show significant caries as a possible source of the infection.

Radiographic presentation

As the name implies, radiographs will likely show an irregular, moth-eaten pattern of osteolysis. An advanced suppurative osteomyelitis will show osteolysis at the inferior border of the mandible. Very advanced cases may show a pathologic fracture. In some chronic cases, subperiosteal bone formation will be seen as a fuzzy bone formation on the surface of the cortex.

Differential diagnosis

Without a good medical history, secondary osteomyelitis from osteoradionecrosis or drug-induced osteonecrosis would be the main considerations. Additionally, fistulae from osteopetrosis or florid cemento-osseous dysplasia may be considered clinically and ruled out with radiographs.

Microscopic features

Inflammation in the marrow space with small vessel sludging and/or thrombosis is the diagnostic picture. Necrotic bone may be seen as well as newly regenerated osteoid on the cortical surface. In contrast to both osteoradionecrosis and drug-induced osteonecrosis, viable normal-appearing osteoclasts will be seen.

→

Suggested course of action

Confirm with good radiographs, and culture any exudate. Refer the patient to an oral and maxillofacial surgeon for evaluation and treatment.

Treatment

The source of the infection must be identified and removed, followed by debridement and antibiotics that cover anaerobes, especially *Actinomyces* species. In extensive cases, intravenous antibiotics are used. In refractory cases, a continuity resection may be required.

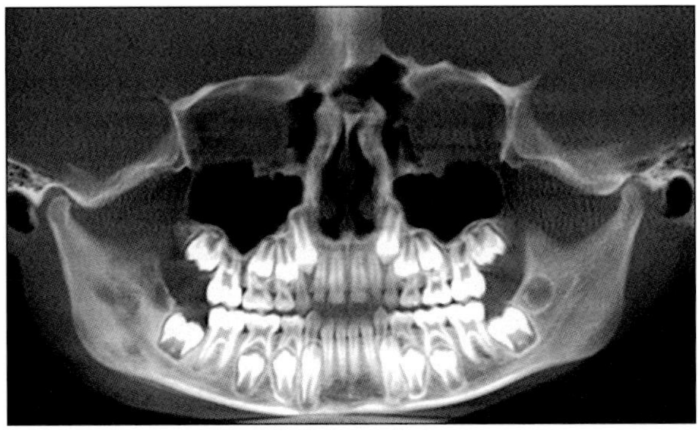

► Granulomatous osteomyelitis in the ramus of a 10-year-old.

Granulomatous Osteomyelitis in Children

Nature of disease

A rare, low-grade osteomyelitis only seen in children where the microscopic appearance reveals well-formed classic epithelioid granulomas similar to those seen in tuberculosis and sarcoidosis.

Predilections

Exclusively seen in children under the age of 12 years. Almost all occur in the ramus of the mandible. No sex or racial predilection is known.

Clinical features

The child is usually asymptomatic or has a dull pain. The ramus may be expanded. There is no mucosal inflammation, fistula formation, or drainage. There is usually no association with teeth.

Radiographic presentation

One or both rami will show a mild expansion and a multilocular radiolucency with somewhat defined borders.

Differential diagnosis

Because of its rarity and mild symptoms, a granulomatous osteomyelitis is not considered with its usual presentation. Instead a Langerhans cell histiocytosis, an odontogenic keratocyst, an odontogenic myxoma, and an ameloblastic fibroma are more realistic considerations.

Microscopic features

Classic granulomas consisting of a center of epithelioid-appearing macrophages surrounded by a ring of lymphocytes are seen amid a background of other lymphocytes.

Suggested course of action

Radiolucencies in the ramus of the mandible or an expansion of bone in a child requires a referral to an oral and maxillofacial surgeon for workup and treatment.

Treatment

Such expansile lesions are explored and debrided by an enucleation procedure. The finding of granulomas then suggests an atypical mycobacterium, although such has never been cultured or proven. Therefore, usually an observation period without antibiotics is undertaken or treatment with rifampin is used empirically.

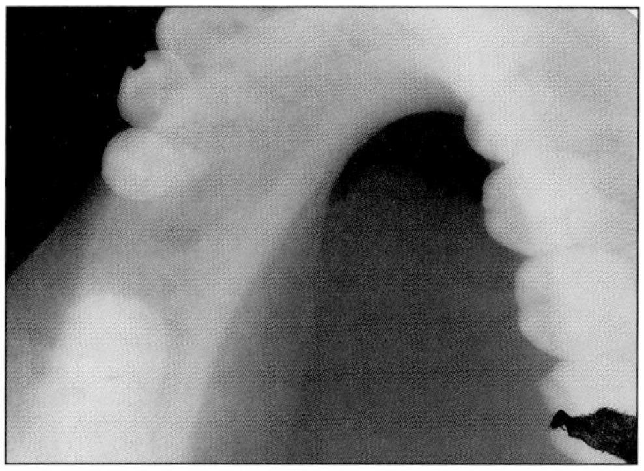

► Garré osteomyelitis showing uniform extracortical bone and a suggestion of a layering effect.

Garré Osteomyelitis

Nature of disease

A limited and localized infection due to a low-virulence bacteria in an immune-competent host with an adequate blood supply, which will stimulate the periosteum to lay down extracortical bone.

Predilections

Most common in children and teenagers and rare over the age of 25 years. No sex or racial predilection is known. It occurs mostly in the mandible and is extremely rare in the maxilla, but it has occurred in long bones.

Clinical features

Most present as an asymptomatic expansion. Rare cases may have dull pain. The expansion is hard with no erythema or pus. Most occur associated with an abscessed tooth. Rare cases may be secondary to trauma causing a stimulation of the periosteum via a subperiosteal hematoma.

Radiographic presentation

Layers of extracortical bone best seen on occlusal radiographs or axial CT scans are often noted. The extracortical bone will arise from an intact cortex and have a ground-glass or onionskin appearance. If an abscessed tooth is the etiology, a radiolucency may be seen around that tooth.

Differential diagnosis

The diseases on a differential diagnosis representing a similar presentation are much more concerning than Garré osteomyelitis. These include osteosarcoma, Ewing sarcoma, chronic sclerosing osteomyelitis, and fibrous dysplasia.

Microscopic features

A normal-appearing cortex will be seen to have parallel layers of bone 25 to 100 microns thick outside the cortex. These layers may be connected by trabecular struts of a similar thickness. An outer layer of periosteum with inflammatory cells will rim the extracortical bone.

Suggested course of action

Obtain right-angle occlusal radiographs or CT scans. Examine for a source of infection and remove it. Refer to an oral and maxillofacial surgeon for confirmation or a second opinion.

Treatment

Removal of any obvious source of infection and antibiotics such as phenoxymethylpenicillin or doxycycline for 5 days.

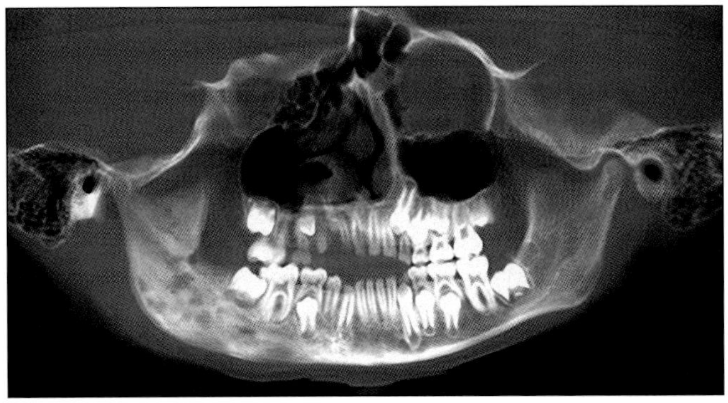

► Diffuse sclerosis and interruption of the inferior border of the mandible in a chronic sclerosing osteomyelitis.

Chronic Sclerosing Osteomyelitis

Nature of disease

An extremely painful osteomyelitis of the mandible caused by a mutualistic infection of *Actinomyces* species together with *Eikenella corrodens* or other carbon dioxide–producing bacteria. The ingress of these bacteria may come from tonsillar crypts, a third molar pericoronitis, a failing root canal treatment, or less likely an apical abscess.

Predilections

Occurs equally in adults and children with no sex or racial predilection.

Clinical features

The patient is often seen by multiple practitioners with no diagnosis made. Pain will mostly be constant, but periods of quiescence may occur as well. The pain is severe and deep-seated. The mandible will be expanded but is only slightly tender to palpation. The mucosa is normal in appearance and texture, with no fistulae or lymphadenopathy. A degree of trismus is present in many cases.

Radiographic presentation

A diffuse sclerosis within the marrow space of the mandible is characteristic. Small areas of radiolucency within the sclerosis are frequent. Periosteal extracortical bone formation is frequently seen as well. Symmetric expansion of each cortex is also noted. CT scans may show edema and/or fibrosis in the masseter and medial pterygoid muscles.

Differential diagnosis

Although the severe pain will point to a diagnosis of chronic sclerosing osteomyelitis, the radiograph may suggest fibrous dysplasia, Paget disease, a severe anemic state, or an early mild case of osteopetrosis.

Microscopic features

Dense bone and fibrosis are usually seen. Organisms are sparse but may be seen as *Actinomyces* species appearing as basophilic mycelia adherent to a bone surface or as small colonies.

Suggested course of action

Refer to an oral and maxillofacial surgeon for workup and treatment.

Treatment

Nonsurgical management with long-term antibiotics (eg, phenoxymethylpenicillin or doxycycline) and hyperbaric oxygen achieves control of the symptoms and limits its extent. In persistent and severely painful cases (50% to 60%), a continuity resection is required to resolve the disease and the pain.

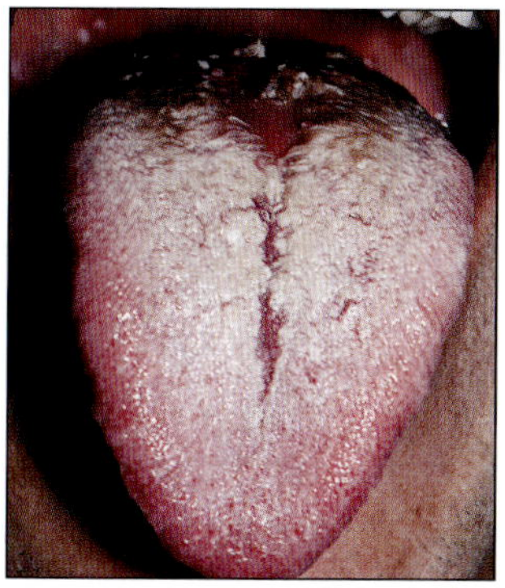

► Black hairy tongue.

Black Hairy Tongue

Nature of disease

A superficial colonization and infection of the dorsum of the tongue with bacteria that produce a black pigment (chromogenic bacteria).

Predilections

No specific age, sex, or racial predilection is known. It occurs more commonly in individuals with a sensitive gag reflex.

Clinical features

The dorsum of the tongue will indeed appear to have brown/black hairlike proliferations of the filiform papillae. Areas of a red atrophic appearance from denudations of filiform papillae at the midline may be seen. Mild pain on swallowing and gagging may be present as well.

Radiographic presentation

None.

Differential diagnosis

The location and color of black hairy tongue is distinctive. However, candidiasis and hairy leukoplakia may be considered if the black pigmentation is not prominent.

Microscopic features

Because black hairy tongue remains a clinical recognition diagnosis, biopsy specimens are rare. Those obtained have shown elongation of the filiform papillae, in which colonies of gram-positive microorganisms reside. The underlying connective tissue shows a mixed inflammatory infiltrate.

Suggested course of action

Black hairy tongue responds well to antibiotics and tongue brushing. Prescribe phenoxymethylpenicillin 500 mg four times daily for 5 days and tongue brushing with 0.12% chlorhexidine. For penicillin-allergic patients, doxycycline 100 mg once daily may be substituted. In refractory cases, refer to an oral medicine specialist or an oral and maxillofacial surgeon.

Treatment

Antibiotic therapy and tongue brushing as noted above are effective in nearly all cases. Refractory cases may require culture and sensitivity testing followed by intravenous antibiotics.

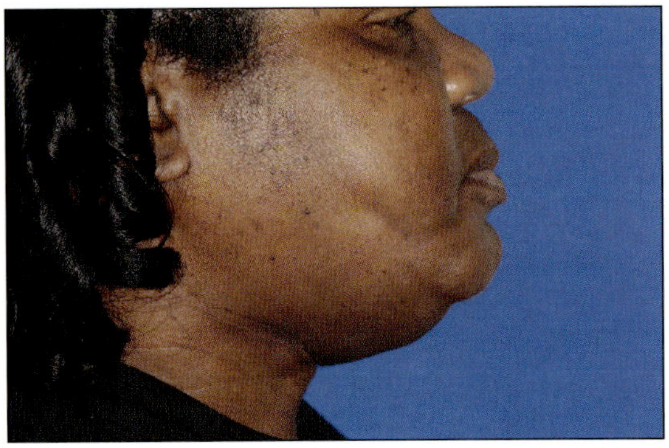

► Fibrosis with trismus in a case of cervicofacial actinomycosis.

Cervicofacial Actinomycosis

Nature of disease

A soft tissue infection caused by one of the several species of *Actinomyces*, of which *Actinomyces israelii* is the most common. It is characterized by chronicity and fibrosis, giving it its historical name of "lumpy jaw." Note: *Actinomyces* is a common pathogen directly responsible (or as a co-pathogen) for most cases of osteomyelitis of the jaw, and it is well known to cause secondary bone infections in the exposed bone from osteoradionecrosis and drug-induced osteonecrosis. These infections are not referred to specifically as *cervicofacial actinomycosis.*

Predilections

There is no age, sex, or racial predilection.

Clinical features

The patient will present with firm fibrotic masses within the fascia and lymph nodes of the neck. The masseter and medial pterygoid muscles are often fibrotic as well, producing trismus. The masses are usually only mildly painful or painless and are fixed to the surrounding tissue. A source of infection, usually odontogenic, is generally found. Most commonly a cracked tooth, pulpal pathology, or a failing root canal treatment is found to be the source of infection or, more rarely, cryptic tonsils, as *Actinomyces* is well known to reside in tonsillar crypts.

Radiographic presentation

Plain radiographs may show the portal of entry of the *Actinomyces*. However, CT scans and MRI scans will show the soft tissue hyperdensity indicative of fibrosis as well as any abscess cavity within the soft tissues. Frequently, the masseter and medial pterygoid muscles are noted to be enlarged and hyperdense, indicative of a diffuse fibrosis.

Differential diagnosis

On initial presentation, the patient's trismus and fibrosis will suggest radiation fibrosis and traumatic myositis ossificans. Trismus should also suggest a possible carcinoma within the pterygomandibular space.

Microscopic features

The fibrosis will be represented by dense acellular collagen. Scattered inflammatory cells may be noted. However, the pathognomonic feature is that of a basophilic-staining colony of *Actinomyces* organisms surrounded by neutrophils. This is known as a *sulfur granule*. Note: Today sulfur granules are very rarely seen clinically. In the past, more advanced and long-term cases produced macroscopic yellow flecks during drainage and debridement procedures, leading to the term *sulfur granules*. Today *sulfur granules* usually refer to this microscopic finding. →

Suggested course of action

Accomplish a thorough oral examination with radiographs, looking for a definitive focus of infection. Refer to an oral and maxillofacial surgeon for further workup and treatment.

Treatment

Removal of the focus of infection and debridement is crucial. Antibiotics of the penicillin type via a PICC line for 3 months is recommended. If the infection advances or persists, a more extensive debridement is required to remove fibrotic tissue, and intravenous antibiotics should be continued. Note: *Actinomyces* is incapable of penicillin resistance and should be used in all cases except in patients allergic to penicillin. Alternative antibiotics for the penicillin-allergic patient are doxycycline, cefoxitin, and vancomycin.

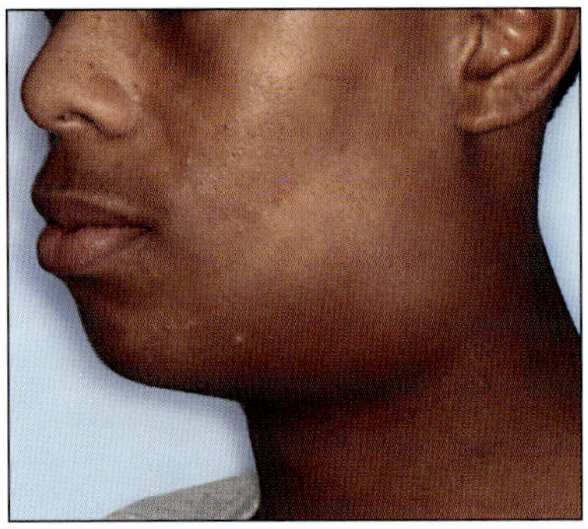

► Cat-scratch disease lymph node mass.

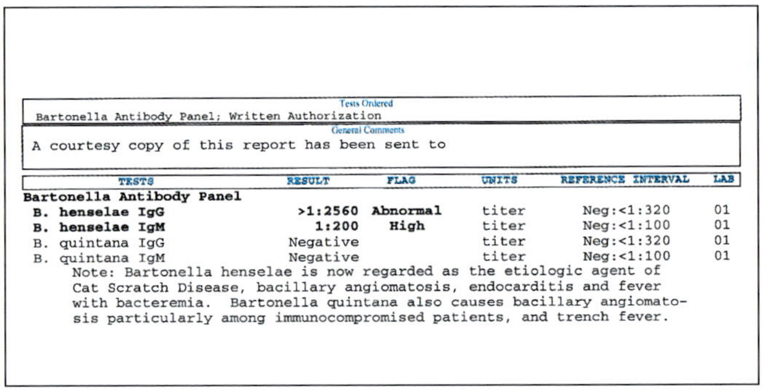

Tests Ordered
Bartonella Antibody Panel; Written Authorization

General Comments
A courtesy copy of this report has been sent to

TESTS	RESULT	FLAG	UNITS	REFERENCE INTERVAL	LAB
Bartonella Antibody Panel					
B. henselae IgG	**>1:2560**	**Abnormal**	titer	Neg:<1:320	01
B. henselae IgM	**1:200**	**High**	titer	Neg:<1:100	01
B. quintana IgG	Negative		titer	Neg:<1:320	01
B. quintana IgM	Negative		titer	Neg:<1:100	01

Note: Bartonella henselae is now regarded as the etiologic agent of Cat Scratch Disease, bacillary angiomatosis, endocarditis and fever with bacteremia. Bartonella quintana also causes bacillary angiomatosis particularly among immunocompromised patients, and trench fever.

► Cat-scratch antibody test positive for cat-scratch disease.

Cat-Scratch Disease

Nature of disease

A necrotizing lymphadenitis caused by an infection from the microorganism *Bartonella henselae.*

Predilections

Can occur at any age but seen mostly in children and young adults. No sex or racial predilection is known. There is a strong association with kittens and cats younger than 1 year.

Clinical features

The involved lymph nodes will present as a firm, painless, lobulated mass of lymph nodes adhered together. Only 50% of patients are actually scratched by a cat, but nearly all have been around young cats. Additionally, if the patient has been scratched, the location of the lymphadenitis is usually not in the drainage field of the scratch. In late-stage cases, the lymph nodes may undergo liquefactive necrosis, presenting as a mildly painful abscess that may also drain pus.

Radiographic presentation

Cat-scratch disease will not be seen on plain radiographs. A medical CT scan will identify a hyperdense mass that may have a central area of hypodensity if liquefactive necrosis is present.

Differential diagnosis

Adherent, painless cat-scratch lymph nodes will appear identical to those of squamous cell carcinoma and tuberculous lymphadenitis. Other considerations are Hodgkin and non-Hodgkin lymphoma and infectious mononucleosis.

Microscopic features

A dense inflammatory infiltrate is seen between germinal centers that often have a central area of breakdown (necrosis).

Suggested course of action

Obtain a serum cat-scratch antigen test for *Bartonella henselae.* (Note: Cat scratch cases usually do not show a lymphocytosis.) A positive cat-scratch antigen value in a dilution equal to or greater than 1:320 is diagnostic. Refer to an infectious disease specialist or an oral and maxillofacial surgeon for definitive treatment.

Treatment

Although many cases resolve without treatment, most are treated with erythromycin or doxycycline to prevent liquefaction, necrosis, and drainage. In cases of necrosis and clinical abscess, incision and drainage is not recommended. Instead, complete removal of the necrotic lymph node is preferred.

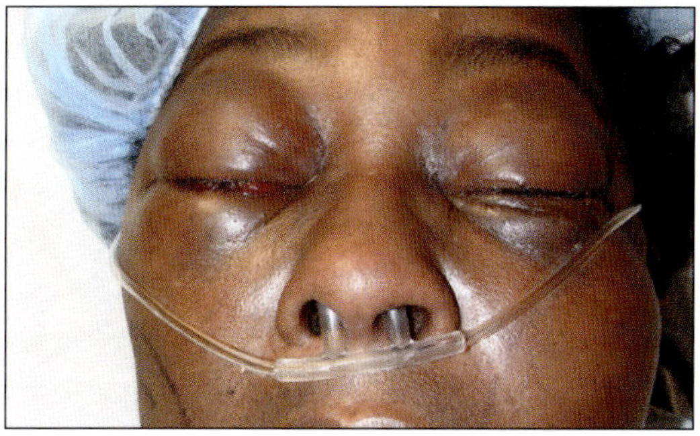

► Proptosis, orbital edema, and lid paralysis seen in cavernous sinus thrombosis.

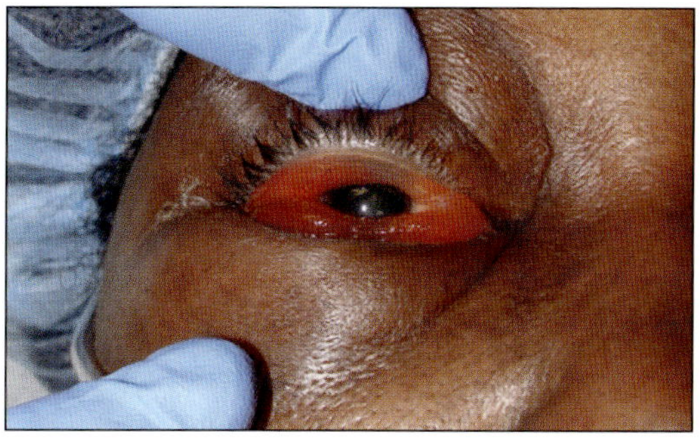

► Fixed and dilated pupil (ophthalmoplegia) and chemosis of the conjunctiva in cavernous sinus thrombosis.

Cavernous Sinus Thrombosis

Nature of disease

A life-threatening disease in which an infected thrombosis, usually with staphylococcal organisms, produces a subset of dramatic symptoms that can lead to death if unresponsive to treatment.

Predilections

No specific age, sex, or racial predilection is known.

Clinical features

Most patients will be somewhat lethargic with ocular edema and proptosis. In its early development, one or both eyes will exhibit internal strabismus due to loss of abducens nerve (cranial nerve VI) function. As the infection progresses, cranial nerves III, IV, and V passing through the cavernous sinus become involved as well, creating ophthalmoplegia and loss of corneal sensation. Fever and tachycardia occur commonly as well.

Radiographic presentation

Plain radiographs may elucidate the source of the infection such as an abscessed maxillary tooth or a maxillary sinusitis. However, CT scans will identify an opacified cavernous sinus, ocular edema, and exophthalmia.

Differential diagnosis

Orbital cellulitis and meningitis will present a picture similar to an early cavernous sinus thrombosis. A retrobulbar tumor or a brain tumor may present a picture similar to the later stages of a cavernous sinus thrombosis.

Microscopic features

No biopsy specimens have been taken except at autopsy, which identified a blood clot containing numerous gram-positive bacteria.

Suggested course of action

Search for a source of infection (eg, apical abscess, periodontal abscess, other infections around the maxilla and facial skin) and, if feasible, remove it. Send the patient immediately to a hospital emergency room for workup, evaluation, and treatment.

Treatment

Any obvious source of infection is removed if it has not already been identified and removed. Intravenous antibiotics using multiple drugs effective against staphylococci such as vancomycin, amoxicillin with clavulanate (Unasyn, Pfizer), and cefotaxime together with metronidazole for anaerobic coverage for other species of microorganisms are used. Anticoagulation therapy using heparin or Lovenox (Sanofi Aventis) may also be used in some cases.

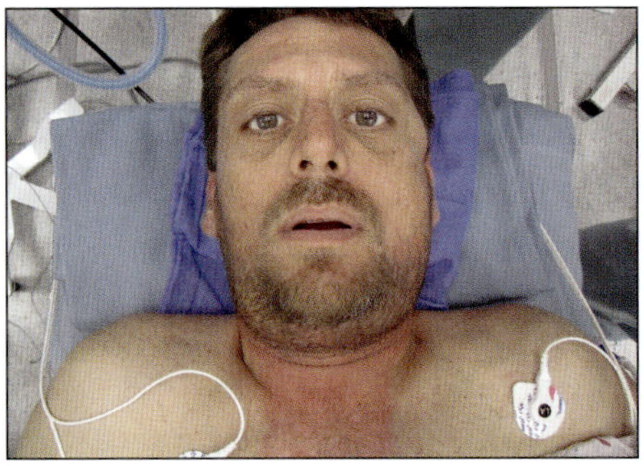

► Neck edema, dysphagia, bilateral space infections, and difficulty breathing in a patient with Ludwig angina.

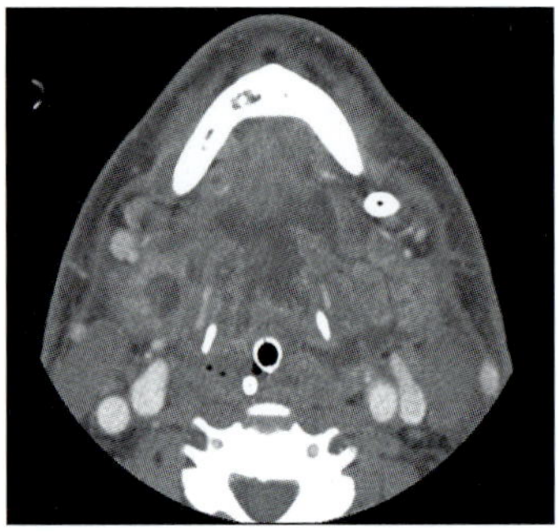

► Cellulitis, abscesses, and a closed airway around an endotracheal tube in a patient with Ludwig angina.

Ludwig Angina

Nature of disease

A life-threatening bacterial fascial space infection caused by a mixed infection from anaerobic streptococcal organisms and various other anaerobes (ie, *Moraxella*, *Eikenella*, *Bacteroides*). The severe cellulitis and abscess formation may obstruct the upper airway, leading to dyspnea and stridor and may advance to a suffocation death.

Predilections

No specific sex or racial predilection is known. Children are rarely seen with Ludwig angina. However, the late teenage years and early 20s are the times of increased case numbers, presumably due to third molar–related infections.

Clinical features

The patient will exhibit a bilateral facial swelling. The floor of the mouth will be elevated, and the tongue will be displaced posteriorly and elevated as well. Pain and difficulty swallowing will be reported by the patient. Drooling will be readily observed. Difficulty breathing is an ominous sign of an impending airway obstruction requiring immediate action (ie, intubation or tracheostomy).

Radiographic presentation

Plain radiographs may show the source of the infection (eg, an abscessed tooth, a periodontal abscess/pericoronitis, a salivary gland sialolith, or a failing root canal treatment). CT scans will show a significant soft tissue cellulitis and/or abscesses encroaching on the airway space.

Differential diagnosis

A true Ludwig angina involves the submandibular and lateral pharyngeal spaces bilaterally as well as the sublingual space across the midline and the retropharyngeal space. Other fascial space infections not involving all of these spaces may be considered.

Microscopic features

Pus and tissue specimens will identify gram-positive cocci and gram-negative rods and may also show necrotic tissue.

Suggested course of action

Assess the airway and the patient's ability to breathe. Call 911 for immediate help and have the patient transported to an emergency room with medical or emergency-trained personnel in attendance.

→

Treatment

The first and foremost treatment is to secure an airway via intubation or preferably via a tracheostomy. All fascial spaces are incised, drained, and irrigated with either large volumes of 0.12% chlorhexidine, 3% hydrogen peroxide, or half-strength Dakin solution. Intensive multidrug antibiotics such as amoxicillin with clavulanate (Unasyn, Pfizer) and metronidazole or clindamycin are prescribed. For the penicillin-allergic patient, vancomycin may be substituted for the penicillin.

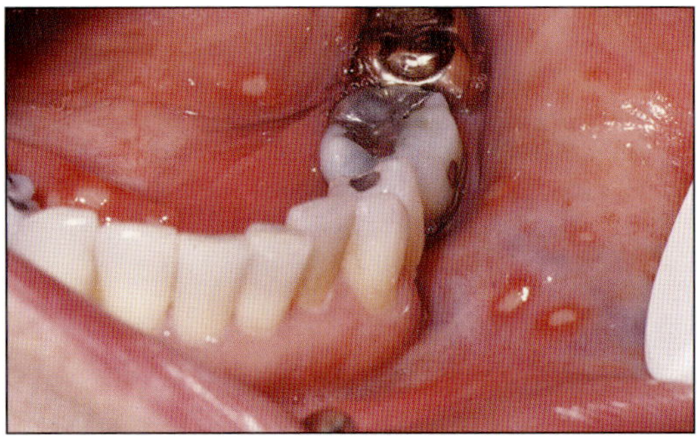

► Minor aphthous stomatitis.

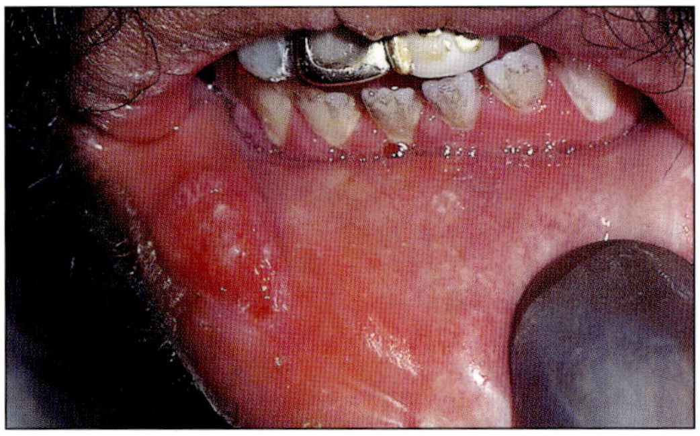

► Major aphthous stomatitis.

Aphthous Stomatitis

Nature of disease

Specific painful oral ulcers called *canker sores* that develop and last for 5 to 14 days possibly caused by a leukoclastic vasculitis where autoantibodies to either *Streptococcus sanguinis* or mucous membrane epithelium elicit an intense localized neutrophil response.

Predilections

No specific age, sex, or racial predilection is known.

Clinical features

Aphthous stomatitis is seen in two clinical forms:

1. Minor aphthous stomatitis in which discrete, yellow fibrin-based ulcers periodically appear. The patient may report a prodromal stage of pruritis or mild pain prior to the emergence of the ulcer. These ulcers will often have a red periphery around their fibrin base.
2. Major aphthous stomatitis (also called *Sutton's aphthae*) relates to larger and more numerous ulcers, some of which last for several months.

Radiographic presentation

None.

Differential diagnosis

Recurrent herpes vesicles that rupture may appear similar to aphthous ulcers. The ulcers of Behçet syndrome will appear much like those of major aphthous stomatitis, and the oral lesions of hand, foot, and mouth disease will appear much like those of minor aphthous stomatitis. Both can be ruled out by the other signs and features of each disease.

Microscopic features

The ulcers are only rarely biopsied. When specimens are obtained, a punched-out crater is seen. The ulcer's surface is usually infiltrated with neutrophils, whereas the deeper portions contain lymphocytes and macrophages.

Suggested course of action

1. Minor aphthous stomatitis can be treated with topical silver nitrate, phenol cautery, or 0.12% chlorhexidine lavage, which will shorten the course. Reassure the patient of the self-limiting nature of aphthous ulcers with and without treatment.
2. Major aphthous stomatitis may be treated by the nonspecialist dental provider or referred to an oral medicine specialist or an oral and maxillofacial surgeon.

Treatment

Major aphthous stomatitis responds best to antibiotics of the tetracycline family and prednisone therapy. Alternatively, topical 0.3% tacrolimus may be used.

Rheumatic Fever with Risk for Infective Endocarditis

Nature of disease

A disease that begins with a beta-hemolytic streptococcal pharyngitis usually from *Streptococcus pyogenes* that stimulates antibodies to streptolysin O and streptodornase. These antibodies can then cross-react with collagen, particularly in heart valves, to create tissue damage.

Predilections

Rheumatic fever mostly affects children between 5 and 15 years of age, with no sex or racial predilection.

Clinical features

The child will complain of a sore throat and may have dysphagia and fever initially. About 2 to 3 weeks later, the anti–streptolysin O and anti–streptococcal DNA antibodies begin the symptoms associated with rheumatic fever, referred to as the *Jones criteria*. With variation, these may include carditis, erythema marginatum on skin, subcutaneous nodules, involuntary rapid jerking movements known as *Sydenham chorea*, arthritis or arthralgia, and fever.

Radiographic presentation

None.

Differential diagnosis

The Jones criteria separate rheumatic fever from other childhood infectious diseases such as other forms of streptococcal pharyngitis, measles (rubeola), German measles (rubella), meningitis, and juvenile rheumatoid arthritis.

Microscopic features

None. The streptococcal pharyngitis and the Jones criteria used to diagnose rheumatic fever are all clinical and laboratory studies.

Suggested course of action

Children with a significant pharyngitis or children who have recently had pharyngitis who develop weakness, fatigue, fever, and some of the Jones criteria need to be immediately referred to their pediatrician or to an infectious disease specialist.

Treatment

A 10-day course of penicillin and prednisone is the usual treatment. Some cases of persistent symptoms require a longer course of therapy. In penicillin-allergic patients, erythromycin is used. Because many children are reluctant to take or are noncompliant with oral antibiotics, long-lasting intramuscular

⟶

Rheumatic Fever with Risk for Infective Endocarditis *(cont)*

benzathine penicillin 1.2 million units may be used as a single dose, or sulfadiazine 1 g by mouth just one time is used.

Note

Infective endocarditis can occur years later related to a bacteremia that settled microorganisms on the damaged heart valves to create obstructive vegetations. The most common organisms are *Streptococcus viridans*, *Streptococcus mutans*, and *Streptococcus mitis*. Because infective endocarditis can occur related to oral infection and invasive dental procedures, it is prudent for today's dental care provider to be familiar with the American Heart Association (AHA) recommendations on antibiotic prophylaxis to prevent infective endocarditis.

AHA prophylaxis regimen to prevent infective endocarditis during dental procedures

		Regimen (single dose 30–60 min before procedure)	
Situation	***Agent***	***Adults***	***Children***
Oral	Amoxicillin	2 g	50 mg/kg
Unable to take oral medication	Ampicillin **or**	2 g IM or IV	50 mg/kg IM or IV
	Cefazolin or ceftriaxone	1 g IM or IV	50 mg/kg IM or IV
Allergic to penicillins or ampicillin (oral regimen)	Cephalexin[a,b] **or**	2 g	50 mg/kg
	Clindamycin **or**	600 mg	20 mg/kg
	Azithromycin or clarithromycin	500 mg	15 mg/kg
Allergic to penicillins or ampicillin and unable to take oral medication	Cefazolin or ceftriaxone[b] **or**	1 g IM or IV	50 mg/kg IM or IV
	Clindamycin	600 mg IM or IV	20 mg/kg IM or IV

IM, intramuscular; IV, intravenous.

[a] Or other first- or second-generation oral cephalosporin in equivalent adult or pediatric dosage.

[b] Cephalosporins should not be used in an individual with a history of anaphylaxis, angioedema, or urticaria with penicillins or ampicillin.

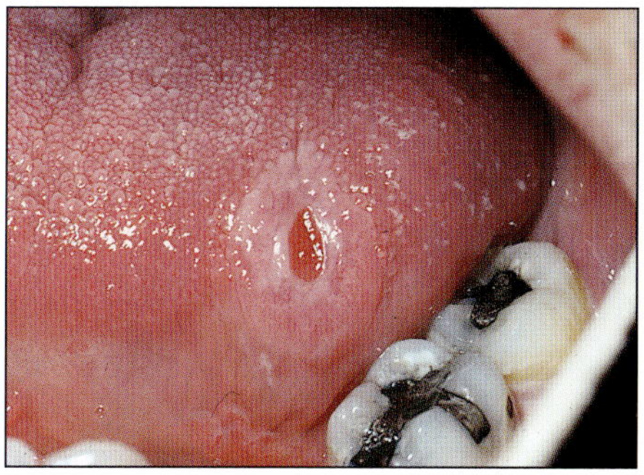

► Chancre of primary syphilis.

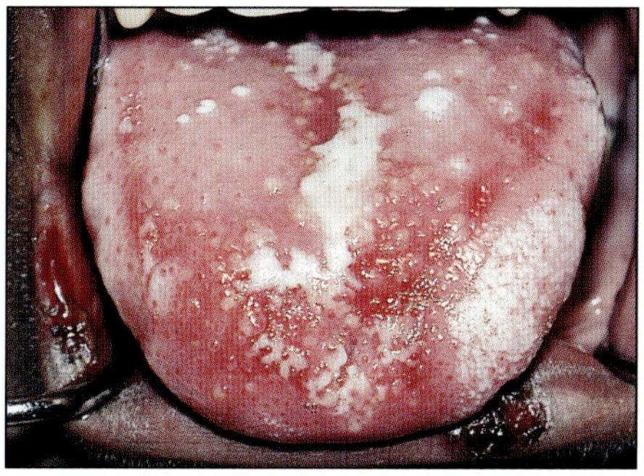

► Mucositis of secondary syphilis.

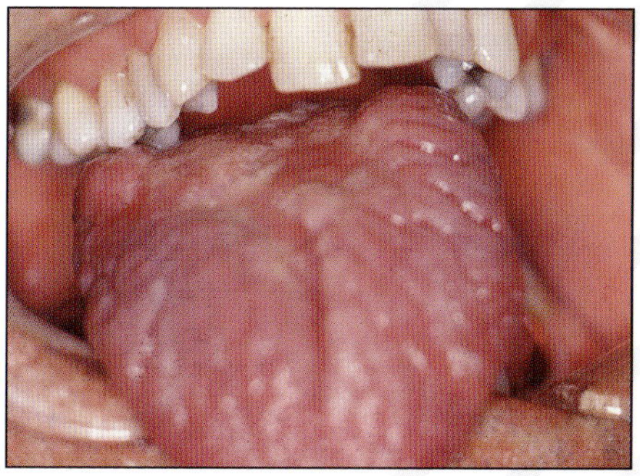

► Interstitial glossitis of tertiary syphilis.

Syphilis

Nature of disease

A specific sexually transmitted infection due to *Treponema pallidum* that, if untreated, will progress through three stages: primary syphilis (an ulcer referred to as a *chancre*), secondary syphilis (a systemic skin and/or oral mucosal eruption), and tertiary syphilis (a widespread involvement of destructive lesions and multiorgan involvement including the brain and spinal cord. A congenital syphilis also occurs from transplacental transmission from an infected mother.

Predilections

Acquired syphilis is more common in adult men. Congenital syphilis occurs equally between male and female newborns. No racial predilection is known.

Clinical features

- Primary syphilis: The chancre is a localized, only mildly tender, clean ulcer at the point of inoculation. The ulcer is usually found in the genital area but may also appear on the tongue and/or lips. Regional lymphadenopathy may accompany the chancre.
- Secondary syphilis: A diffuse macular skin rash that may also form numerous painless, round to ovoid, erythematous areas on the oral mucosa known as *mucous patches.*
- Tertiary syphilis: May present in several ways such as an interstitial glossitis, an oronasal fistula (gumma) or ataxia (tabes dorsalis), paralysis, or aortic aneurysms.
- Congenital syphilis: The classic Hutchinson triad (interstitial keratitis, eighth nerve hearing loss, and Hutchinson teeth comprising "screwdriver" central incisors and mulberry molars) may be seen in part or completely along with rhagades (perioral creases) and a saddle nose deformity from loss of the nasal septum and vomer.

Radiographic presentation

None.

Differential diagnosis

An oral chancre will appear similar to a traumatic ulcer, a squamous cell carcinoma, or an oral fungal lesion of histoplasmosis or coccidioidomycosis. The oral lesions of secondary syphilis will suggest candidiasis, pemphigus, or lichen planus. The oral lesions of tertiary syphilis will be suspicious for carcinomas, lymphoma, and various infections. Congenital syphilis is usually apparent but may be confused with fetal alcohol syndrome or various developmental syndromes (ie, Goldenhar, Pierre Robin).

→

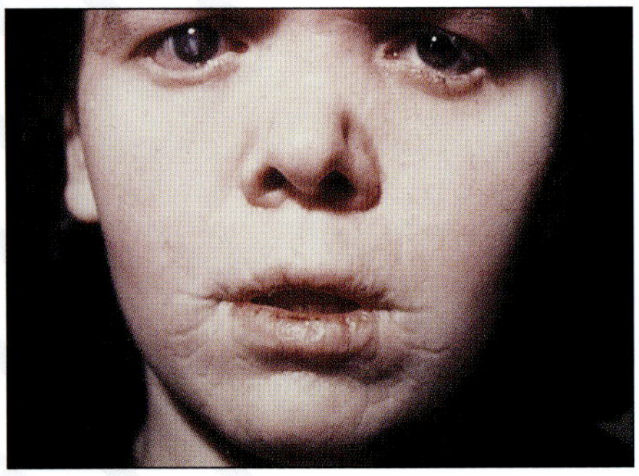

► Rhagades of congenital syphilis.

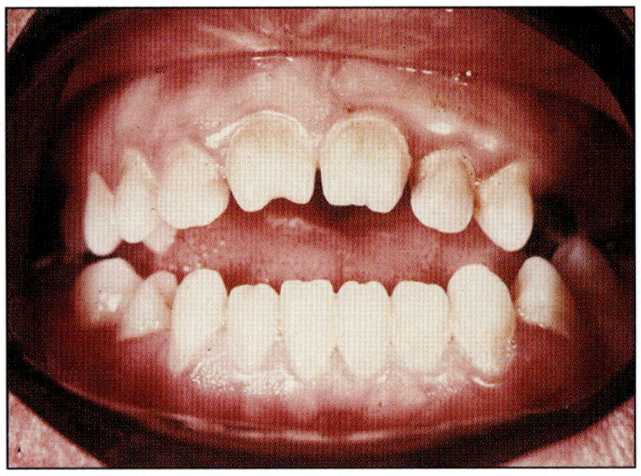

► "Screwdriver" incisors of congenital syphilis.

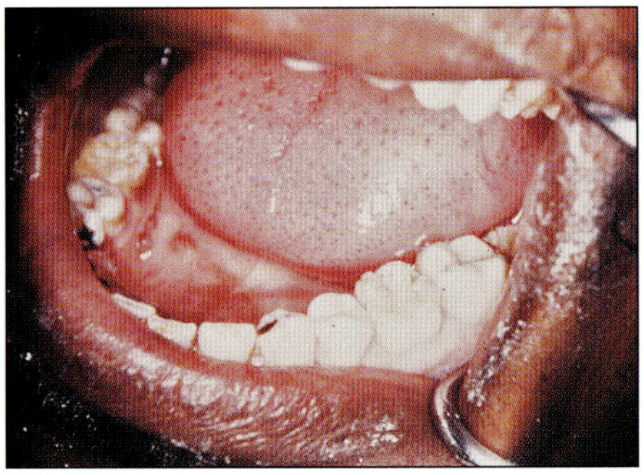

► Mulberry molars of congenital syphilis.

Syphilis *(cont)*

Microscopic features

Primary, secondary, and congenital syphilis are characterized by a proliferative endarteritis as seen by swelling and proliferation of endothelial cells with a dense perivascular infiltration of plasma cells. Tertiary syphilis is characterized by the formation of classic epithelioid granulomas as seen by discrete round collections of epithelial-appearing macrophages surrounded by a concentric ring of lymphocytes. Some Langhans giant cells may also be seen.

Suggested course of action

Recognition of an any stage of syphilis requires a referral to an infectious disease specialist.

Treatment

Primary and secondary syphilis are treated with 1.2 to 2.4 million units of benzathine penicillin delivered intramuscularly in one dose. For penicillin-allergic patients, oral doxycycline 100 mg twice daily by mouth or erythromycin 500 mg four times daily for 14 days is effective. Congenital syphilis is treated with weight-adjusted dosages of the same antibiotics. Tertiary and neurosyphilis are treated with 2.4 million units of benzathine penicillin delivered intramuscularly three times over a 7-day period followed by additional antibiotics for 28 days: penicillin or doxycycline (if the patient is allergic to penicillin). There is not an effective substitute for intramuscular penicillin for these stages.

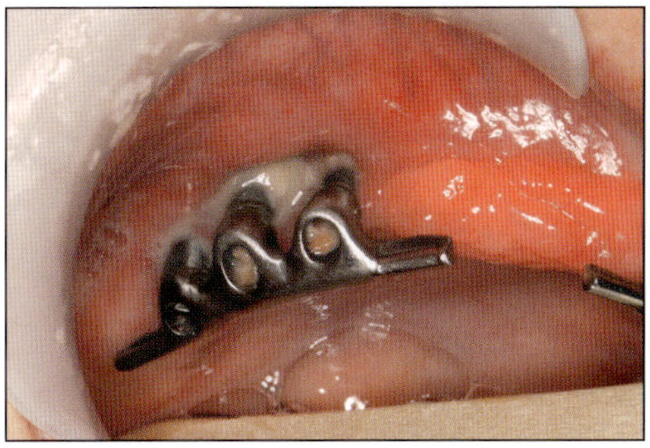

► Suppurative maxillary sinusitis.

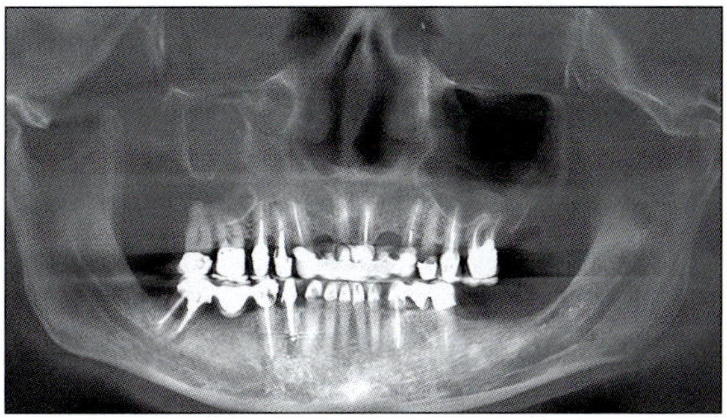

► Opacifications of the maxillary sinus in a patient with suppurative maxillary sinusitis.

Suppurative Maxillary Sinusitis

Nature of disease

Maxillary sinusitis other than the self-limiting component of an upper respiratory infection (common cold) is mostly caused by extension of an odontogenic infection, osteoradionecrosis, or drug-induced osteonecrosis.

Predilections

It is rare in children. No sex or racial predilection is known.

Clinical features

The patient will report nasal congestion. The mucosa over the sinus may be tender to palpation. A nasal drainage or at times an oroantral fistula with drainage may be present. If secondary to osteoradionecrosis or drug-induced osteonecrosis, exposed bone will be present as well.

Radiographic presentation

Panoramic radiographs and cone beam CT scans will show a diffuse opacification of the involved sinus. An air-fluid level may also be seen.

Differential diagnosis

The most important differential is that of a tumor in the maxillary sinus. A large number of benign and malignant tumors will cause a radiographic opacification of the maxillary sinus. In addition, an allergic rhinitis or a common cold causing a reactive sinus membrane should also be considered.

Microscopic features

Numerous mucus-filled collections (mucoceles) will be seen in the sinus membrane, often incorrectly referred to as *sinus polyps*, together with a mixed inflammatory infiltrate beneath the basement membrane.

Suggested course of action

Look for and treat any source of odontogenic infection that may be the cause of the sinusitis. Refer to an oral and maxillofacial surgeon or an otorhinolaryngologist.

Treatment

If a focal source of infection is identified, it is removed, and a course of antibiotics is prescribed, usually amoxicillin 500 mg three times daily or doxycycline 100 mg twice daily (for the penicillin-allergic patient) for 10 to 14 days. In refractory cases, either a Caldwell-Luc sinus debridement or a nasal endoscopic sinus debridement is used, followed by the aforementioned antibiotic regimen.

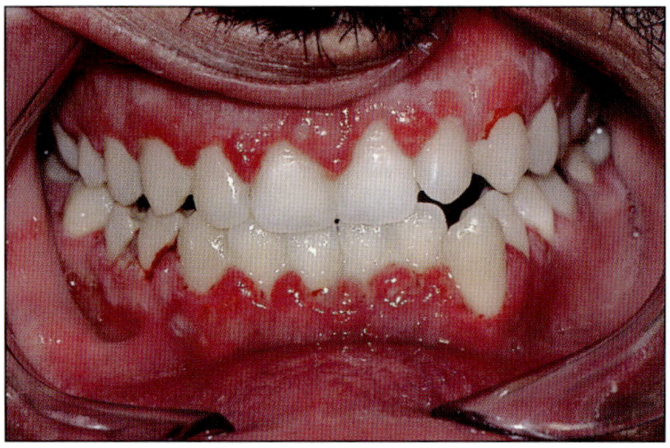

► Acute necrotizing ulcerative gingivitis/periodontitis.

Acute Necrotizing Ulcerative Gingivitis/ Periodontitis

Nature of disease

A rapid-onset, painful bacterial infection of the gingiva caused primarily by *Fusobacterium* species in combination with spirochetes.

Predilections

Most commonly seen in the age range of 15 to 35 years. No sex or racial predilection is known.

Clinical features

Pain and foul odor will be evident. The gingiva will be red, puffy, and friable. Some of the gingival papillae will be lost and replaced by a gray pseudomembrane representing necrosis.

Radiographic presentation

Most cases will show normal alveolar bone height, while others will show horizontal and vertical periodontal bone loss possibly preexisting the acute infection.

Differential diagnosis

The clinical presentation of acute herpetic gingivostomatitis will closely parallel that of acute necrotizing ulcerative gingivitis and should be considered. Otherwise, pemphigus, erosive lichen planus, and a lichenoid drug eruption may mimic acute necrotizing ulcerative gingivitis to a certain extent.

Microscopic features

Acute necrotizing ulcerative gingivitis/periodontitis is a clinical recognition diagnosis without specimens for microscopy.

Suggested course of action

Debride the sloughing necrotic gingiva under local anesthesia and irrigate with either 3% hydrogen peroxide or 0.12% chlorhexidine followed by a 5-day course of either phenoxymethylpenicillin 500 mg four times daily or doxycycline 100 mg twice daily in the penicillin-allergic patient.

Treatment

Local debridement and a 5-day course of antibiotics as noted above are effective in resolving this infection.

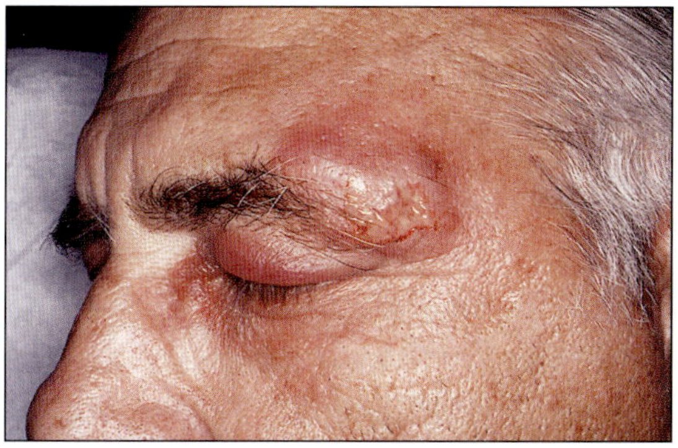

► Skin abscess in nocardiosis.

Nocardiosis

Nature of disease

An uncommon primary pulmonary infection caused by either the soil bacteria *Nocardia asteroides* or *Nocardia brasiliensis* in which an occasional dissemination results in an oral or skin nodule.

Predilections

More common in adults who work in professions that bring them into contact with soil or soil products. Also more common in patients with chronic illness states, steroid use, and immune deficiency states. No specific sex or racial predilection is known.

Clinical features

Oral and cutaneous lesions will be present as mildly tender abscesses with fibrosis and induration. Drainage may also be present. The patient may have a productive cough, fever, and decreased breath sounds indicative of a pulmonary infection. The patient may also report fatigue, weight loss, and night sweats.

Radiographic presentation

Nocardia infections in the head and neck are uncommon and are limited to soft tissue. However, a chest radiograph or CT scan will show pulmonary infiltrates and/or a pleural effusion.

Differential diagnosis

Nocardia infections are sufficiently rare so as to exclude them from most differential lists. However, actinomycosis, skin metastasis from a cancer, and epidermoid cysts should be considered along with the more common lung infections that seed into the oral tissues and facial skin, such as histoplasmosis and coccidioidomycosis.

Microscopic features

Necrotic tissue is seen in which gram-positive filamentous colonies are seen in a sunray pattern, giving rise to the term "ray fungus" when it is actually a bacterium. The organisms are also weakly acid-fast.

Suggested course of action

Oral and/or facial skin abscesses should be referred to an oral and maxillofacial surgeon for workup and treatment.

Treatment

Oral and/or facial skin abscesses are drained, and specimens are taken for culture and histopathology. Both the oral/skin lesions and the pulmonary lesions are treated with intravenous trimethoprim/sulfamethoxazole (Bactrim, Roche) every 6 hours for 1 month, after which oral trimethoprim/sulfamethoxazole is given for 5 months.

Diphtheria

Nature of disease

A serious pharyngeal infection caused by *Corynebacterium diphtheriae* that before common childhood immunizations was a life course or life-threatening infection for children. It is transmitted via airborne water droplets from infected individuals.

Predilections

Mostly children. No sex or racial predilection is known.

Clinical features

The nonimmunized individual will initially present with fever, malaise, and a complaint of a sore throat. Symptoms will then progress to a higher fever, weakness, and cervical lymphadenopathy. The chronic diphtheria pseudomembrane created by the organisms' exotoxin leads to necrosis of the pharyngeal epithelium and may cause upper airway or bronchial obstruction, which can lead to a suffocation death.

Radiographic presentation

None.

Differential diagnosis

Other pharyngitis conditions such as streptococcal pharyngitis, adenovirus pharyngitis, and infectious mononucleosis should be considered.

Microscopic features

The corynebacteria do not invade the pharynx. They exert their pathogenesis via their exotoxin, which creates an intense submucosal inflammatory picture with hyperemia of blood vessels and edema. Epithelial cells in various stages of necrosis may also be seen.

Suggested course of action

Because nearly all children today are immunized with the diphtheria-pertussis-tetanus (DPT) vaccine, diphtheria is not likely to be suspected. However, a serious pharyngitis requires deferral of elective dental care and a referral to the patient's pediatrician.

Treatment

In confirmed nonimmunized cases, diphtheria horse serum antitoxin 40,000 to 60,000 units is given simultaneously with intravenous aqueous penicillin G 20 million units every 6 hours.

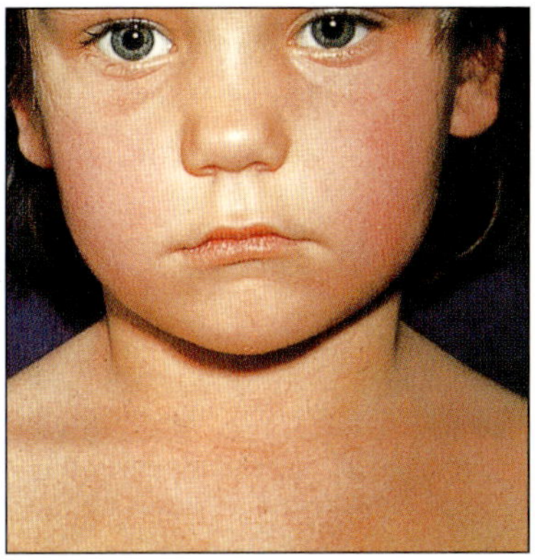

► Red macular skin rash seen in scarlet fever.

Scarlet Fever

Nature of disease

Today, a rare bacterial infection caused by group A beta-hemolytic streptococci (*Streptococcus scarlatina* or *Streptococcus pyogenes*) that produces a unique red macular skin rash and a red swollen tongue by virtue of its erythrotoxin elaboration.

Predilections

Mostly children and young adults. No sex or racial predilection is known.

Clinical features

The child or young adult will present with fever, a sore throat, and headache. The red macular skin rash may appear on the face but will be more prominent in the axillary and groin areas. The tongue will be swollen with reddened fungiform papillae standing out against a white coat on the tongue. This is referred to as "raspberry tongue."

Radiographic presentation

None.

Differential diagnosis

Other infections such as nonspecific streptococcal pharyngitis, infectious mononucleosis, and pseudomembranous pharyngitis as well as diphtheria should be considered.

Microscopic features

Tissue specimens are rarely taken. If one is taken, it will show a nonspecific inflammatory cell infiltrate with prominent endothelial lysis, dilation of small blood vessels, and hyperemia.

Suggested course of action

Throat cultures of suspicious cases should be taken and a referral made to an infectious disease specialist.

Treatment

Penicillin is the drug of choice. Either phenoxymethylpenicillin 500 mg orally four times daily for 10 days or one intramuscular dose of benzathine penicillin 1.2 million units. For penicillin-allergic patients, oral erythromycin 500 mg four times daily or 40 mg/kg per day for 10 days for children is prescribed.

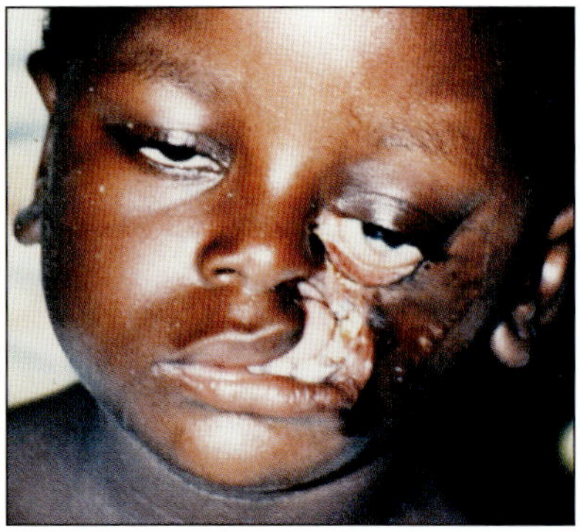

► Tissue loss and deformity resulting from noma.

Noma

Nature of disease

A tissue-necrosing secondary bacterial infection in a health-compromised individual. It is often seen as a complication of malnutrition and measles in Africa but can also be seen as a complication of dysentery, leukemia, chemotherapy, and immunosuppressive drugs.

Predilections

More common in underdeveloped countries and in children. When it occurs in adults, it is mostly as a complication of cancer therapy or immunosuppression. No sex or racial predilection is known.

Clinical features

The usual child or teenager will present with a gangrenous black soft tissue slough emitting a sour odor and leaving a contracted deformity. In its early stages, a painful ulcer develops that progresses to spontaneous tissue breakdown. Underlying bone and tooth roots often become exposed.

Radiographic presentation

If extensive, the noma will progress to an osteomyelitis showing an irregular moth-eaten osteolysis.

Differential diagnosis

Malignancies such as leukemia and lymphomas may also cause such severe tissue loss. Additionally, necrotizing fasciitis is well known to necrose large segments of skin and fascia and should be considered.

Microscopic features

Tissue necrosis predominates along with acute inflammation mostly consisting of neutrophils.

Suggested course of action

Recognition of an impending or progressing noma requires an immediate referral to an emergency room, preferably within a major medical center, and an infectious disease consultation.

Treatment

Noma is treated by controlling or reversing the underlying disease that established the conditions for noma to develop. Nutritional support sometimes via a gastrostomy (PEG) tube is needed. The necrotic tissue is debrided, and intensive multidrug antibiotic therapy is provided. If hyperbaric oxygen therapy is available, it is used as well. Tissue flap reconstruction can be considered after the disease process is arrested and all areas of involvement have healed.

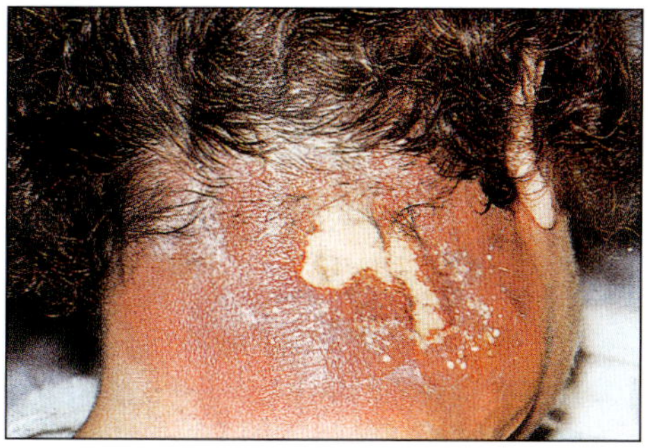

► Rapidly advancing erythema and central necrosis seen early in a necrotizing fasciitis.

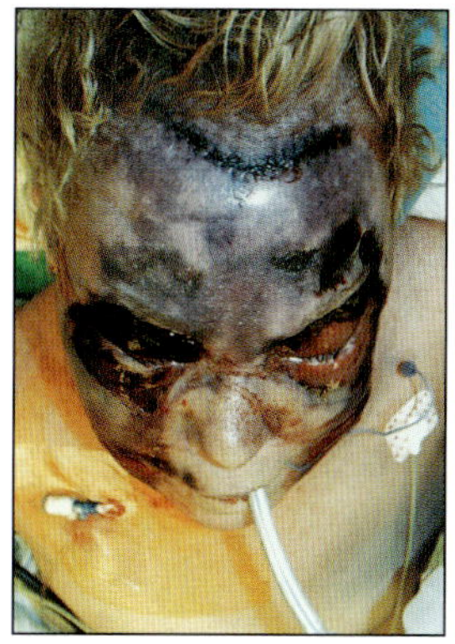

► Necrotizing fasciitis with mottled and discolored skin along with some areas of frank necrosis and epithelial slough. The ballooning-out of the skin is due to gas formation. (Courtesy of Dr Curt Schalit.)

Necrotizing Fasciitis

Nature of disease

A rapidly progressing subcutaneous infection of skin and fascia due to a synergistic infection involving streptococci and *Bacteroides* species.

Predilections

Mostly adults. More common in patients with type 1 diabetes and immunocompromised individuals. No sex or racial predilection is known.

Clinical features

Involvement of the neck and face will present with mottled skin and crepitus from gas bubbles in the subcutaneous compartment. The skin may be cyanotic or diffusely erythematous. As it progresses, large areas of full-thickness skin are sloughed off, exposing underlying muscles, which has given rise to the term "flesh-eating bacteria." If unresponsive to treatment or if treatment is delayed, weakness progresses to coma and death.

Radiographic presentation

Plain radiographs and CT scans will show tissue edema and prominent gas bubble collections.

Differential diagnosis

Dramatic skin necrosis such as occurs in necrotizing fasciitis may also be seen in noma, some leukemias, immunoblastic lymphoma, and paraneoplastic pemphigus.

Microscopic features

Tissue necrosis with severe inflammation, mostly of neutrophils, is seen together with a mixed gram-positive and gram-negative bacterial population.

Suggested course of action

Recognize the rapidly progressive course of a probable necrotizing fasciitis. Call 911 for immediate help, and transport the patient to an emergency room.

Treatment

Aggressive treatment with intravenous aqueous penicillin G 2 million units every 4 hours plus metronidazole 500 mg every 8 hours and hyperbaric oxygen therapy are the mainstays of treatment, along with surgical debridement and repeated irrigation.

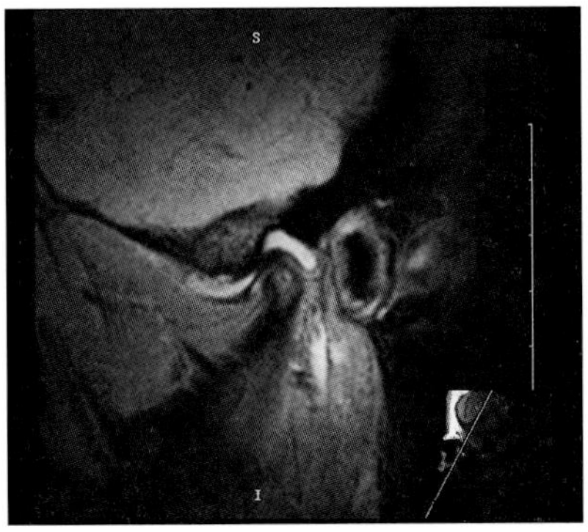

► A septic temporomandibular joint from a rare case of gonococchal arthritis.

Gonorrhea

Nature of disease

A sexually transmitted disease caused by *Neisseria gonorrhoeae* that mainly affects the genitourinary tract but can involve oropharyngeal tissue and joints (gonococcal arthritis) including the temporomandibular joint.

Predilections

Oropharyngeal gonococcal infections are more common in women and homosexual men. Genital gonorrhea is more common in heterosexual men. There is no racial predilection. Adults are mostly affected.

Clinical features

Genital gonorrhea will present in men with a complaint of burning upon urination (dysuria) and urinating pus (pyuria). In women, dysuria also occurs along with vaginitis. Oropharyngeal gonorrhea is associated with nonspecific pain on swallowing (dysphagia). The rare temporomandibular joint with gonococcal arthritis will be swollen and painful to palpation as well as upon opening and will have a restricted opening.

Radiographic presentation

The rare temporomandibular joint arthritis is best imaged with an MRI scan, which will show a very enhanced water content and a swollen joint indicative of joint effusion.

Differential diagnosis

The oropharyngeal involvement is nonspecific. Therefore, streptococcal pharyngitis, adenovirus pharyngitis, and infectious mononucleosis may be considered. If gonococcal arthritis involves the temporomandibular joint, one may consider the more common anterior disc dislocation, capsulitis, or a disc perforation.

Microscopic features

Gonorrhea of the oropharyngeal tissues is seen as a mild acute inflammation of mostly neutrophils.

Suggested course of action

Cases suspicious for oropharyngeal gonorrhea should be referred to an infectious disease specialist, and all but emergency dental care should be deferred until treatment is completed.

Treatment

The most effective treatment for all strains of *Neisseria gonorrhoeae* is a single intramuscular dose of ceftriaxone (Rocephin, Roche).

► Early contractions of extraocular muscles producing an upward gaze, and contractions of the muscles of mastication producing trismus.

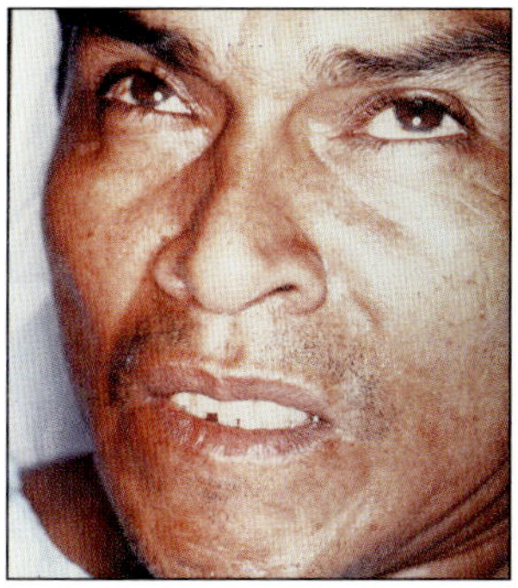

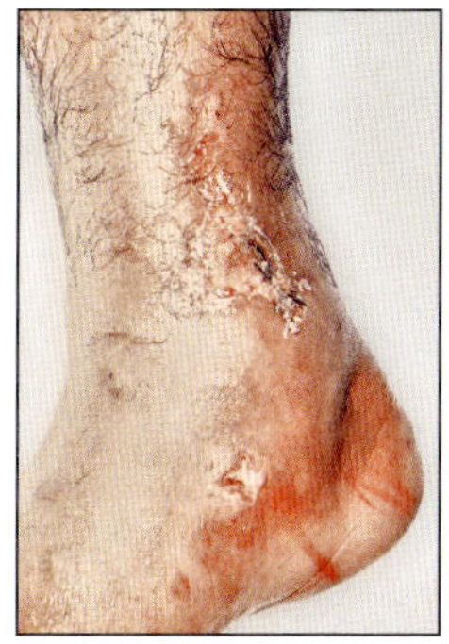

► A contaminated penetrating wound is the usual initiating event in tetanus.

Tetanus

Nature of disease

A life-threatening infection due to *Clostridium tetani* that produces the neurotoxin tetanospasmin, which creates overactive muscle activity and spasms. The *Clostridium* portal of entry is mostly via a penetrating wound or via contaminated needles from intravenous drug abuse.

Predilections

Mostly unvaccinated adults. No sex or racial predilection is known. Some newborns also develop tetanus prior to vaccination.

Clinical features

Initially, the patient will complain of double vision (diplopia) and, soon thereafter, a stiff neck and trismus. Left untreated, the tetanospasmin toxin's concentration builds to involve larger muscle groups, resulting in spasm of the extensor muscles of the back, creating a "wrestler's bridge" posture called *opisthotonos*. As it progresses to involve the diaphragm, breathing is halted, and death ensues.

Radiographic presentation

A CT scan may show gas bubbles in the soft tissue around the penetrating wound. Otherwise, there are no radiographic features.

Differential diagnosis

The initial muscle spasms and stiff neck will suggest meningitis, poisons such as strychnine, or a phenothiazine overdose. In the intravenous drug user, various designer drugs that have muscle spastic properties should be considered.

Microscopic features

The initial wound will only show a limited tissue necrosis, hyperemia, and inflammatory infiltrates mostly of neutrophils.

Suggested course of action

Cases with trismus, diplopia, stiff neck complaints, and a history of a penetrating wound (eg, a nail, fishhook, knife, etc) require an evaluation in an emergency room. Call 911 for immediate help, and transport the patient to an emergency room as tetanus can rapidly progress.

Treatment

Patients immediately receive 5,000 units of tetanus immune globulin delivered intramuscularly. The penetrating wound is debrided and irrigated, and cultures are taken. Intravenous metronidazole 500 mg three times daily is the standard antibiotic regimen. Hyperbaric oxygen is also used if the patient is sufficiently stable. In cases that have progressed to large muscle group spasms and for diaphragm involvement, a tracheostomy is performed, the patient's muscles are relaxed with paralytic agents, and breathing is supported by a ventilator.

Botryomycosis

Nature of disease

A rare bacterial infection of internal organs that may disseminate to cause an infection of the oral mucosa and facial soft tissues. Note: The causative organisms are not a fungus as the name implies but rather generally include *Staphylococcus aureus*, *Pseudomonas aeruginosa*, and *Escherichia coli*.

Predilections

Most commonly seen in chronically ill individuals, the elderly, or debilitated patients. No sex or racial predilection is known.

Clinical features

The oral and maxillofacial area involvement will present with indurated soft tissue swelling of facial skin or oral mucosa. The tissue will become firm and nodular.

Radiographic presentation

Botryomycosis rarely involves bone. However, a case involving the mandible will present an irregular osteolysis as seen in osteomyelitis.

Differential diagnosis

The indurated nodular nature of botryomycosis will suggest cervical facial actinomycosis or an infiltrating malignancy. Additionally, nodular fasciitis and aggressive fibromatosis may also be considered.

Microscopic features

Similar to actinomycosis, an influx of neutrophils is seen surrounded by a thick fibrous tissue component.

Suggested course of action

Refer to an oral and maxillofacial surgery for further workup and treatment.

Treatment

Large, disfiguring lesions are debrided or excised followed by intensive long-term (6 months or more) antibiotic treatment. If methicillin-resistant *Staphylococcus aureus* (MRSA) is cultured, intravenous vancomycin (Vancocin, Eli Lilly) 500 mg twice daily is used. Otherwise, other culture-specific antibiotics are used or added to the vancomycin.

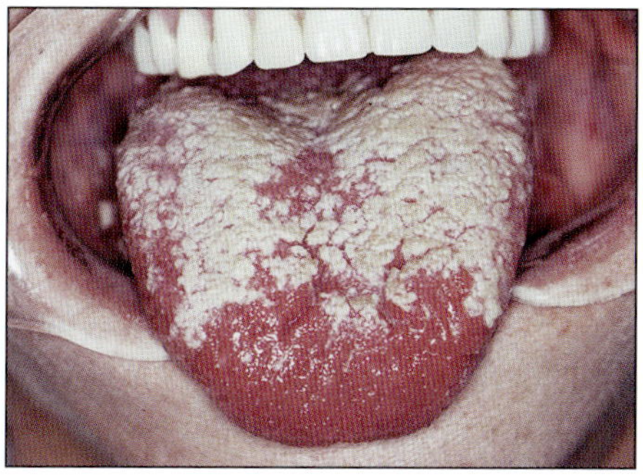

► Thrush.

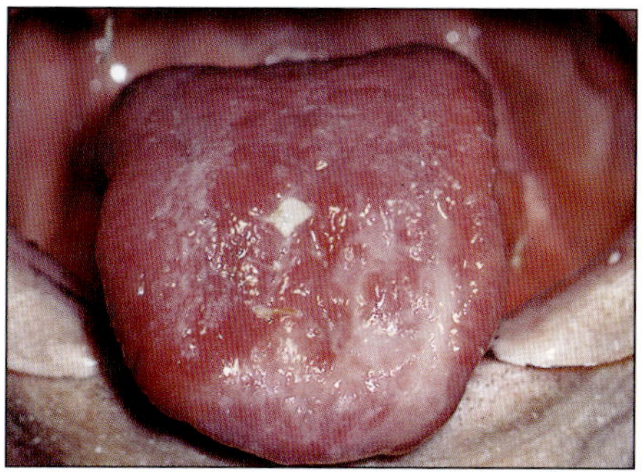

► Atrophic glossitis.

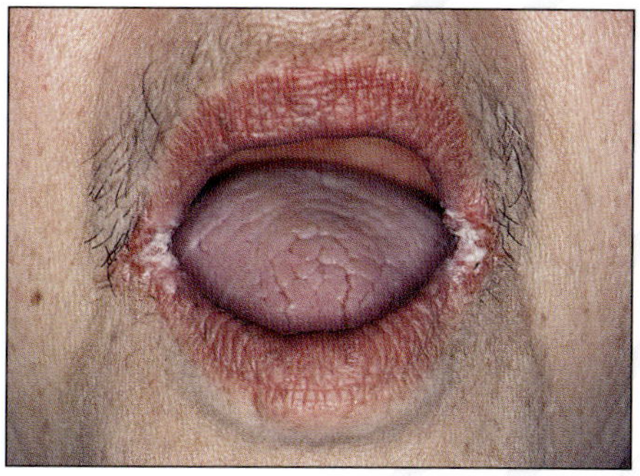

► Angular cheilitis.

Fungal Diseases

Candidiasis

Nature of disease

A fungal (yeast) colonization and/or actual invasive infection by one of the many species of *Candida*, the most common of which is *Candida albicans*.

Predilections

There is no specific age, sex, or racial predilection. However, it is more often seen as an opportunistic infection in someone prone to develop it, including *(1)* children whose immune system is not complete; *(2)* older individuals with age-related reduced immune function; *(3)* patients who were recently on antibiotics; *(4)* patients who underwent radiation therapy; *(5)* patients undergoing chemotherapy; *(6)* patients with diseases that affect the immune system (eg, leukemia, HIV); *(7)* patients with trauma from ill-fitting dentures; and *(8)* patients with warm, moist creases at the commissures of the mouth with reduced occlusal vertical dimension.

Clinical features

There are many clinical presentations of candidiasis:

1. Classic thrush with white *Candida* colonies able to be removed with a tongue depressor
2. Angular cheilitis (perlèche), in which red-white painful lesions on the commissures of the mouth result from a loss of occlusal vertical dimension
3. Median rhomboid glossitis represented by a rhomboid or diamond-shaped, flat red patch on the dorsum of the tongue
4. Hyperplastic candidiasis, which cannot be removed with a tongue depressor and looks similar to leukoplakia
5. Inflammatory hyperplasia under an ill-fitting denture
6. Atrophic glossitis, where the *Candida* has resulted in loss or flattening of the filiform papillae
7. Mucocutaneous candidiasis, which is a severe and more widespread involvement of skin and other mucous membranes
8. Systemic disseminated candidiasis from a candidemia, most often from a central venous line or catheter

Radiographic presentation

None.

Differential diagnosis

In its various presentations, the differential diagnosis will change. The most significant differential is to consider leukoplakia, epithelial dysplasia, squamous cell carcinoma, and lichen planus. →

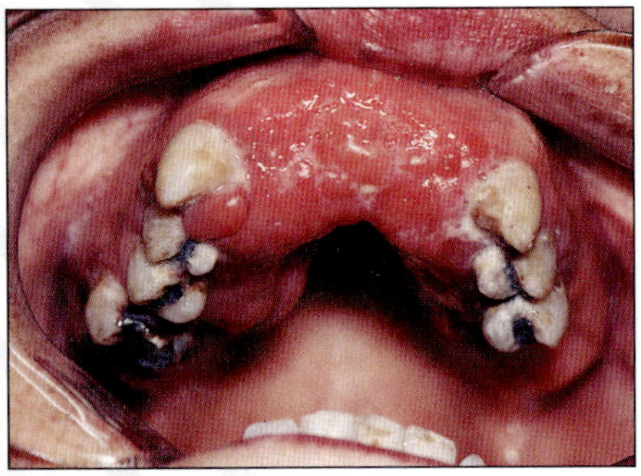

► Inflammatory hyperplasia.

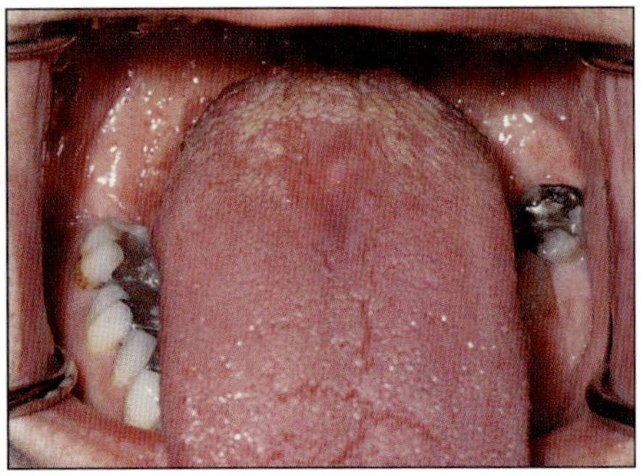

► Median rhomboid glossitis.

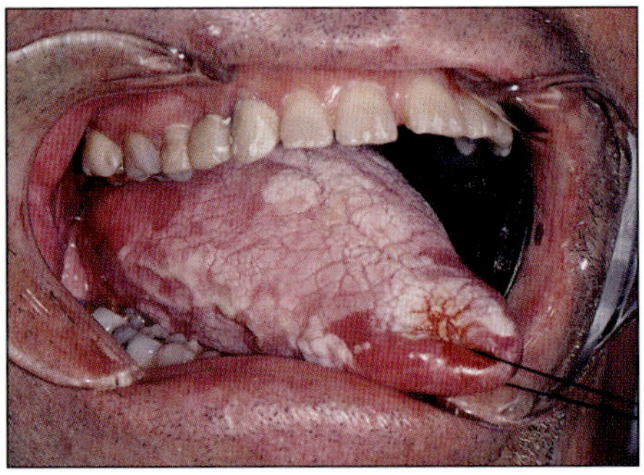

► Hypertrophic candidiasis.

Candidiasis *(cont)*

Microscopic features

Candida are nonseptate hyphae that can be highlighted by a periodic acid-Schiff stain or a silver stain. With these stains, the hyphae will be seen on the mucosal surface and also vertically oriented and burrowing through the epithelial layer. Neutrophils are also often seen within the epithelial layer, presumably in response to the *Candida*. Beneath the basement membrane, a lymphocytic-histiocytic inflammatory infiltrate will be seen.

Suggested course of action

Treat oral lesions initially with oral nystatin suspension 100,000 units/mL using 5-mL swish and spit. Skin and commissure lesions may be treated with nystatin powder. Refractory cases are best referred to an oral medicine specialist or an oral and maxillofacial surgeon.

Treatment

Refractory cases often need systemic as well as topical anti-*Candida* treatment. In such cases, fluconazole 100 mg daily for 5 to 7 days or ketoconazole 200 mg twice daily is used. In the rare systemic or disseminated candidiasis, intravenous micafungin or amphotericin B may be required.

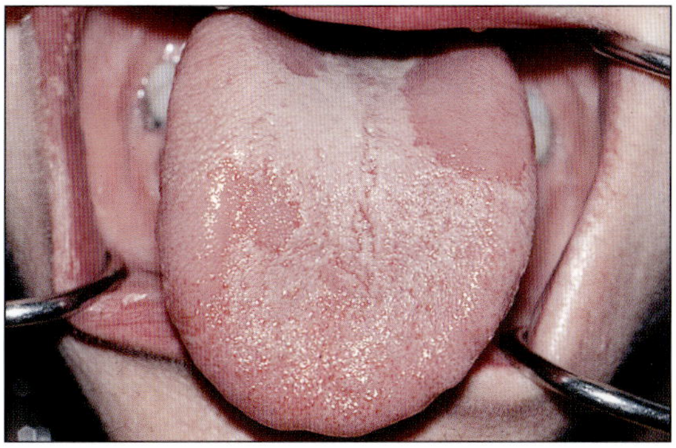

► Benign migratory glossitis.

Benign Migratory Glossitis

Nature of disease

An asymptomatic and innocuous condition involving the tongue in which smooth red areas absent of filiform papillae are contrasted against the textured pale areas of the normal dorsum of the tongue. These red areas will resolve and then appear in another position on the tongue dorsum, hence giving it a migratory appearance over time.

Predilections

Adults mostly. There is no sex or racial predilection.

Clinical features

In a single one-time examination, a portion of the tongue dorsum will appear as normal textured and pale white together with flat, smooth red areas.

Radiographic presentation

None.

Differential diagnosis

Asymptomatic red-white surface lesions on the dorsum of the tongue may be seen in atrophic candidiasis, lichen planus, and, more rarely, in systemic lupus erythematosus and squamous cell carcinoma.

Microscopic features

Narrow, elongated rete pegs are seen between connective tissue papillae that approach a thin surface epithelium. Beneath the basement membrane, an inflammatory infiltrate is usually seen.

Suggested course of action

Reassure the patient of the nonpremalignant nature of benign migratory glossitis and that it does not represent any known systemic disease.

Treatment

None required.

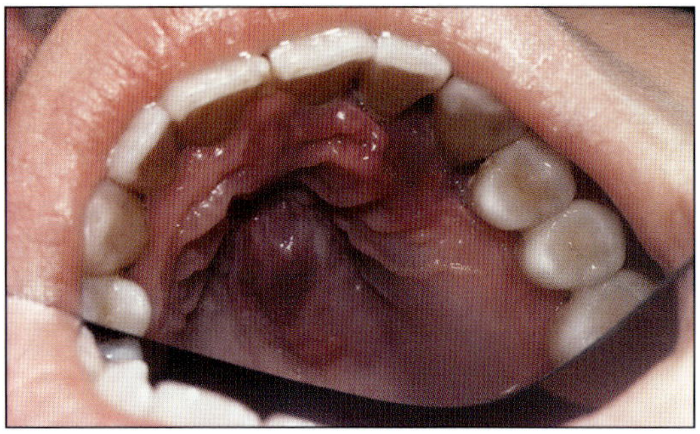

► Soft, fleshy oral lesions from pulmonary histoplasmosis.

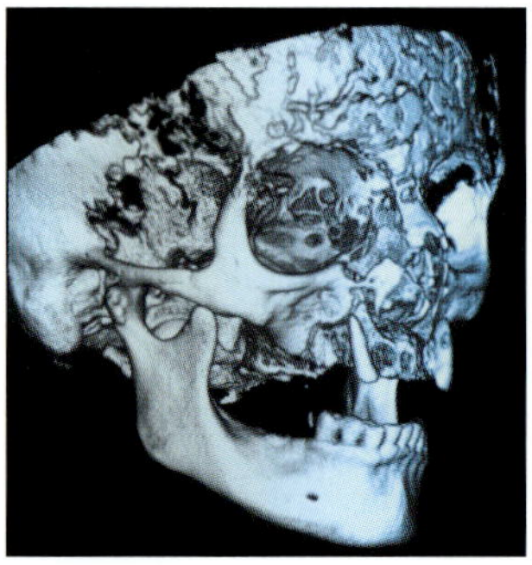

► Advanced untreated histoplasmosis with bone necrosis.

Histoplasmosis

Nature of disease

Primarily a pulmonary infection due to *Histoplasma capsulatum* in which oral lesions may develop from blood-borne routes or via coughed-up sputum.

Predilections

Related as endemic in the Mississippi and Ohio valleys, it now increasingly occurs outside these areas due to travel. Affects mostly adults. There is no sex or racial predilection.

Clinical features

Oral lesions present as mildly painful, red, fleshy tissue nodules or as ulcers. The patient may report a chronic productive cough, weakness, fatigue, and shortness of breath (dyspnea). Oral lesions are mostly seen on the tongue or palatal mucosa.

Radiographic presentation

The alveolar bone may be seen to be eroded under a clinical oral lesion. Chest radiographs and CT scans of the lungs will show hilar adenopathy, interstitial fibrosis, and focal radiodense masses.

Differential diagnosis

A fleshy oral lesion together with a chronic lung illness suggests other fungal lesions such as coccidioidomycosis and blastomycosis as well as tuberculosis. Additionally, squamous cell carcinoma and a simple pyogenic granuloma should be considered.

Microscopic features

Histoplasmosis is more readily diagnosed by histopathology than by culture methods. The low-power views will show noncaseating granulomas, whereas the high-power views will show the small, round *Histoplasma* organisms within macrophages. Each organism will have a clear halo around it.

Suggested course of action

Defer all but emergency dental care, and refer the patient to an infectious disease specialist.

Treatment

Oral histoplasmosis lesions as well as the lung lesions are treated with either oral itraconazole (Sporanox, Janssen) 200 to 400 mg daily for 7 months or the lipid preparation of intravenous amphotericin B (Abelcet, Enzon).

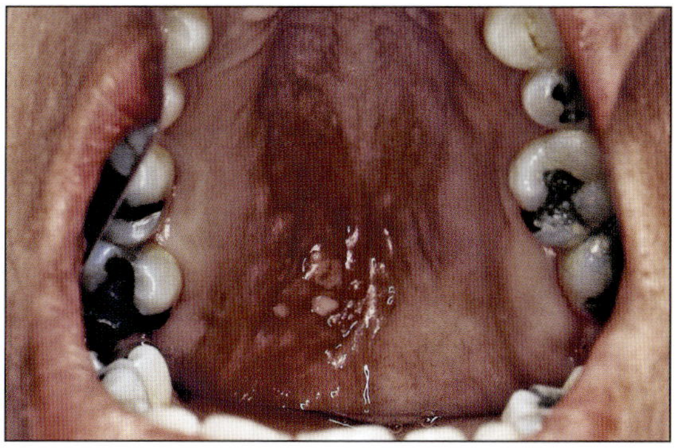

► Coccidioidomycosis of the palate secondary to pulmonary coccidioidomycosis.

Coccidioidomycosis

Nature of disease

A primary fungal lung infection that may disseminate infection to the oral mucosa from blood-borne routes or via coughed-up sputum.

Predilections

Endemic in the San Joaquin Valley of California, but cases can occur elsewhere due to travel. It is found much more often in Filipinos and somewhat more often in black individuals of African heritage. Adult men are more frequently affected than women.

Clinical features

Oral lesions will appear as mildly tender, friable soft tissue nodules or ulcerations. The patient may have a productive or dry cough or a recent history of a nonspecific pneumonitis diagnosis. Weakness and fatigue may be present as well.

Radiographic presentation

Chest radiographs and CT scans will show a hilar adenopathy along with a scarred lung parenchyma and possibly a pleural effusion.

Differential diagnosis

A fleshy and friable oral soft tissue lesion together with a history of a pneumonitis or present lung symptoms will suggest other pulmonary fungal diseases such as histoplasmosis and blastomycosis or tuberculosis. Additionally, a pyogenic granuloma and squamous cell carcinoma will appear similar and should be considered.

Microscopic features

The diagnosis of coccidioidomycosis is more readily made by histopathology than by culture methods. In contrast to the small size of histoplasmosis organisms, the sporangia of coccidioidomycosis are very large. They will be much larger than a macrophage and will have a double refractive capsule containing budding new organisms referred to as *endospores*. These features are best seen with silver stains.

Suggested course of action

Defer all but emergency dental care, and refer the patient to an infectious disease specialist.

Treatment

Coccidioidomycosis is treated with either oral itraconazole (Sporanox, Janssen) 100 mg twice daily or the lipid preparation of intravenous amphotericin B (Abelcet, Enzon).

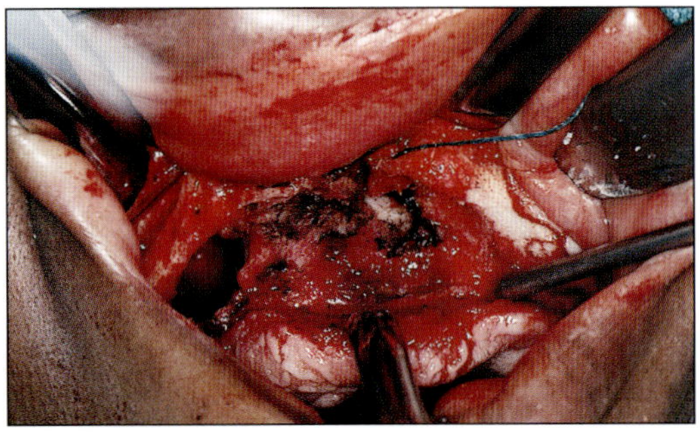

► Discolored black necrotic sequestra in the maxilla from mucormycosis.

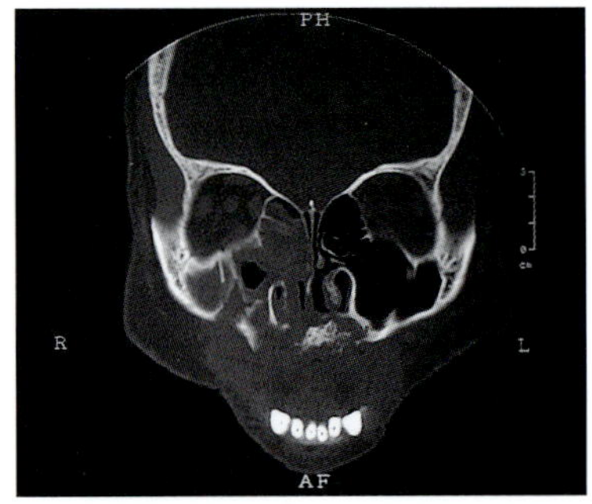

► Osteolysis and extensive maxillary and ethmoid sinus infection in mucormycosis.

Mucormycosis

Nature of disease

A severe fungal infection of the maxilla, maxillary sinuses, and nasal vault due to an otherwise nonpathogenic soil fungus of the Mucorales family, including genera *Absidia*, *Mucor*, or *Rhizopus*. This usually nonpathogenic organism becomes an opportunistic invader of the maxilla in poorly controlled diabetes and immunosuppressed individuals.

Predilections

Mostly adults. More than 90% occur in patients with poorly controlled insulin-dependent diabetes, while the remaining 10% occur in HIV patients, transplant-related immunosuppressed patients, patients with chronic renal failure or leukemia, and on rare occasion, individuals in good health. No age, sex, or racial predilection is known.

Clinical features

Patients will present with a swollen, painful maxilla often with exposed black-colored necrotic bone. Granulation tissue will abound, and bony sequestra and mobile teeth are often noted. Orbital swelling may also be seen.

Radiographic presentation

Plain radiographs and CT scans will identify osteolysis, sequestra, and defects from lysed bone. The air spaces of one or both maxillary sinuses will be opacified. The ethmoid sinuses may also be opacified. In severe cases, brain involvement may be seen as streaks of increased soft tissue density intracranially.

Differential diagnosis

Other diseases that cause destruction of the palate or the maxillary sinuses include the extranodal natural killer/T-cell lymphoma (formerly called *midline lethal granuloma*), a nasopharyngeal carcinoma, tertiary syphilis, and high-grade mucoepidermoid cancers.

Microscopic features

An intense mixed inflammatory infiltrate is seen together with bone and soft tissue necrosis. The *Mucor* organisms are made to be readily seen with either a silver stain or a periodic acid-Schiff stain as T- or Y-shaped organisms.

Suggested course of action

Suspicious cases should be referred to an oral and maxillofacial surgeon for workup and treatment.

Treatment

Treatment is focused on controlling the diabetes or other chronic illness state, surgical debridement, and lipid intravenous amphotericin B (Abelcet, Enzon). Hyperbaric oxygen is also very useful in treating mucormycosis.

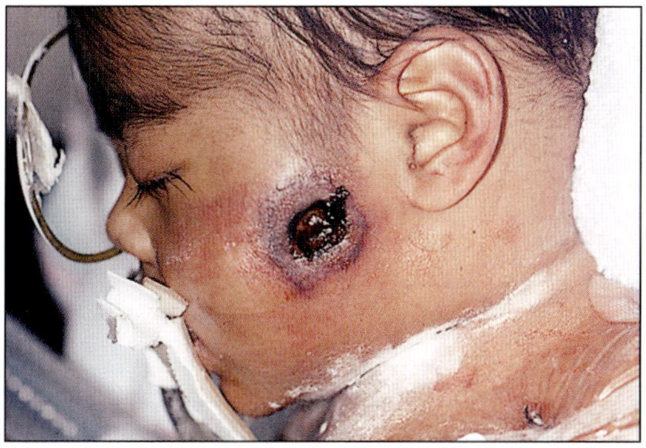

► Black-colored ulcer from *Aspergillus niger* in an immunocompromised transplant patient.

Aspergillosis

Nature of disease

A fungal infection usually of the maxillary sinuses/nasal cavity or external ear caused by *Aspergillus niger* or *Aspergillus fumigatus*.

Predilections

More common in immunocompromised individuals, particularly transplant patients and around foreign bodies. No age, sex, or racial predilection is known.

Clinical features

A common clinical presentation is that of a tender external ear canal and pinna. In this scenario, black colonies of *A niger* develop from loss of the protective cerumen and provoke inflammation (otitis externa). Another clinical presentation is a chronic maxillary sinusitis with swelling and pain. At times the nasal bones and cartilage are destroyed, producing a deformity. In some transplant patients, a black ischemic skin lesion develops.

Radiographic presentation

The otitis externa presentation will not have any radiographic features. However, the maxillary involvement presentation will show a soft tissue opacification of the maxillary as well as the ethmoid air spaces. Osteolysis of the maxillary walls, vomer, and nasal bone may be seen in long-standing cases.

Differential diagnosis

For the otitis externa presentation, a *Pseudomonas* infection should be considered due to its frequency as well as a dry ear known as "swimmer's ear" from loss of cerumen from water immersion. The maxillary sinus presentation requires a consideration for other sinus infections including mucormycosis and *Klebsiella* sinusitis. Additionally, maxillary sinus cancers and lymphomas as well as drug-induced osteonecrosis and osteoradionecrosis may be considered if supported by the history.

Microscopic features

Small blood vessel thrombosis and occlusion are seen amid colonies of branching hyphae best seen with silver stains or a periodic acid-Schiff stain.

→

Aspergillosis *(cont)*

Suggested course of action

The external otitis presentation can be treated with acetic acid/aluminum acetate ear drops (Domeboro Otic, Bayer). However, a referral to an otorhinolaryngologist is recommended to check for damage to the external ear or tympanic membrane. Any maxillary sinus infection such as *Aspergillus* sinusitis should be referred to either an oral and maxillofacial surgeon, an otorhinolaryngologist, or an infectious disease specialist.

Treatment

External otitis is treated with irrigation and the acetic acid/aluminum acetate ear drops. The maxillary sinus infection is much more concerning and persistent. It is treated with debridement and an acetic acid lavage followed by itraconazole (Sporanox, Janssen) 200 mg twice daily for 2 weeks or longer.

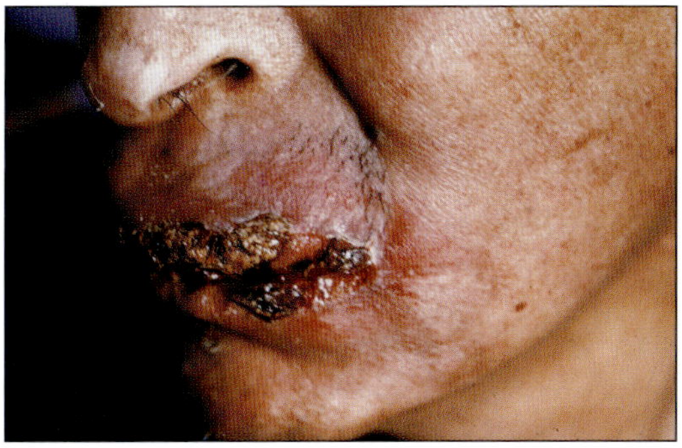

► Lip lesions in blastomycosis.

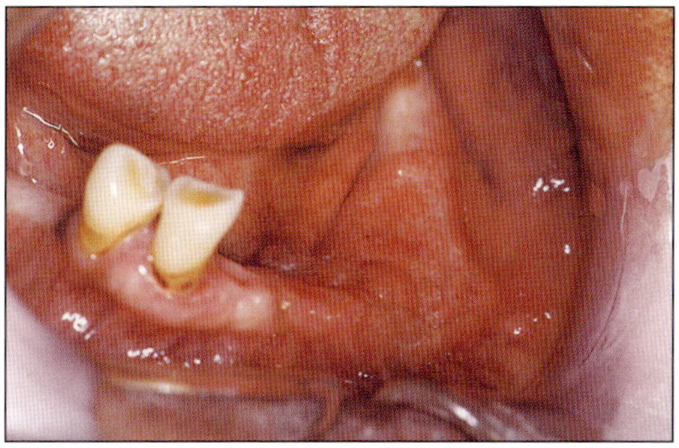

► Red oral mucosal lesion in an individual with blastomycosis.

Blastomycosis

Nature of disease

A primary pulmonary fungal infection that can disseminate to develop oral or facial skin lesions due to *Blastomyces dermatitidis*.

Predilections

More common in South American than North America. Although it was once separated into a North American blastomycosis and a South American blastomycosis, today it is recognized as a single disease entity. It is mostly seen in adults. No sex or racial predilection is known.

Clinical features

Oral lesions will present as red, fleshy nodules. Some will appear verrucoid. Pain is minimal. Facial skin lesions are more verrucoid with rolled borders and usually cover a large surface area and are disfiguring. Patients will also likely have a productive cough and complain of chest pain. Fever and chills are intermittent.

Radiographic presentation

Oral and facial lesions are limited to soft tissue. Chest radiographs and chest CT scans will likely show pleural effusions, hilar adenopathy, and foci of increased soft tissue density.

Differential diagnosis

The presentation of blastomycosis is similar to that of histoplasmosis and coccidioidomycosis and may also resemble Wegener granulomatosis.

Microscopic features

Oral and skin lesions often show an abscess formation with numerous neutrophils. In some cases, classic noncaseating epithelioid granulomas are apparent.

Suggested course of action

Defer all but emergency dental care, and refer the patient to an infectious disease specialist.

Treatment

The chronic and disfiguring nature of blastomycosis requires aggressive therapy with either itraconazole (Sporanox, Janssen) 200 mg daily for 3 months or the lipid form of intravenous amphotericin B (Abelcet, Enzon).

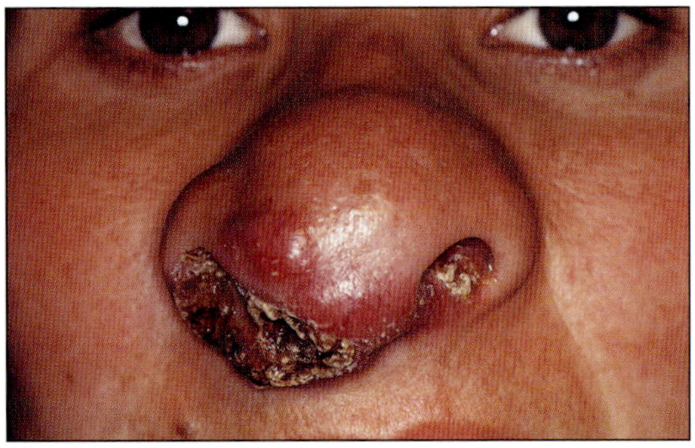

► Nasal lesion of rhinoscleroma. (Courtesy of Dr Roman Carlos.)

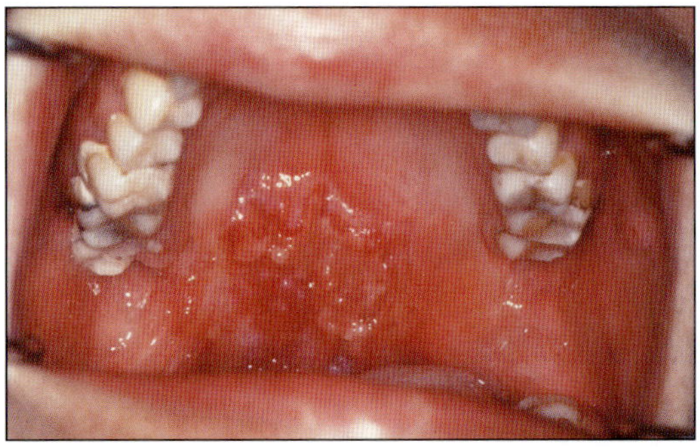

► Palatal lesion of rhinoscleroma. (Courtesy of Dr Roman Carlos.)

Rhinoscleroma

Nature of disease

A bacterial granulomatous infection of the nasal mucosa and skin over the nose caused by *Klebsiella rhinoscleromatis.*

Predilections

Uncommon in North America and more common in Egypt, Central America, and Indonesia. No age, sex, or particular racial predilection is known.

Clinical features

Patients will present with red, crusting masses within the nasal cavity causing nasal obstruction. The skin of the nose will be edematous, or lesions will emerge through the nasal cavity onto the skin of the nose. In some cases, identical lesions are seen in the maxillary gingiva and palate.

Radiographic presentation

CT scans will identify the usually large soft tissue mass in the nasal cavity as well as any destruction of the nasal septum, nasal cartilage, vomer, or nasal bones.

Differential diagnosis

The nasal target of rhinoscleroma will suggest a rhinophyma (hyperplasia and hypertrophy of the sebaceous cells in the skin of the nose), a juvenile angiofibroma if the patient is a young male, a nasal squamous cell carcinoma, or a mucormycosis.

Microscopic features

Granulomatous inflammation will be present with large pale-staining macrophages containing *Klebsiella* organisms referred to as *Mikulicz cells* and amorphous deposits of immunoglobulin from plasma cells called Russell bodies.

Suggested course of action

Defer all but emergency dental care, and refer the patient to an infectious disease specialist.

Treatment

Ciprofloxacin 750 mg twice daily or doxycycline 100 mg twice daily for 3 months slowly resolves the infection.

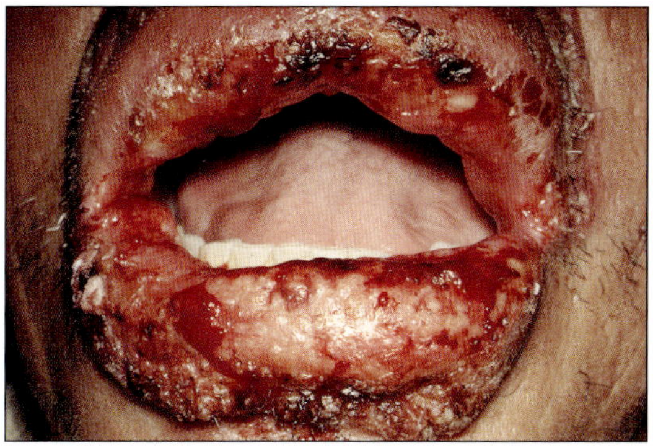

► Mucocutaneous leishmaniasis.

Parasitic Diseases

Leishmaniases

Nature of disease

A group of parasitic infections caused by one of several species of the genus *Leishmania*. All are transmitted by sandfly bites except visceral leishmaniasis (Kala-Azar), which is transmitted by human-to-human contact.

Predilections

There is no specific age, sex, or racial predilection. However, each of the several forms is seen more commonly in a geographical area:

1. New World leishmaniasis, caused by *L mexicana*, is found in Central America and Mexico.
2. Mucocutaneous leishmaniasis, caused by *L braziliensis*, is found in Central and South America.
3. Old World cutaneous leishmaniasis:
   - A: *L tropica* is found in the Middle East and South Central Asia.
   - B: *L major* is found in the deserts of the Middle East and Africa.
   - C: *L aeithiopica* is found in Ethiopia and Kenya.
4. Visceral leishmaniasis is found in China, Bangladesh, other parts of Asia, Ethiopia, and Kenya.

Clinical features

The clinical presentation will vary with the specific *Leishmania* species involved. Generally, oral and skin ulcers develop that progress into papillomatous nodules and tissue loss, leading to scarring and disfigurement. The visceral form produces a protruding abdomen, fever, chills, and weight loss.

Radiographic presentation

None.

Differential diagnosis

The disfiguring skin lesions of the mucocutaneous form of leishmaniasis will suggest leprosy, tuberculosis of the skin (lupus vulgaris), skin basal cell and squamous cell carcinomas, and mycosis fungoides.

Microscopic features

Large macrophages in which the leishmania organism can be seen will be apparent amid a lymphocytic plasmacytic infiltrate. →

Leishmaniases *(cont)*

Suggested course of action

Defer all but emergency dental care. Refer the patient to an infectious disease specialist.

Treatment

Old World leishmaniasis usually resolves spontaneously. New World leishmaniasis is treated with sodium antimony gluconate 20 mg/kg per day or with paromomycin (Humatin, Pfizer) 250 mg by mouth three times daily.

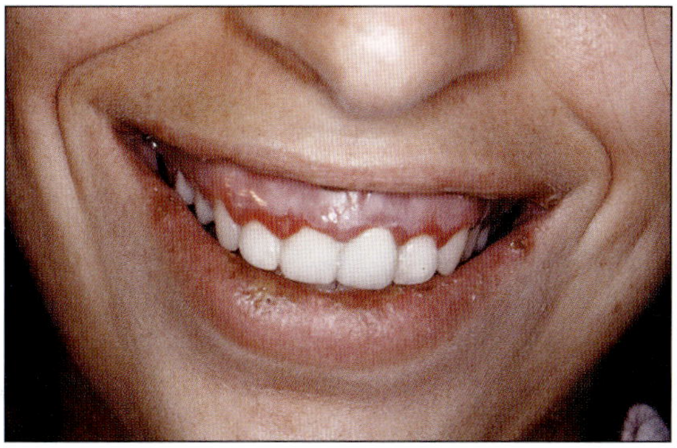

► Primary herpetic gingivostomatitis.

Viral Diseases

Primary Herpetic Gingivostomatitis

Nature of disease

A painful viral infection of the gingiva and oral mucosa caused by herpes simplex virus 1 (HSV-1), which enters the gingiva/oral mucosa via a direct airborne water-droplet vector.

Predilections

Mostly seen in children and young adults. No sex or racial predilection is known.

Clinical features

The individual will present with painful vesicular ulcerative lesions on the gingiva and oral mucosa. The person will often be drooling, and a noticeable foul odor will be present. Although the lesions will start out to be vesicular, they soon rupture, producing a necrotic fibrin-based ulcer and the thick, foul-smelling exudate.

Radiographic presentation

None.

Differential diagnosis

Painful gingival/oral mucosal lesions in children and young adults may also be seen in acute necrotizing ulcerative gingivitis/periodontitis, pemphigus, erosive lichen planus, and erythema multiforme if targetoid skin lesions are also present.

Microscopic features

Biopsies representative of herpes lesions must be taken in the vesicular stage before rupture. The floor of the vesicle will show a ballooning degeneration of cells with large nuclei that have irregular contours and chromatin displaced to the periphery. The connective tissue beneath the vesicle will show an intense nonspecific inflammatory infiltrate of predominantly neutrophils.

Suggested course of action

Assure parents and patients that primary herpetic gingivostomatitis is a local viral infection that will resolve within 10 days due to patient-synthesized antiviral antibodies produced in response to the infection. If tolerated or with anesthesia, a gentle lavage with 3% hydrogen peroxide, saline, or 0.12% chlorhexidine may provide some relief. Otherwise, supportive care with antipyretics, hydration, and a bland diet help somewhat. If secondary bacterial infection is suspected, phenoxymethylpenicillin or doxycycline in weight-adjusted doses can also be used.

Treatment

The methods noted above are all that is usually required for this self-limiting disease. In severe or prolonged cases, valacyclovir 15 mg/kg three times daily can shorten the course and reduce symptoms.

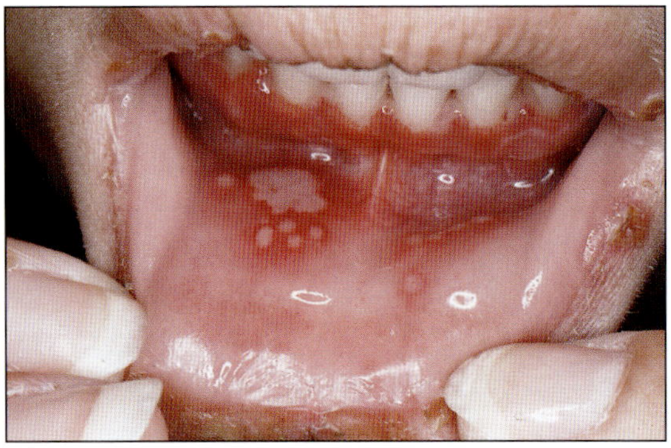

► Recurrent herpes lesions.

Recurrent Herpes

Nature of disease

A reactivation and migration of herpes simplex virus 1 (HSV-1) from the gasserion ganglion to the periphery, where it proliferates and infects the local epithelium around nerve endings, producing blisters that burst into ulcers.

Predilections

Has a predilection for the lower lip vermilion at the vermilion skin junction and to a lesser extent the lateral border of the tongue and the palatal mucosa. Occurs mostly in adults and has no sex or racial predilection. Recurrent herpes lesions are known to be more common in immunosuppressed individuals (eg, transplant patients, HIV patients, patients on immunosuppressive drugs).

Clinical features

Lesions may be preceded by a burning or itching sensation in the area to be involved (prodrome). This is followed by vesicles that will rupture into painful ulcers known as "cold sores." They are often triggered by sun exposure, physical or psychologic stress, cold temperatures, or infections elsewhere in the body.

Radiographic presentation

None.

Differential diagnosis

A single or multiple painful vesicles and/or ulcerations on the lower lip or other areas of the oral mucosa may also be seen in pemphigus, erosive lichen planus, herpes zoster (possibly as a component of Ramsay Hunt syndrome), and erythema multiforme if skin lesions are also present.

Microscopic features

Recurrent herpes lesions will appear identical to those in primary herpetic gingivostomatitis—that is, ballooning degeneration of epithelial cells at the floor of any vesicle and somewhat in the adjacent epithelium. The cells will appear to have swollen nuclei that have an irregular contour with the disrupted chromatin marginated at the periphery. The connective tissue beneath the vesicle will likely show a nonspecific inflammatory process rich in neutrophils. ⟶

Suggested course of action

With single or mild lesions, this self-limiting disease requires no action. In cases of multiple or more painful and bothersome lesions, topical agents can be used, such a penciclovir 1% cream (Zovirax, GlaxoSmithKline). Prevention protocols for the patient with repeated outbreaks are best referred to an infectious disease specialist or to practitioners in oral medicine or oral and maxillofacial surgery who are known to treat recurrent herpes patients.

Treatment

In those cases of frequent or more severe and functionally impairing outbreaks, oral acyclovir 200 mg five times daily starting at the beginning of an outbreak and continuing for 10 days or valacyclovir (Valtrex, GlaxoSmithKline) 1,000 mg three times daily for 7 days is effective in aborting or limiting the course.

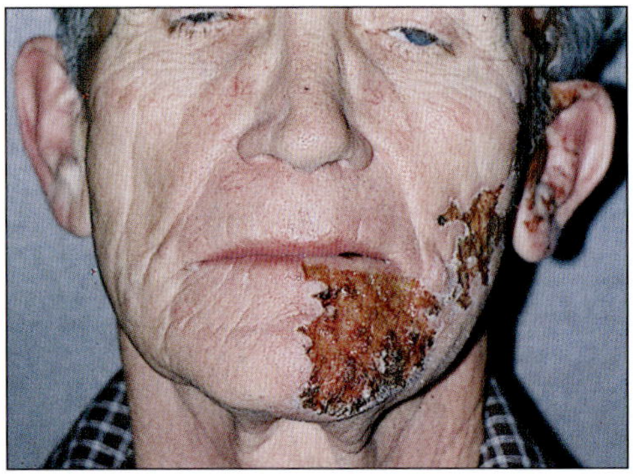

► Typical unilateral crusty lesions of herpes zoster.

Herpes Zoster (Shingles)

Nature of disease

A reactivation of the latent varicella zoster virus (VZV) from a resolved chickenpox infection during childhood. Dormant VZV in ganglia become activated and migrate down a nerve sheath to infect epithelial cells at the terminal nerve endings. Note: When a herpes zoster infection involves more than one cranial nerve distribution (ie, trigeminal nerve plus facial nerve, or vagus nerve, or glossopharyngeal nerve), it is termed *Ramsay Hunt syndrome.*

Predilections

Adults with a history of childhood chickenpox. There is no sex or racial predilection, but it is seen somewhat more commonly in unvaccinated individuals with an immune status alteration such as lymphomas, HIV infection, or leukemia and those on immunosuppressant drugs and other chemotherapies. The chest wall is the most common site, followed by the ophthalmic division of the trigeminal nerve.

Clinical features

A prodrome of itching and mild pain often precedes the emergence of more painful vesicles and pustules over a known nerve distribution. The skin becomes necrotic and develops a surface crust. Pain becomes progressively more intense, and the individual frequently experiences episodic bursts of pain. In the oral cavity, bone beneath lesions often becomes exposed. In the fully developed herpes zoster, a distinct midline demarcation is seen.

Radiographic presentation

Despite exposure of bone at times, radiographic features are not usually seen. As the herpes zoster resolves and the exposed surface bone becomes resorbed and covered by granulation tissue, a surface irregularity may be seen on a cone beam CT scan.

Differential diagnosis

Herpes zoster is clinically distinctive. In mild cases of only oral involvement, a herpes simplex infection or a focal candidiasis may be considered.

Microscopic features

The skin and oral lesions will show ballooning degeneration of epithelial cells with swollen nuclei, disrupted chromatin, and intranucelar inclusion bodies. In the ganglion of the involved nerve distribution, ganglion cells will be swollen with intranuclear inclusion bodies. Some large neurons may be seen to become necrotic, and the ganglion itself will be infiltrated by lymphocytes, plasma cells, and macrophages.

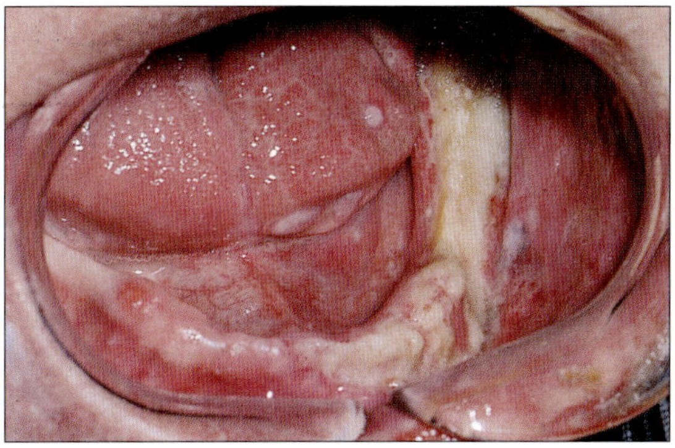

► Unilateral mucosal slough exposing the mandibular alveolus and lesions of the left hemitongue in a patient with herpes zoster.

Suggested course of action

Suspected cases should be referred to an infectious disease specialist.

Treatment

Because herpes zoster is a serious disease known to frequently result in sequelae such as postherpetic neuralgia, encephalitis, and severe scarring, it is treated intensely. Local wound care and antibiotics to treat secondary bacterial skin or mucosal infections supplement antiviral treatment with either acyclovir 800 mg five times daily, famciclovir 500 mg three times daily, or valacyclovir 1 g three times daily for 10 days. Carbamazepine 200 mg four times daily or gabapentin 600 mg twice daily is used to treat herpes zoster pain as well as postherpetic neuralgia. Frequently, prednisone is added to the antiviral treatment to reduce the skin and mucosal necrosis.

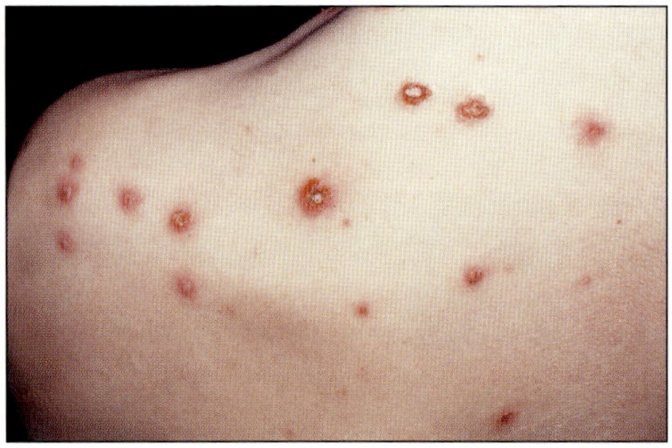

► Painful pustules from chickenpox.

Chickenpox (Varicella)

Nature of disease

A transmissible childhood skin infection that may also uncommonly form oral lesions caused by a DNA virus known as the *varicella zoster virus* (VZV).

Predilections

Children between the ages of 4 and 10 years are most commonly affected. There is no sex or racial predilection. Lesions develop mostly on the trunk and facial skin.

Clinical features

Painful red pustules develop on the trunk and facial skin 5 to 10 days after exposure to the virus via water droplet contact. Chills, fever, malaise, and headache are common. The child is often irritable due to the constant pain. In later stages, the lesions will develop a crust before healing.

Radiographic presentation

None.

Differential diagnosis

Other painful childhood diseases should be considered such as rubeola (measles); rubella (German measles); and hand, foot, and mouth disease. Additionally, erythema multiforme (particularly erythema multiforme major, also known as *Stevens-Johnson syndrome*) should be considered.

Microscopic features

Biopsy specimens are rarely taken. However, those that are taken show an identical picture to that seen in herpes simplex infections—that is, ballooning degeneration of epithelial cells with disrupted nuclei and chromatin marginated to the periphery of the nuclear membrane. The surrounding connective tissue will be seen to have a nonspecific inflammatory response with neutrophils predominating.

Suggested course of action

Nonvaccinated individuals (other patients, staff, etc) should be isolated from the infected child and should avoid direct contact. Only true dental emergencies should be treated during the course of infection, using barrier precautions, and all instruments should be separated for immediate sterilization. Disposable gowns should be used if possible; otherwise, any gowns used during treatment should be removed and replaced with fresh ones before other patients are seen.

Treatment

No treatment is required for this self-limiting disease other than supportive care. However, for immunocompromised individuals and women in the third trimester of pregnancy, intravenous acyclovir 30 mg/kg daily over 10 days or intravenous foscarnet (Foscavir, AstraZeneca) 20 mg/kg as a loading dose followed by 120 mg/kg three times daily for 2 weeks is often used.

Infectious Mononucleosis

Nature of disease

A viral infection involving the pharynx and cervical lymph nodes caused by the Epstein-Barr virus, which is human herpesvirus 4. Called the "kissing disease" in the 1960s, it is transmitted by direct saliva contact.

Predilections

Most common in teenagers and young adults. No sex or racial predilection is known.

Clinical features

The individual will be acutely ill will fever, chills, and malaise. He or she will complain of a sore throat and difficulty swallowing. There will be prominent, tender, bilateral cervical lymphadenopathy. In some cases, palatal or gingival inflammation and petechiae will be present. Photophobia and neck stiffness add to the plethora of symptoms in some cases.

Radiographic presentation

None.

Differential diagnosis

The picture of a weak young individual with bilateral cervical lymphadenopathy will suggest Hodgkin lymphoma, Ludwig angina, and other pharyngitis-based diseases such as streptococcal pharyngitis and rheumatic fever.

Microscopic features

Cervical lymph nodes will exhibit follicular hyperplasia with abnormal shapes from overproliferating lymphoblasts. Some focal areas of necrosis within the lymph node may be seen together with a collection of macrophages.

Suggested course of action

Refer to the patient's primary care provider or to an infectious disease specialist.

Treatment

Infectious mononucleosis is a self-limiting viral disease that is treated with supportive care (ie, antipyretics, analgesics, hydration, and rest).

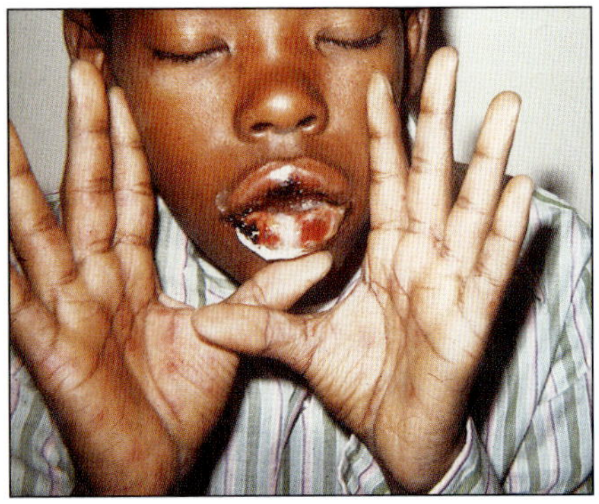

► Hand and mouth lesions in hand, foot, and mouth disease.

Hand, Foot, and Mouth Disease

Nature of disease

A viral infection caused by coxsackievirus A16, so named after Coxsackie, New York, where the virus was first identified. It is transmitted by either airborne water droplets or oral-fecal spread. The virus seems to proliferate better in areas of cooler temperature, thus focusing its systemic spread to the hands, feet, and mouth.

Predilections

Mostly affects children under 5 years of age. It occurs more frequently during the summer months. There is no sex or racial predilection.

Clinical features

Children will be seen to have oral vesicles early in the course. However, most often by the time they are seen by a practitioner, the vesicles have ruptured to form yellow fibropurulent ulcers that are only mildly painful. The skin of the hands and feet will more likely show vesicles due to their greater epithelial layer thickness. These will eventually rupture to form a targetlike lesion.

Radiographic presentation

None.

Differential diagnosis

Children with mildly symptomatic oral as well as skin lesions may also be seen in erythema multiforme minor, varicella (chickenpox), rubeola (measles), and rubella (German measles).

Microscopic features

Epithelial and subepithelial vesicles are seen together with ballooning degeneration of the epithelium and a dense inflammatory infiltrate in the reticular dermis and submucosa predominantly consisting of neutrophils.

Suggested course of action

Suspected cases should be referred to an infectious disease specialist or the patient's primary care physician.

Treatment

No specific treatment is required beyond supportive care for this self-limiting disease in which symptoms and lesions will resolve within 2 weeks.

Herpangina

Nature of disease

A viral infection caused by coxsackieviruses A and B. It will develop rapidly, producing a sore throat (dysphagia) and high fever after direct water-droplet/saliva contamination.

Predilections

Occurs almost exclusively in children under the age of 10 years. No sex or racial predilection is known. It affects the pharynx posterior to the anterior tonsillar pillars.

Clinical features

The child will be obtunded and have a fever of 103°F to 105°F. The pharynx will have 1- to 2-mm gray-white vesicles, producing the symptom of dysphagia. Pharyngeal and soft palate petechiae are frequently seen as well. Ulcers are less commonly seen.

Radiographic presentation

None.

Differential diagnosis

Pharyngeal lesions with dysphagia and fever with no skin lesions may also be seen in streptococcal pharyngitis, tonsillitis, and, although very rarely seen today due to vaccinations, diphtheria.

Microscopic features

Lesions are rarely biopsied. However, those that are biopsied show intraepithelial vesicles with a submucosal mixed inflammatory infiltrate.

Suggested course of action

Suspected cases should be referred to an infectious disease specialist or to the patient's primary care provider.

Treatment

No specific treatment is required other than antipyretics, hydration, analgesics, and rest. If a streptococcal pharyngitis cannot be ruled out or occurs as a secondary infection, phenoxymethylpenicillin 250 mg four times daily for 10 days is prescribed. For the penicillin-allergic child, erythromycin ethyl succinate 200 to 400 mg four times daily for 10 days is prescribed.

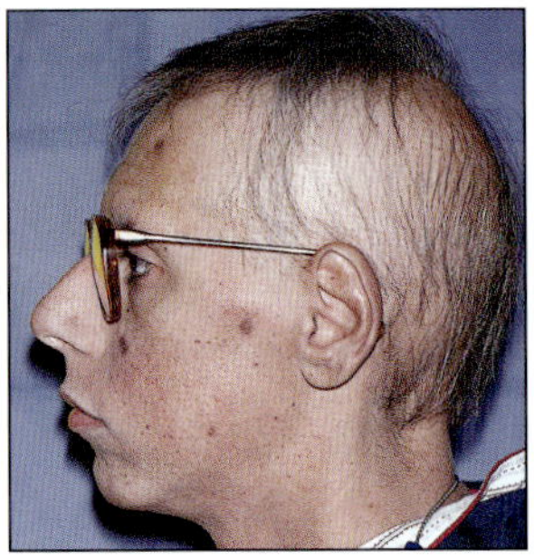

► Hair and weight loss in a patient with AIDS.

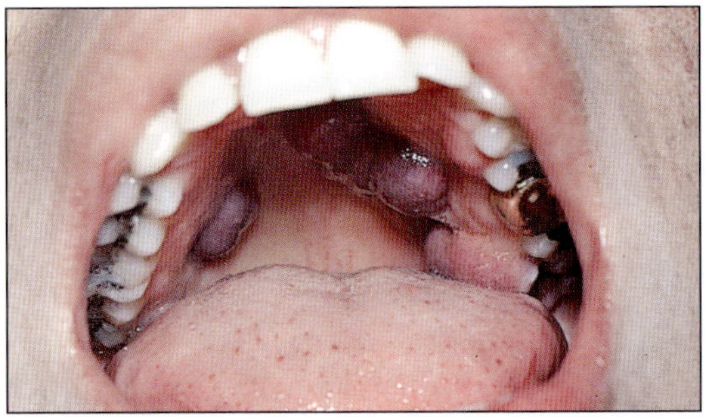

► Although rare today, some AIDS patients still develop Kaposi sarcoma.

HIV/AIDS

Nature of disease

A viral disease first recognized in 1980 that targets the CD4 lymphocyte and eventuates into lymph node destruction and a severe immune deficiency. The causative virus today is termed *human immunodeficiency virus* (HIV). Untreated, it progresses from HIV infection to acquired immunodeficiency syndrome (AIDS) when the CD4 cell count is less than 200/mm^3 or about 14% of the usual number of these T-helper cells.

Predilections

There is no specific age, sex, or racial predilection. It is more common in men who have sex with other men, followed by intravenous drug users, people in heterosexual relationships, and blood transfusion patients, in that order.

Clinical features

Early HIV infection will be a nonspecific flulike presentation with mildly tender lymphadenopathy that develops 2 to 3 weeks after infection and resolves over another 2 weeks. This is followed by a progressive loss of CD4 cells and immune function over the years, which, if left untreated, may produce any of the following: candidiasis, pneumocystis carini pneumonia, HIV lymphadenitis, Kaposi sarcoma (Note: This is rare today because the HIV virus is not the cause of Kaposi sarcoma. In years past, secondary viruses such as cytomegalovirus were included in the infected inoculum.), hairy leukoplakia, HIV gingivitis/periodontitis, or HIV parotitis.

Radiographic presentation

None.

Differential diagnosis

Early cases will be similar to a common cold or flu. As the immune deficiency becomes apparent, immunosuppressive therapy, leukemias, lymphomas, and multiple myeloma become considerations.

Microscopic features

In hairy leukoplakia, thin surface projections of epithelium with a thick layer of parakeratin are seen. In HIV parotitis, a lymphoepithelial cyst will be seen with germinal centers and hyperemic vessels in the connective tissue wall.

Suggested course of action

Provide needed and comprehensive dental care using standard full barrier techniques. Refer the patient to an infectious disease specialist for workup, monitoring, and treatment. →

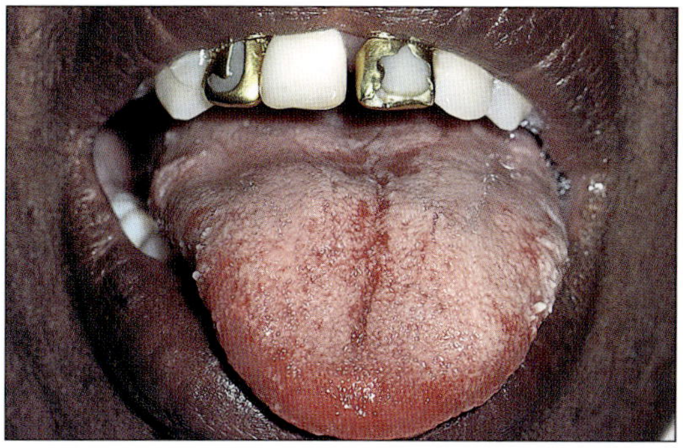

► Hairy leukoplakia not pathognomonic but frequently seen in AIDS patients.

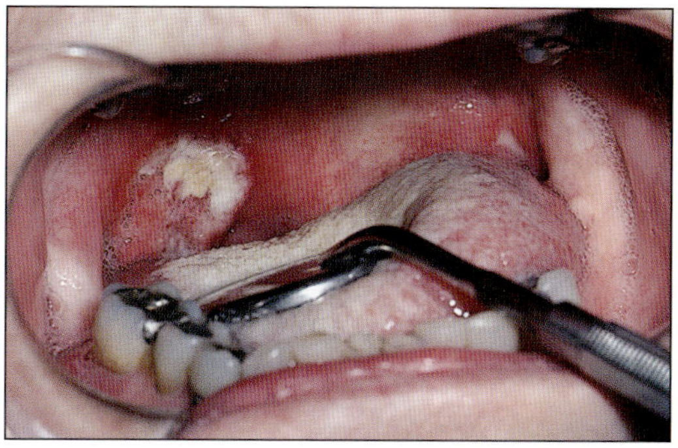

► Nonspecific aphthous-like ulcer in an AIDS patient.

Treatment

Today HIV infection can usually be halted and/or controlled to an undetectable viral load. The standard care with some variation is called *highly active antiretroviral therapy* (HAART). It consists of three specific HIV-targeted drugs: nucleoside analogs, protease inhibitors, and non-nucleoside reverse transcriptase inhibitors.

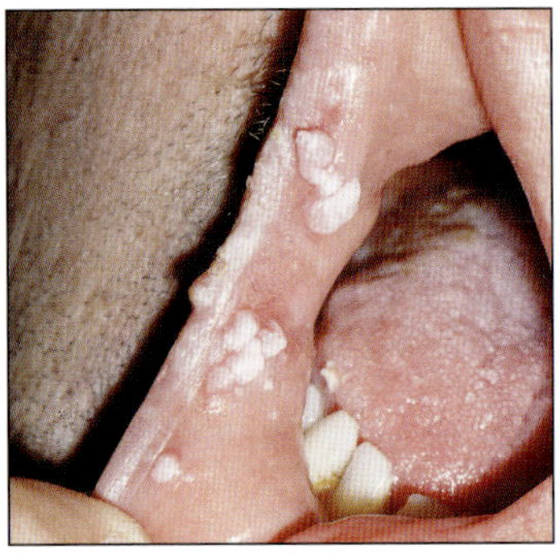

► Oral lesions of condyloma acuminata.

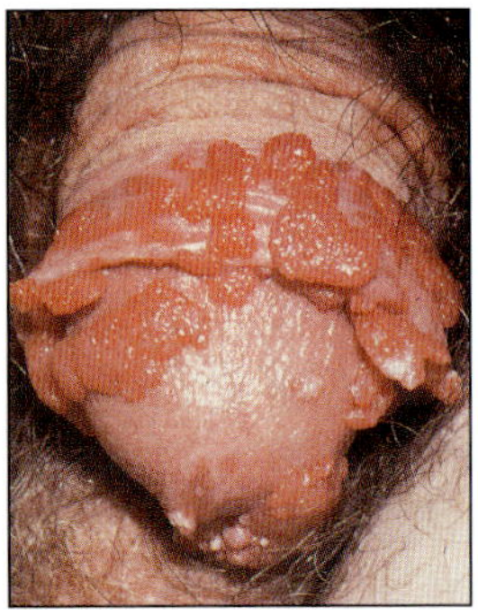

► Genital lesions of condyloma acuminata are often transmitted to the oral cavity.

Condyloma Acuminata (Venereal Warts)

Nature of disease

Condyloma acuminata is caused by DNA human papillomavirus (HPV) 6 and 11. It is highly transmissible by direct surface-to-surface contact.

Predilections

Ninety percent occur in men, with most occurring in men between 15 and 40 years of age. No racial predilection is known.

Clinical features

Oral lesions appear in clusters and are white with a sessile base. They will occur mostly around the commissures and lip vermillion. Less commonly, some may be seen in the floor of the mouth and tongue. These arise from either hand-to-mouth transmission from concomitant genital lesions or from oral sex. Skin lesions look similar but generally have a more red-white appearance and are found on the glans penis in men and the labia or vulva in women. Anal lesions also occur related to anal sex.

Radiographic presentation

None.

Differential diagnosis

Single or a few lesions may appear as the nonvenereal wart (verruca vulgaris) or squamous papillomas. Clusters of lesions will appear similar to a verrucous carcinoma or an exophytic squamous cell carcinoma.

Microscopic features

Lesions will have a marked acanthosis with broad, elongated rete ridges but without hyperparakeratosis or hyperkeratosis. Frequent mitoses are seen, and some nuclei will have a perinuclear halo suggestive of a viral involvement.

Suggested course of action

Suspicious lesions require protective barrier techniques for the dental provider, dental hygienist, and staff. The patient's history should be reviewed related to genital lesions and behavioral risks, and the patient should be referred to either an infectious disease specialist or a dermatologist.

Treatment

All areas with lesions require treatment. This can be accomplished with a CO_2 laser, cryotherapy, topical 25% podophyllum resin, topical 50% trichloroacetic acid, or imiquimod 5% cream. Refractory lesions may require excision.

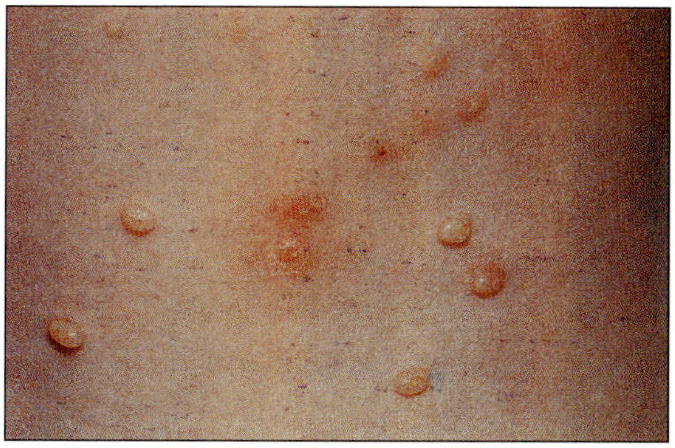

► Circular rings and a central caseous plug are seen in molluscum contagiosum.

Molluscum Contagiosum

Nature of disease

A skin disease caused by an unclassified pox virus that produces single or multiple small, dome-shaped papules.

Predilections

Mostly affects immune-competent children and young adults but has occurred at all ages. Occurs with a more prolonged course in immune-compromised individuals. There is no sex or racial predilection.

Clinical features

Early lesions will be firm and flesh colored. Most begin on the hands, face, abdomen, and/or genital area. Mature lesions are gray in color and develop a caseous center. Transmission is by direct surface-to-surface contact.

Radiographic presentation

None.

Differential diagnosis

Molluscum contagiosum will appear similar to cystic acne or a folliculitis. Individual lesions may appear similar to a solitary keratoacanthoma. The more common presentation of multiple lesions will mimic syndromes in which multiple keratoacanthomas occur (ie, Muir-Torre syndrome, Ferguson-Smith syndrome in children, and Grzybowski syndrome in adults).

Microscopic features

A crateriform appearance of acanthotic epithelium in which a central component of enlarged, ballooned epithelial cells with large viral inclusions compressing the nucleus will be seen.

Suggested course of action

Suspicious cases should be referred to a dermatologist or infectious disease specialist.

Treatment

Molluscum contagiosum is self-healing and requires no specific treatment unless a quickened healing time is required or the patient is immune compromised. In those instances, topical 25% podophyllum or topical 5% imiquimod cream applied three to five times weekly for 4 to 8 weeks is effective.

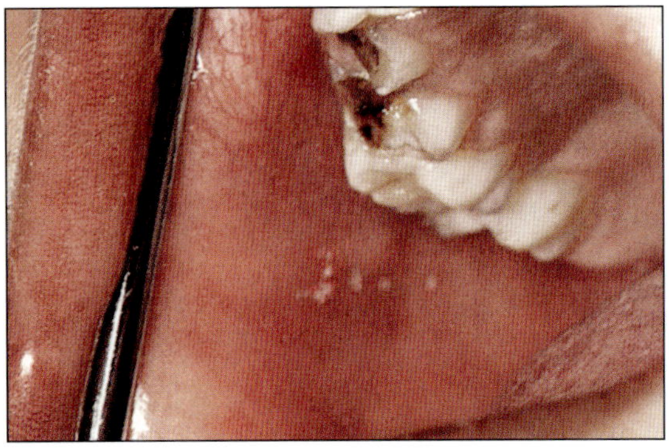

► Koplik spots seen with measles (rubeola).

Measles (Rubeola)

Nature of disease

A childhood viral infection caused by a DNA paramyxovirus and transmitted by airborne water droplets.

Predilections

Targets unvaccinated children under 12 years of age. No sex or racial predilection is known.

Clinical features

The child will have a high fever (103°F to 105°F), nasal stuffiness with sneezing, and a sore throat. The child will be irritable and in pain. In some cases, a prodrome of a skin rash or small oral white spots (Koplik spots) may herald the onset of signs and symptoms such as pinhead-sized papules and red blotches.

Radiographic presentation

None.

Differential diagnosis

Other childhood diseases should be considered such as varicella (chickenpox), rubella (German measles), and scarlet fever.

Microscopic features

Mucosal and skin lesions will identify epithelial cells with central vacuolization leading to hyperkeratosis and necrosis. The connective tissue will be edematous and hyperemic with an infiltrate of lymphocytes and macrophages. If lymphoid tissue is studied, a peculiar multinucleated giant cell is seen (Warthin-Finkeldey giant cell) within lymphoid hyperplasia.

Suggested course of action

Defer all but emergency dental care, and refer the patient to his or her pediatrician. If emergency dental care is required, use disposable masks and gowns and barrier techniques.

Treatment

Measles is self-limiting in 2 weeks but requires supportive care to reduce the potential for measles complications (ie, encephalitis, pneumonia, etc). This includes hydration, antipyretics, analgesics, and rest. Note: Measles is well known to cause premature labor, spontaneous abortions, and low birth weight. Therefore, isolation of the infected child from unvaccinated women of childbearing age should be undertaken.

Rubella (German Measles)

Nature of disease

A childhood viral infection of skin and the lymphatics caused by a togavirus that is transmitted by airborne water droplets.

Predilections

Unvaccinated children and young adults are mostly affected. No sex or racial predilection is known.

Clinical features

Rubella has a milder presentation than rubeola. The child will have fever, mild malaise, and cervical lymphadenitis, particularly of the posterior cervical chain. The face will have a fine red maculopapular rash appearance. The palate and pharynx will be erythematous.

Radiographic presentation

None.

Differential diagnosis

Other childhood and young adult illnesses should be considered such as rubeola (measles), scarlet fever, infectious mononucleosis, and streptococcal pharyngitis.

Microscopic features

None. Specimens are not obtained in rubella. The diagnosis is clinical and can be confirmed by testing the immunoglobulin M antibodies to the togavirus.

Suggested course of action

Defer all but emergency dental care. Refer the patient to his or her pediatrician or primary care provider. If emergency dental care is required, use disposable masks, gowns, and gloves. Note: Rubella is well known to cause birth defects. Isolate women of childbearing age from the patient.

Treatment

Rubella is a short-duration, self-limiting disease that requires only supportive care (ie, hydration, antipyretics, analgesics, and rest). The patient should be isolated from women of childbearing age until the disease is completely resolved.

6

Radiolucent Lesions

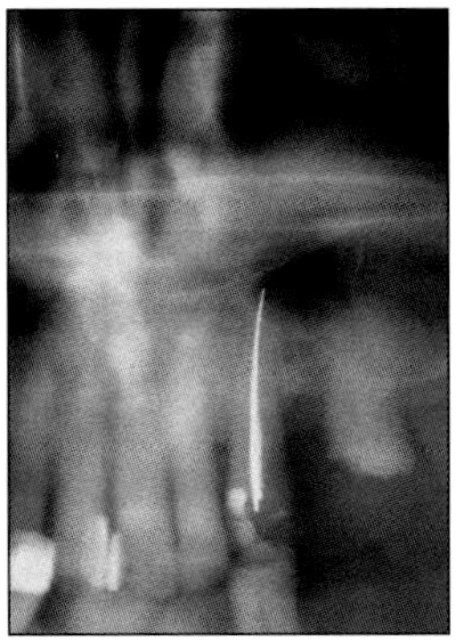

► Apical periodontal cyst (radicular cyst).

Unilocular Radiolucencies

Apical Periodontitis (Radicular Cyst)

Nature of disease

Inflammation at the apex of an erupted tooth due to bacterial toxins that leach out of the apex from a pulpitis. If rests of Malassez are stimulated, they can proliferate and form a lumen termed an *apical* or *radicular cyst.*

Predilections

No age, sex, or racial predilection is known.

Clinical features

May be chronic and asymptomatic. If acute, the tooth will be painful, particularly to percussion. The tooth may be elevated in the socket. If sufficient apical necrosis occurs, it may lead to a fistula and on rare occasions an osteomyelitis.

Radiographic presentation

A unilocular radiolucency at the apex of the involved tooth. The lucency may appear only as a widening of the periodontal ligament space or as a larger, well-defined, or even irregular radiolucency.

Differential diagnosis

Apical periodontitis is radiographically distinct. In rare situations, sublingual or submandibular salivary lingual cortical gland depressions, osteoporotic bone marrow defects, or early odontogenic tumors and central malignancies may be considered.

Microscopic features

Acute and chronic inflammatory cells will be present. The preponderance of specific cells will be dependent on the acuteness or chronicity of the lesion. Odontogenic epithelial rests may be seen within the inflammatory cell milieu; occasionally, these epithelial rests will form a lumen to form a periapical cyst.

Suggested course of action

If the tooth is restorable, consider root canal therapy. If not, extraction of the involved tooth is required.

Treatment

Root canal therapy or extraction of the involved tooth.

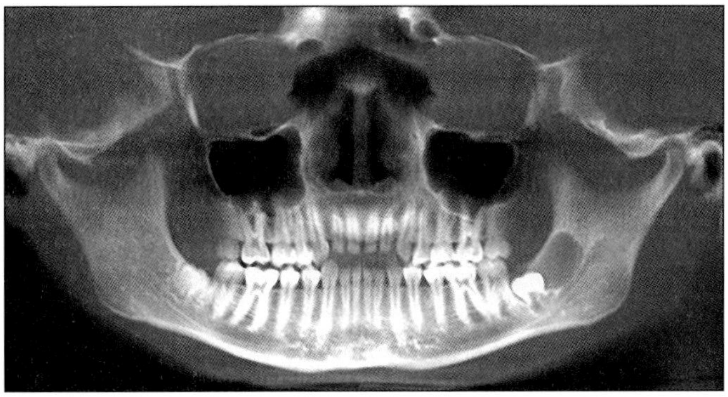

► Dentigerous cyst.

Dentigerous Cyst

Nature of disease

All cysts are defined as a pathologic cavity lined by epithelium. A dentigerous cyst is lined by reduced enamel epithelium after crown formation and disintegration of the stellate reticulum.

Predilections

More common in teenagers and young adults. The incidence diminishes with age. No sex or racial predilection is known.

Clinical features

Usually a painless expansion of the involved jaw. An expected tooth is clinically absent, with no paresthesia or anesthesia. Rarely, pain or drainage is noted if the cyst has perforated through the oral mucosa or after a biopsy.

Radiographic presentation

An expansile unilocular radiolucency associated with an unerupted tooth that is displaced apical to the alveolus. Adjacent teeth may be displaced. The mandibular canal is usually displaced toward the inferior border. In the maxilla, the associated tooth may be displaced into the maxillary sinus with a soft tissue opacity occupying the sinus air space.

Differential diagnosis

Other cysts that may be associated with an unerupted tooth are to be considered, such as ameloblastomas developing with a cyst, an adenomatoid odontogenic cyst, and an odontogenic keratocyst.

Microscopic features

A lumen that is lined by squamous epithelium supported by a connective tissue wall. Cholesterol clefts from cellular and nuclear membranes may be present. Amorphous collections of hyaline termed *Rushton bodies* may also be seen.

Suggested course of action

Aspiration, exploration, and incisional biopsy, or referral to an oral and maxillofacial surgeon.

Treatment

Enucleation and curettage.

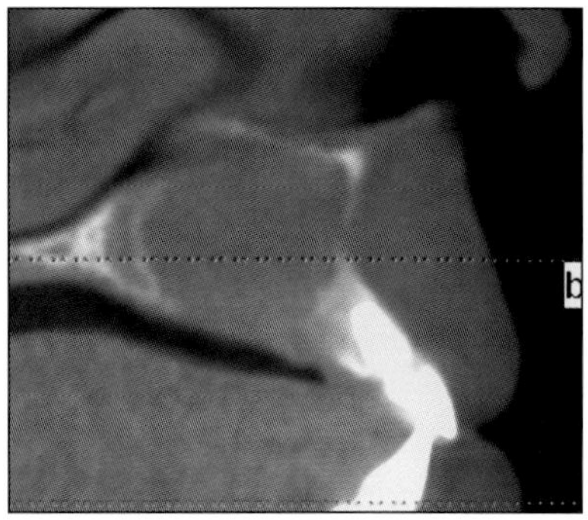

► Small incisive canal cyst.

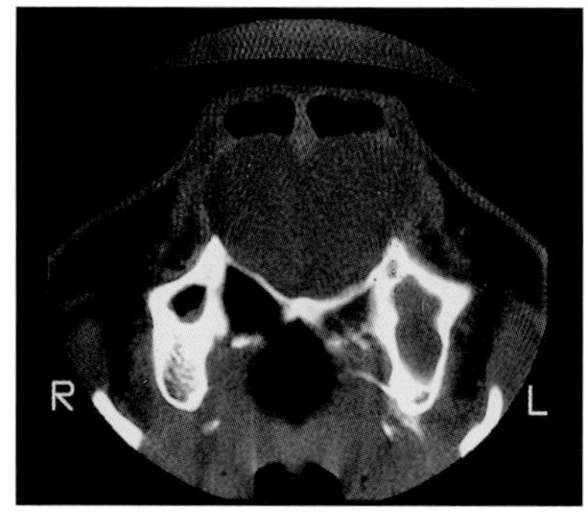

► Large incisive canal cyst with characteristic heart shape.

Incisive Canal Cyst

Nature of disease

A pathologic cavity lined by epithelium from the primitive sphenopalatine duct from embryogenesis.

Predilections

Seen mostly in adults. No sex or racial predilection is known.

Clinical features

Depending on its size, it may present as a small soft tissue enlargement in the incisive papilla or a large midline palatal and/or buccal expansion. Most are painless with no paresthesia. Teeth are not usually displaced.

Radiographic presentation

Small ones will appear as an enlarged incisive canal. The more common larger one will appear as a midline unilocular heart-shaped radiolucency.

Differential diagnosis

Apical cysts, odontogenic keratocysts, and adenomatoid odontogenic cysts are the most important considerations.

Microscopic features

A lumen lined partially by squamous epithelium and partially by pseudostratified columnar epithelium termed *respiratory epithelium*. The connective tissue wall of the cyst often contains blood vessels and nerve fibers from the incisive canal.

Suggested course of action

Pulp test the maxillary incisors to rule out an apical cyst. Then refer to an oral and maxillofacial surgeon.

Treatment

Enucleation and curettage usually via a buccal approach with a palatal splint for support. Unusual cases may be approached by a combined buccal-palatal approach or a palatal approach exclusively.

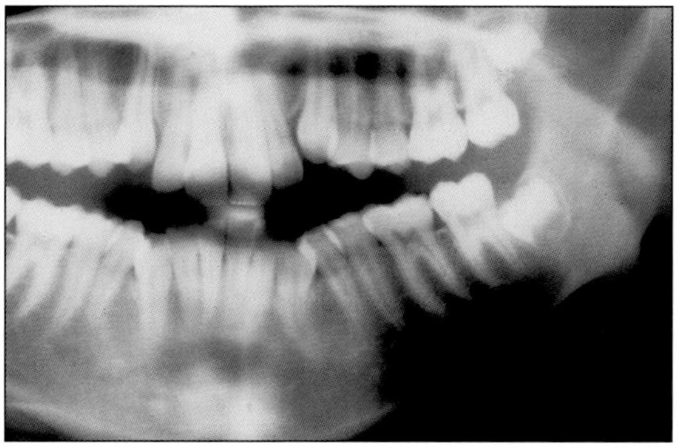

► Idiopathic bone cavity.

Idiopathic Bone Cavity

Nature of disease

A remodeling defect of bone that results in a true empty cavity in bone that is not lined by epithelium and that does not contain any fluid or other contents.

Predilections

A strong predilection for teenagers and young adults. Less common in children and very rare in adults over 40 years. They occur mostly in the midbody of the mandible and are rare to unknown in the maxilla.

Clinical features

Almost always an asymptomatic incidental radiographic finding.

Radiographic presentation

The most common appearance is that of a radiolucency in the midbody of the mandible that scallops between the roots of teeth without displacement of the roots or of the mandibular canal outline. They will have no or only mild expansion and a thinned cortex. Most are unilateral, but they can occur bilaterally on occasion.

Differential diagnosis

A similar clinical and radiographic appearance may be seen with odontogenic keratocysts, ameloblastomas, odontogenic myxomas, and primary or metastatic malignancies.

Microscopic features

None unless a bone biopsy is taken, in which case it may show a thin lining of fibrin or fibroblasts on the inner wall of the cortex.

Suggested course of action

Aspiration followed by exploration, or referral to an oral and maxillofacial surgeon.

Treatment

Aspiration. Note: Blood may be returned due to the negative pressure of the aspiration. To rule out a vascular lesion, aspirate with 1 mL of saline in the syringe. An idiopathic bone cavity will first return a few air bubbles, whereas a vascular lesion will return blood without the preceding air bubbles. If blood is returned, remove the syringe. An idiopathic bone cavity will drip some blood and then stop, whereas a vascular lesion will continue bleeding through the needle hub. Curative treatment is rendered by exploration and curettage of the bony cavity.

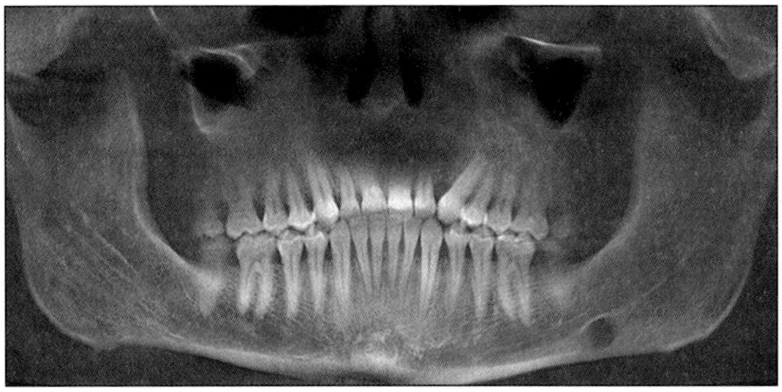

► Lingual submandibular salivary gland depression as seen on a panoramic radiograph.

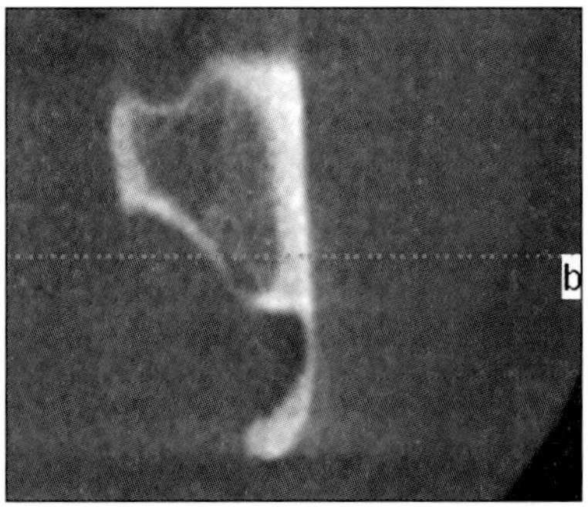

► Lingual submandibular salivary gland depression as seen on a CT scan.

Lingual Submandibular Gland Depression (Staphne Cyst)

Nature of disease

A concave depression in the lingual cortex in the molar region of the mandible caused by the position of the submandibular gland. Note that it is a deformity due to the position and size of the submandibular gland and not a true cyst.

Predilections

No predilection is known.

Clinical features

Always an asymptomatic incidental radiographic finding.

Radiographic presentation

A panoramic radiograph will show a well-outlined, oval, unilocular radiolucent lesion below the level of the mandibular canal. A cone beam CT scan will more accurately identify a concave depression of the lingual cortex.

Differential diagnosis

Idiopathic bone cavities, metastatic deposits, and non-odontogenic tumors such as central schwannomas or mucoepidermoid tumors may show a similar radiographic appearance.

Microscopic features

None.

Suggested course of action

Accomplish a cone beam CT scan or a medical CT scan to confirm or rule out a suspected case.

Treatment

None required.

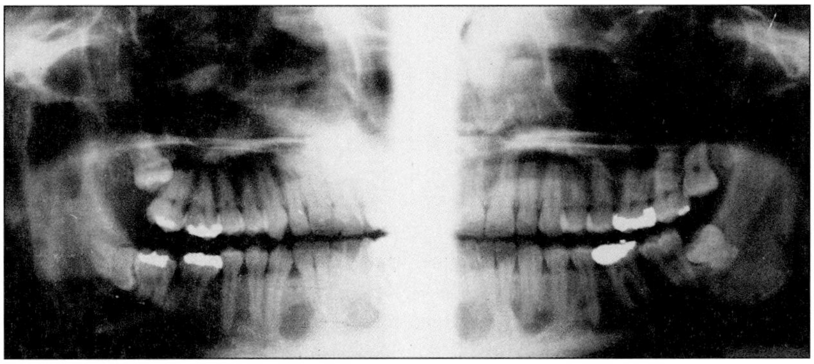

► Bilateral sublingual salivary gland depressions as seen on a panoramic radiograph.

Sublingual Gland Depressions

Nature of disease

Developmental concavities in the lingual cortex of the anterior mandible due to the position and size of the sublingual glands.

Predilections

Very rare. No predilection is known.

Clinical features

Always an asymptomatic incidental radiographic finding.

Radiographic presentation

Well-demarcated unilocular radiolucencies superimposed over the apices of the mandibular incisors and canines. Usually seen as two radiolucencies, one from each gland.

Differential diagnosis

Apical periodontal granulomas or radicular cysts are the more serious considerations. Odontogenic keratocysts, ameloblastomas, and central mucoepidermoid carcinomas may also be considered.

Microscopic features

None.

Suggested course of action

Accomplish a cone bean CT scan or a medical CT scan of suspicious cases to identify or rule out the lingual cortical concave depression.

Treatment

None.

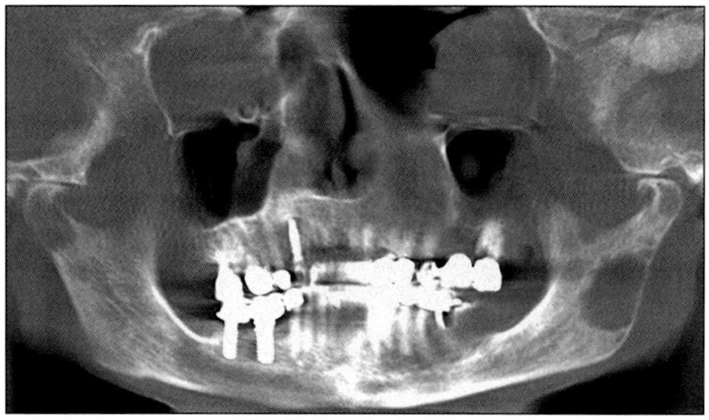

► Bilateral metastasis from a lung cancer.

Metastatic Malignant Deposit

Nature of disease

A proliferation of malignant cells that traveled to the jaws via blood vessels or lymphatics.

Predilections

Most metastatic cancer deposits are in adults over 40 years of age. The primary site origins are the breast (31%), lung (27%), kidney (15%), thyroid (6%), and others (5%).

Clinical features

Many are asymptomatic and are an incidental radiographic finding. Objective anesthesia or paresthesia is common. Bony expansion is also common. Some will be associated with a soft tissue growth emerging from a tooth socket or the alveolar crest.

Radiographic presentation

It will vary. However, most will be a poorly delineated radiolucency that may displace teeth and resorb roots. Rarely, some will show a radiopacity, particularly metastatic breast cancer and some prostate cancers.

Differential diagnosis

The radiographic pattern will also be suggestive of an idiopathic bone cavity, an odontogenic keratocyst, an osteoporotic bone marrow defect, and a lingual salivary gland depression as well as several benign odontogenic tumors and primary site cancers.

Microscopic features

The histopathology will represent or be similar to that of the primary tumor. However, many are poorly differentiated, requiring special stains or genomic analysis to determine the primary tumor site and type.

Suggested course of action

Exploration and incisional biopsy, or referral to an oral and maxillofacial surgeon.

Treatment

The metastatic deposit may be treated as the primary site, usually with chemotherapy. However, local resection or radiotherapy is useful to eliminate pain or functional impairment caused by the metastatic deposit.

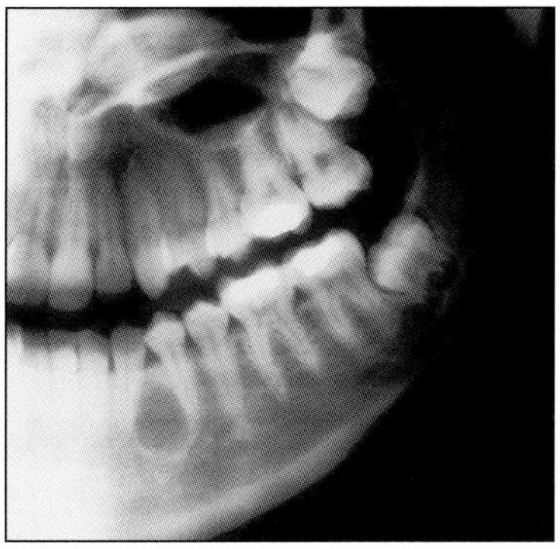

► Lateral periodontal cyst.

Lateral Periodontal Cyst

Nature of disease

A thin-walled cyst arising from epithelial remnants from the breakup of the Hertwig epithelial root sheath (rests of Malassez).

Predilections

Mostly adults, with a slight female predilection. Occurs mostly between the premolars or between the first premolar and canine.

Clinical features

A buccolingual expansion with an intact overlying mucosa between the involved teeth. The expansion may cause divergence of the roots, resulting in tipping of the crowns toward each other. Tooth mobility may be present but is not common.

Radiographic presentation

A unilocular radiolucency between the involved teeth. Roots of the involved teeth are usually divergent. Root resorption may be present but is uncommon.

Differential diagnosis

This location is also a common location for odontogenic keratocysts, adenomatoid odontogenic cysts, and squamous odontogenic tumors. Others to be considered are early ameloblastomas, odontogenic myxomas, and idiopathic bone cavities.

Microscopic features

A thin, cuboidal, epithelial-lined lumen with a loose connective tissue wall. The epithelial lining will have only one to three cell layers for most of the lining, but in some regions the epithelial lining will be much thicker, appearing like a "speed bump" in the lining.

Suggested course of action

Exploration and removal of the lesion for diagnosis and treatment, or referral to an oral and maxillofacial surgeon.

Treatment

Complete removal of the lesion via enucleation and curettage or, in rare instances, a peripheral resection observing 0.5-cm margins, particularly for recurrent cysts.

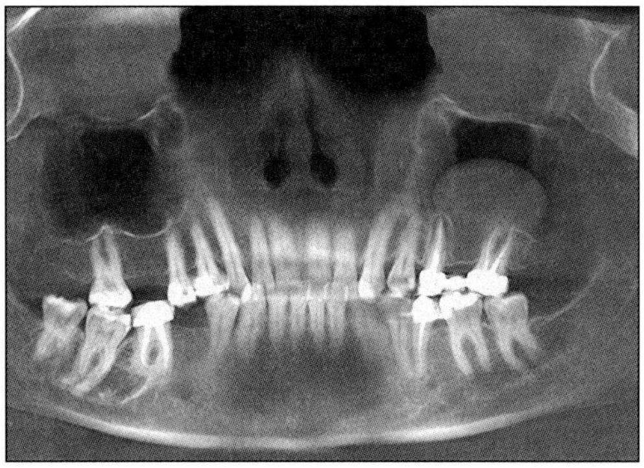

► Residual cyst in the maxilla after a molar extraction.

Residual Cyst

Nature of disease

The persistence or development of a cyst after tooth removal or an attempted cyst removal.

Predilections

None.

Clinical features

Most are asymptomatic incidental radiographic findings. Others will produce an expansion with an intact overlying mucosa.

Radiographic presentation

A unilocular radiolucency in an area of a previous extraction or attempted cyst removal. Obtaining previous radiographs are helpful and will show the presence of the lesion prior to surgery.

Differential diagnosis

Other radiolucent lesions that may persist after an extraction or attempted removal include lingual salivary gland depressions, idiopathic bone cavities and osteoporotic bone marrow defects, as well as unrecognized odontogenic tumors.

Microscopic features

An epithelial-lined lumen with a connective tissue wall. Cholesterol clefts may be present along with collections of hyaline known as *Rushton bodies.*

Suggested course of action

Exploration and removal of the cyst for diagnosis and treatment, or referral to an oral and maxillofacial surgeon.

Treatment

Complete removal via enucleation and curettage.

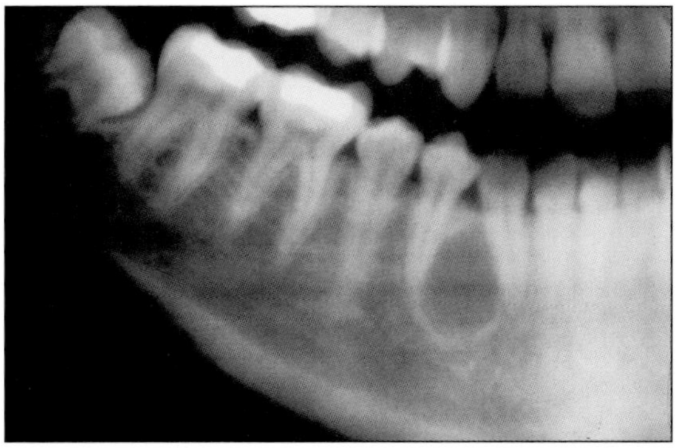

► Unilocular odontogenic keratocyst.

Odontogenic Keratocyst

Nature of disease

Arises from odontogenic epithelium from either dental lamina rests (rests of Serres), the breakup of the Hertwig epithelial root sheath (rests of Malassez), or reduced enamel epithelium after crown development.

Predilections

Slightly more common in the mandibular third molar area. No sex or racial predilection is known.

Clinical features

Most present as a painless expansion in either the maxilla or mandible without objective paresthesia. Rarely they will present with pain and/or trismus if keratin leaks out or if the cyst becomes secondarily infected.

Radiographic presentation

May be multilocular or unilocular. Noted to frequently occur between the premolars. They will displace roots, the sinus floor, the mandibular canal, and adjacent unerupted teeth and may also cause a smooth root resorption. In those arising from reduced enamel epithelium, the associated tooth will be displaced away from the alveolar bone.

Differential diagnosis

If multilocular, one should consider an ameloblastoma, odontogenic myxoma, central giant cell tumor, or a central hemangioma of bone. If between the premolars or between the first premolar and canine, a botryoid odontogenic cyst should be considered. If unilocular and if associated with an unerupted tooth crown, one should consider a dentigerous cyst or an adenomatoid odontogenic cyst if it is in the canine/premolar region. If unilocular and between a first premolar and canine or between premolars, consider a lateral periodontal cyst.

Microscopic features

Epithelial-lined lumen with the specifics of 6 to 10 cells, parakeratin in a corrugated alignment, and a redundant and prominent basophilic staining of the basal cells.

Suggested course of action

Aspiration followed by an incisional biopsy, and/or referral to an oral and maxillofacial surgeon.

Treatment

The mainstay of treatment is a thorough enucleation of the entire cyst. Large unilocular cysts are sometimes marsupialized. Large, destructive cysts or those that have recurred frequently may require a resection.

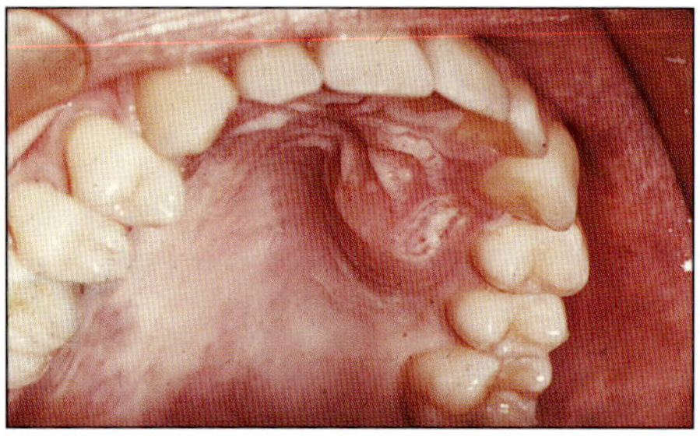

► The maxillary premolar area is a site of predilection for a squamous odontogenic tumor.

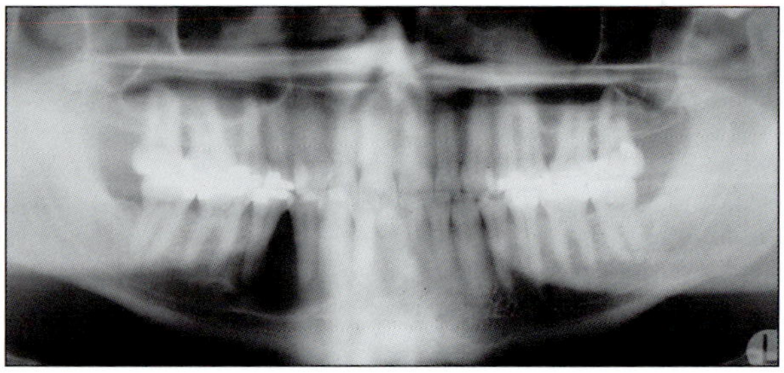

► Squamous odontogenic tumor of the mandible.

Squamous Odontogenic Tumor

Nature of disease

A solid hamartomatous proliferation of odontogenic rests of Malassez.

Predilections

Mostly young adults, with a female predilection. No racial predilection is known. Most occur in the anterior quadrants of the maxilla and a lesser number in the mandibular molar area.

Clinical features

Expansion between involved teeth, with mobility of the teeth and an intact overlying mucosa.

Radiographic presentation

A unilocular radiolucency between and around teeth that extends from the crestal bone to the midroot level or to the apical level or beyond in some cases.

Differential diagnosis

Lateral periodontal cysts and odontogenic keratocysts often present in an identical manner. Other considerations include early ameloblastomas and odontogenic myxomas as well as an apical abscess.

Microscopic features

Nests of odontogenic epithelium or a solid mass of odontogenic epithelium resembling a proliferation of odontogenic rests with squamous differentiation.

Suggested course of action

Pulp test the involved teeth followed by exploration and removal for diagnosis and treatment, or refer to an oral and maxillofacial surgeon.

Treatment

Complete removal of the entire tissue mass via enucleation and curettage.

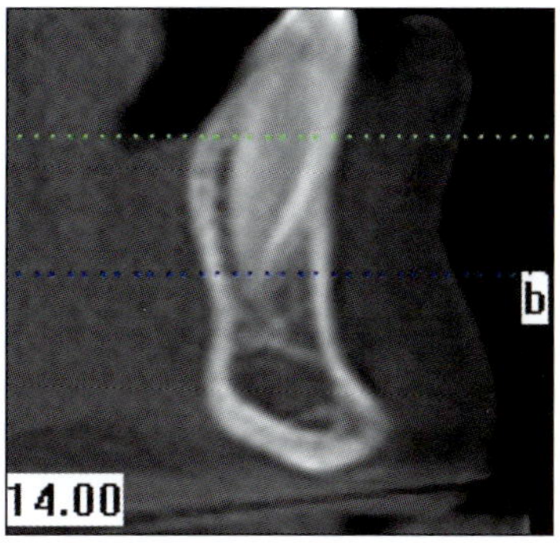

► Osteoporotic bone marrow defect.

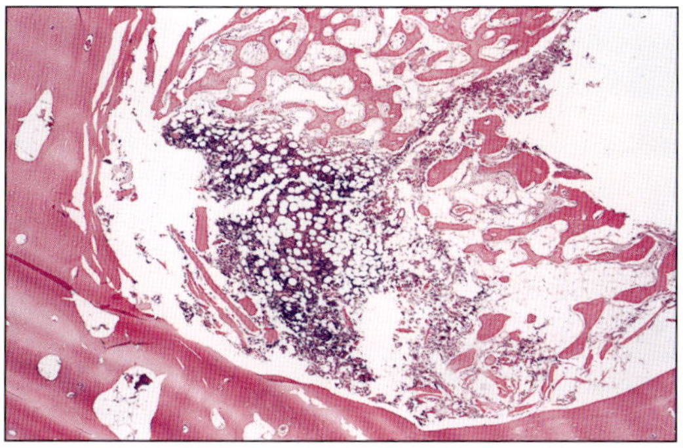

► Normal marrow cells are seen in an osteoporotic bone marrow defect.

Osteoporotic Bone Marrow Defect

Nature of disease

A cavity in bone in which the trabecular bone has given way to creating spaces filled with mostly fatty bone marrow or less commonly cellular bone marrow.

Predilections

Postmenopausal women over the age of 50 years. More common in white and Asian women. Occurs mostly in the posterior mandible and tuberosity of the maxilla.

Clinical features

A painless, asymptomatic incidental radiographic finding.

Radiographic presentation

A poorly delineated unilocular radiolucency without expansion. The cortex may be somewhat thinner in a uniform fashion.

Differential diagnosis

The diseases that can present with a similar picture are more concerning than the osteoporotic defect itself. These include metastatic cancer deposits, idiopathic bone cavities, several odontogenic tumors such as ameloblastomas and odontogenic myxomas, as well as a central mucoepidermoid tumor.

Microscopic features

Rarely are these defects biopsied yielding tissue sufficient to diagnose. However, they are seen as cavitary spaces in which fatty tissue is present along with apparent empty air spaces and a few hematopoietic cells.

Suggested course of action

Exploration to rule out the more concerning diseases on the differential diagnosis or referral to an oral and maxillofacial surgeon.

Treatment

None required. Notes:

1. For patients who complain of pain, look for other sources for their pain. Too often this entity has been misdiagnosed as *neuralgia-inducing cavitational osteonecrosis* (NICO), which is a fraudulent concept and diagnosis. Such misdiagnosis has led to unnecessary and often debilitating procedures.
2. Finding an osteoporotic bone marrow defect in the jaws in a postmenopausal woman may indicate that her osteoporosis needs to be reexamined and a DEXA scan accomplished. Referral to her physician is recommended.

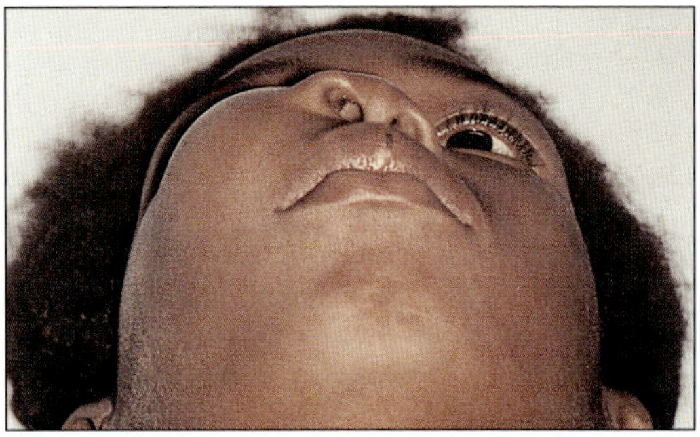

► Expansion from an adenomatoid odontogenic cyst in the maxilla.

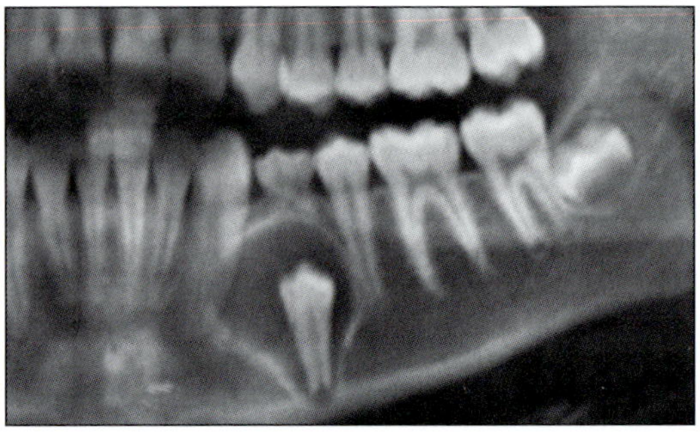

► This adenomatoid odontogenic cyst clearly shows its evolution from the Hertwig epithelial root sheath.

Adenomatoid Odontogenic Cyst

Nature of disease

A proliferation of cells from the Hertwig epithelial root sheath to create a lumen lined with odontogenic epithelium that proliferates into the lumen. Note: The former term *adenomatoid odontogenic tumor* is incorrect. This entity satisfies the definition of a cyst (a pathologic cavity lined by epithelium) and develops and grows as a cyst, not a tumor.

Predilections

More common in females (2:1 with males) and in the maxilla (2:1 with the mandible). Strong predilection for preteens and teenagers as well as for the canine/premolar regions.

Clinical features

A slow-growing, painless expansion in the canine/premolar region of either jaw. In rare cases, the expansion will be of a more rapid onset and will be painful. The mucosa is intact. Either a premolar or a canine tooth might be clinically absent.

Radiographic presentation

A well-delineated, unilocular radiolucent lesion in the canine/premolar region of the involved jaw. In two-thirds of cases, an unerupted canine or premolar is seen within the radiolucency. One should pay particular attention to the outline of the radiolucency. If the border of the radiolucency completely surrounds an unerupted tooth, the diagnosis of an adenomatoid odontogenic cyst should be suspected. If the border of the radiolucency connects to the cementoenamel junction of the tooth crown, a dentigerous cyst is more likely. Fine flecks of calcifications may be present, which are rarely identified on a panoramic radiograph but are better seen on periapical radiographs or cone beam CT scans.

Differential diagnosis

The clinical and radiographic presentation of an adenomatoid odontogenic cyst is very similar to that of a dentigerous cyst. Others that would bear consideration are odontogenic keratocysts, the early phase of an ossifying fibroma, and an ameloblastic fibroma and an odontogenic fibroma. →

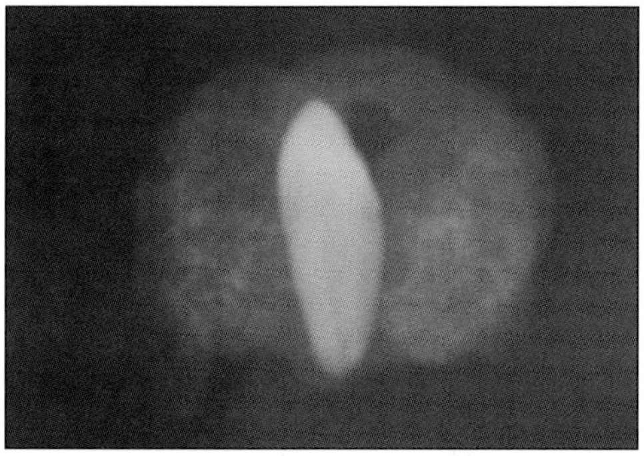

► A specimen radiograph shows the calcified material in the cyst wall.

Microscopic features

The cyst lumen may be completely filled with an intraluminal proliferation of the cyst lining, giving the impression of a solid tumor. However, this proliferation can be traced to a generally thin lining of cuboidal cells in which various areas demonstrate round to oval proliferations into the lumen, in which spaces are seen with a ductlike appearance lined by cuboidal cells. Eosinophilic staining of small flecks within these proliferations are seen and are responsible for the calcifications seen on radiographs. The cyst wall is usually thick and composed of parallel bands of collagen.

Suggested course of action

Referral to an oral and maxillofacial surgeon for definitive treatment.

Treatment

Enucleation of the lesion, which will be shelled out without difficulty. It is recommended to open the gross specimen for evaluation. If the cyst lining is attached at the midroot level rather than the cementoenamel junction, the diagnosis of an adenomatoid odontogenic cyst is confirmed.

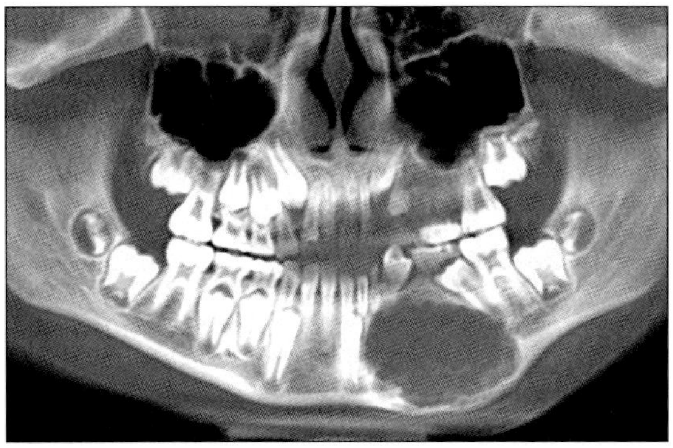

► Odontogenic fibroma.

Odontogenic Fibroma

Nature of disease

A rare, benign odontogenic tumor that arises from mesenchymal cells from the dental papilla.

Predilections

Teenagers and young adults. No sex or racial predilection is known.

Clinical features

A painless expansile mass that may develop in either jaw. The mucosa will be intact. Tooth displacement and tooth mobility are often seen as a result of the mass.

Radiographic presentation

A well-delineated, expansile, unilocular radiolucency will be present. The cortex will be thinned. Tooth displacement, root divergence, and some outlined root resorption may also be seen.

Differential diagnosis

Unilocular radiolucencies encompassing unerupted teeth may also be seen in odontogenic keratocysts and ameloblastic fibromas as well as in the early phase of an ossifying fibroma and some adenomatoid odontogenic cysts and calcifying odontogenic cysts where the calcification is not radiographically apparent.

Microscopic features

A slight to moderate number of fibroblasts is seen with abundant immature collagen production. With the fibrous proliferation, scattered oval or round foci of odontogenic epithelium may be noted.

Suggested course of action

Exploration and incisional biopsy, or referral to an oral and maxillofacial surgeon.

Treatment

Complete removal of the lesion via enucleation and curettage or a peripheral resection observing 0.5-cm margins.

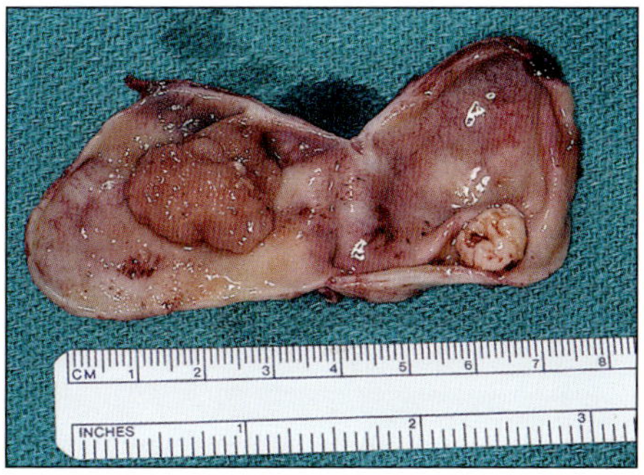

► Ameloblastoma growing out of a cyst lining.

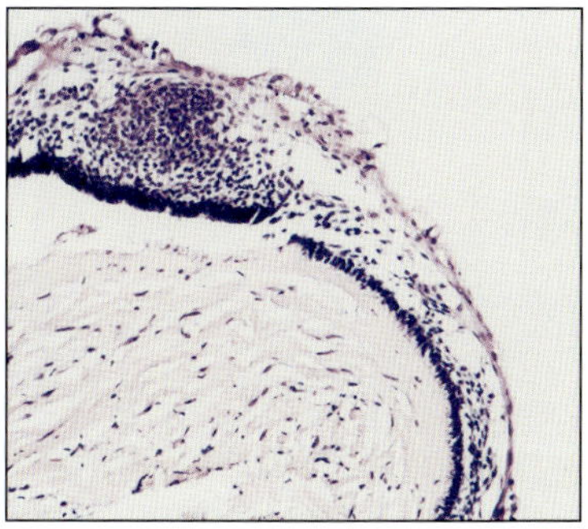

► Mural ameloblastoma.

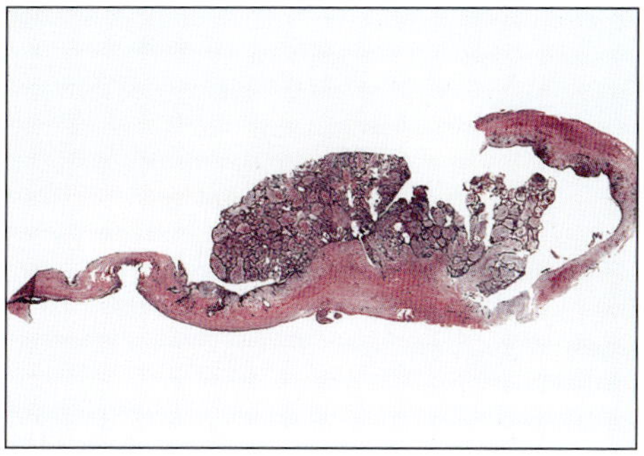

► Intraluminal ameloblastoma.

Ameloblastoma Arising from a Cyst Lining

Nature of disease

The transformation of ameloblasts from the pluripotent lining of a dentigerous cyst, which can grow in either one or a combination of patterns:

1. Mural: Within only the lining of the cyst
2. Intraluminal: Within only the lining and lumen of the cyst
3. Intramural: Within the lining and lumen and into the connective tissue wall of the cyst
4. Transmural: Within the lining and lumen and through the entire thickness of the connective tissue wall of the cyst

Predilections

Mostly seen in teenagers and young adults. There is no known sex or racial predilection.

Clinical features

A painless expansion in either jaw. The overlying mucosa will be intact. Some tooth mobility or displacement may be seen as in a dentigerous cyst. Paresthesia or anesthesia is not present.

Radiographic presentation

Usually a somewhat large, unilocular radiolucency in which an impacted tooth crown is seen displaced and within the radiolucency. The mandibular canal, sinus floor, and teeth may be displaced as in other dentigerous cysts.

Differential diagnosis

The clinical and radiographic presentation will be identical to a dentigerous cyst without ameloblastoma changes. Other considerations include a solid invasive ameloblastoma, a dentigerous origin odontogenic keratocyst, and an adenomatoid odontogenic cyst if the anatomical location is in the canine/premolar area. →

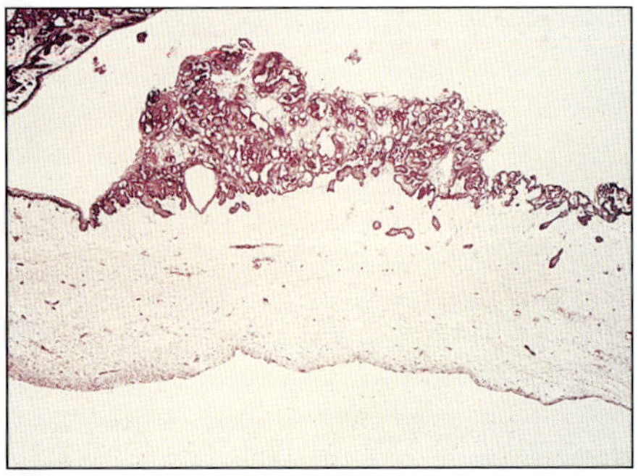

► Intramural ameloblastoma.

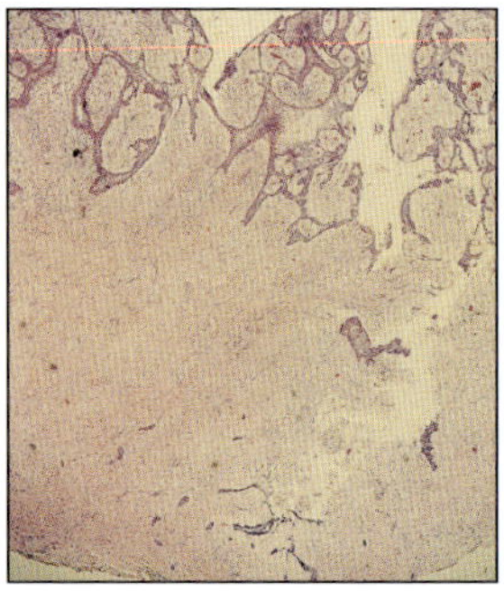

► Transmural ameloblastoma.

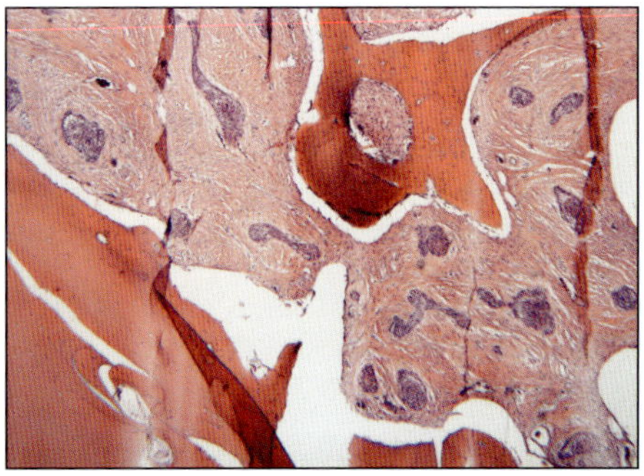

► Invasive ameloblastoma.

Ameloblastoma Arising from a Cyst Lining *(cont)*

Microscopic features

1. Mural: A squamous cell lining that is either in part or completely seen to have cuboidal to columnar cells with reverse polarization.
2. Intraluminal: A squamous cell lining in which a portion is seen to change to a cuboidal or columnar cell lining with reverse polarization. Cells from these transformed areas proliferate into the lumen, often developing islands in which stellate reticulum formation can be seen.
3. Intramural: A squamous cell lining in which a portion is seen to change to a cuboidal or columnar cell lining with reverse polarization, and similar cells are seen to proliferate into the connective tissue wall of the cyst.
4. Transmural: A squamous cell lining in which a portion is seen to change to a cuboidal or columnar cell lining with reverse polarization, and similar cells are seen to proliferate in nests and bands throughout the complete thickness of the connective tissue wall.

Suggested course of action

Aspiration and exploration for incisional biopsy, or referral to an oral and maxillofacial surgeon.

Treatment

Because the finding of an ameloblastoma arising within a dentigerous cyst is a microscopic diagnosis after the cyst is removed, the clinical question for the provider becomes whether further treatment is required. Mural, intraluminal, and intramural proliferation have the surgical margin as the outermost portion of the connective tissue wall. Therefore, these ameloblastoma in situ proliferations are completely removed, requiring no further treatment. A transmural ameloblastoma in situ leaves tumor at the marginal edge, in which invasion into bone cannot be ruled out. Therefore, a return to surgery to remove 0.5 to 1.0 cm of surrounding bone is recommended.

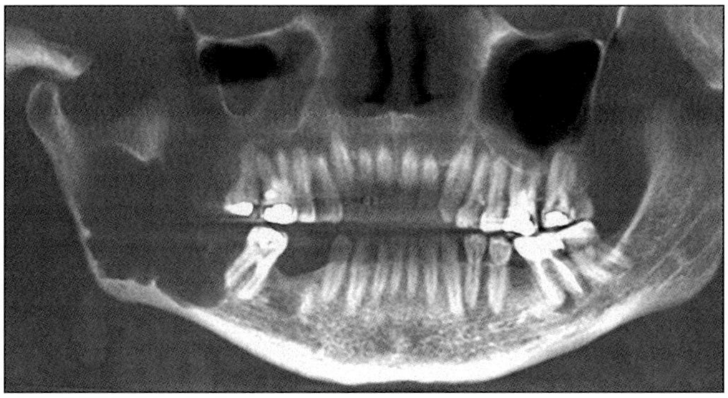

► Central schwannoma of the mandible.

Central Schwannoma

Nature of disease

A benign neoplastic proliferation of Schwann cells that line the outside of a nerve bundle.

Predilections

Schwannomas are most commonly soft tissue neoplasms. They rarely occur centrally in the mandible from the inferior alveolar nerve. There is no known age, sex, or racial predilection.

Clinical features

A painless expansion of the jaw. The mucosa is intact. Teeth may be displaced. Because schwannomas develop from the epineurium on the outside of the nerve bundle, the mandibular canal may be displaced rather than widened. Paresthesia or anesthesia is not usually present.

Radiographic presentation

A usually large (≥ 3 cm), oval, unilocular radiolucency that is well demarcated within bone. The cortices will be uniformly thinned and expanded. A soft tissue density will be implied by a good-quality, well-contrasted radiograph. Although teeth may be displaced by the mass, there is no direct association with a tooth. Very large and long-standing schwannomas may be seen to have scattered calcifications.

Differential diagnosis

Due to the rarity of a central schwannoma of bone, it is usually not a consideration on a differential diagnosis. Instead, odontogenic keratocysts, residual cysts, ameloblastomas, and the early phase of an ossifying fibroma are to be considered.

Microscopic features

A fibrous capsule is present. Within the capsule, spindle cells in palisading columns termed *Antoni A cells* amid small blood vessels and randomly placed spindle cells termed *Antoni B cells* are seen. Between palisading columns of the Antoni A cells, there is often an amorphous eosinophil-stained substance. This arrangement is termed a *Verocay body*.

Suggested course of action

Exploration and incisional biopsy, and/or referral to an oral and maxillofacial surgeon.

Treatment

Pericapsular excision of the mass. Note: The tumor can usually be observed to arise from the inferior alveolar neurovascular bundle. It can then often be excised from the stalk, preserving the neurovascular bundle and therefore its nerve sensation.

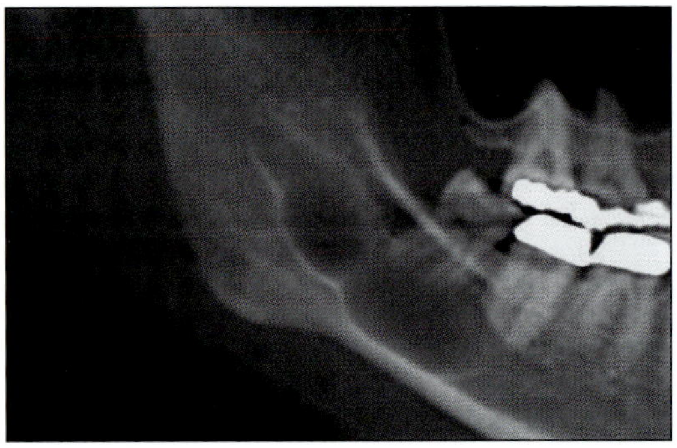

► Central neurofibroma of the mandible.

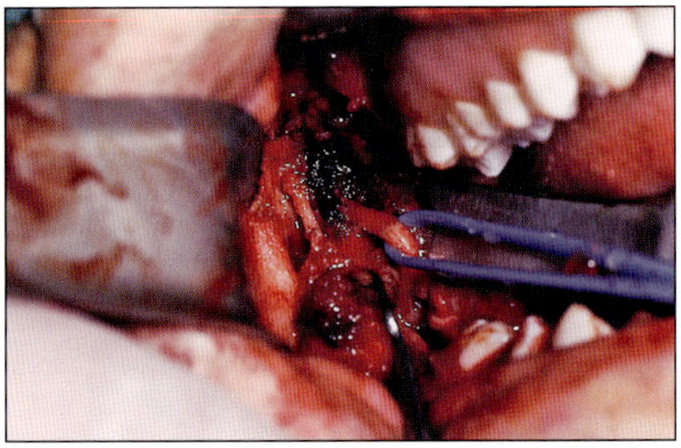

► The inferior alveolar nerve is seen entering the neurofibroma mass.

Central Neurofibroma

Nature of disease

Often a large but hamartomatous proliferation of neurofibroblasts from within a nerve bundle.

Predilections

Occurs more frequently in the mandible. No age, sex, or racial predilection is known.

Clinical features

An expansile unilocular lesion with an intact cortex. Large lesions will cause tooth mobility and displacement. Pain and/or paresthesia is not usually present.

Radiographic presentation

Usually an oblong or tapered unilocular radiolucency with indistinct borders. Teeth may be displaced, and roots may be partially resorbed. The mandibular canal may be widened and seem to go into the radiolucency or may be part of it.

Differential diagnosis

Unless the patient has signs of or has been diagnosed with hereditary neurofibromatosis type 1, a neurofibroma would not be a primary consideration. Central hemangiomas, arteriovenous malformations, ameloblastomas, odontogenic myxomas, odontogenic keratocysts, and a metastatic malignant deposit would be the major considerations.

Microscopic features

Spindle-shaped fibroblasts are haphazardly arranged amid collagen fibers in loose arrangement along with numerous small blood vessels. The mass will be unencapsulated. A plexiform pattern is often seen.

Suggested course of action

Exploration and incisional biopsy, and/or referral to an oral and maxillofacial surgeon.

Treatment

Because neurofibromas are hamartomas rather than true continually growing neoplasms, they can be removed in a subtotal fashion. Most can be removed by enucleation and curettage. Larger ones may require a resection observing 0.5-cm margins. It should be noted that neurofibromas arise from within the nerve bundle. Therefore, the parent nerve must be sacrificed. Neurofibromas are very vascular and unencapsulated, which at times makes them impossible to totally remove. The prudent surgeon often prepares type and screened blood for a possible transfusion prior to surgery.

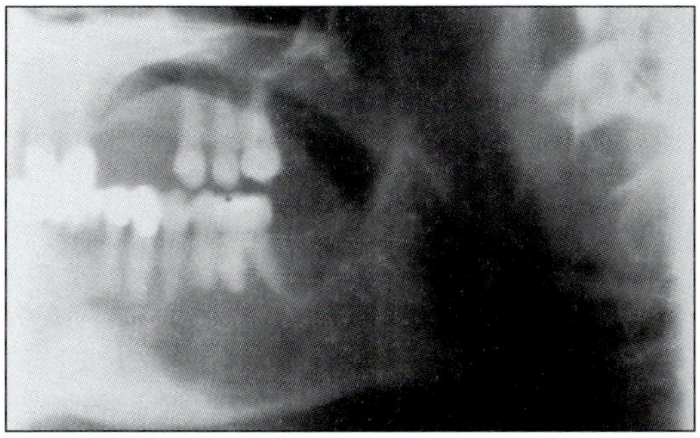

► Radiolucency from a "brown tumor" of hyperparathyroidism.

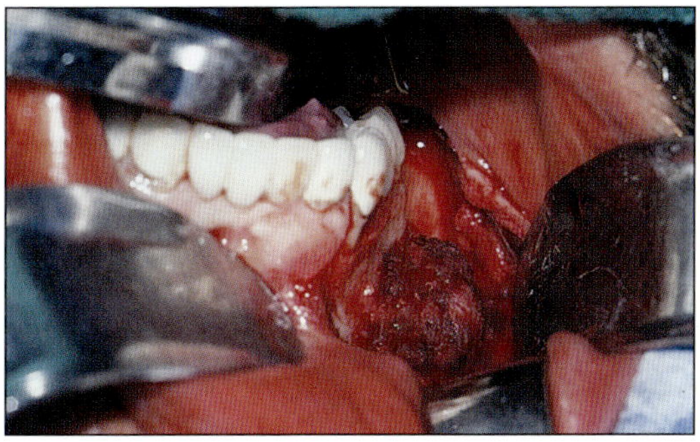

► A "brown tumor" of hyperparathyroidism will indeed be red-brown in color.

Primary Hyperparathyroidism

Nature of disease

Primary hyperparathyroidism results mostly from hyperplasia and oversecretion of parathormone from one or more of the four parathyroid glands. Rarely does it result from a benign parathyroid adenoma and rarer still from a parathyroid carcinoma. The oversecretion of parathormone activates osteoclasts, which results in bone-resorption cavities filled with giant cells (osteoclasts), hypercalcemia, hypophosphatemia, and hypercalciuria.

Predilections

More common in women and those over 50 years of age.

Clinical features

Related to the jaws, mildly expansile radiolucencies filled with a red-brown soft tissue called "brown tumors" may be seen. Patients may complain of constipation, fatigue, bone pain, thirst, nausea, and vomiting due to hypercalcemia. Occasionally, tooth mobility unrelated to periodontal disease is observed.

Radiographic presentation

Brown tumors may be unilocular or multilocular. The lamina dura may be absent, and the trabecular bone pattern may be generally ill defined.

Differential diagnosis

The differential diagnosis revolves around radiolucencies with hypercalcemia. Therefore, multiple myeloma, sarcoidosis, small cell carcinoma of the lung, and adrenal insufficiency are considerations.

Microscopic features

A fibroblastic stroma of plump fibroblasts, multinucleated giant cells, and extravasated red blood cells indistinguishable from a central giant cell tumor.

Suggested course of action

Incisional or excisional biopsy that identifies these aforementioned microscopic features, or referral to an oral and maxillofacial surgeon. Follow up with serum calcium determination; if above 10.5 mg/dL, refer the patient to a general surgeon for definitive workup and treatment.

Treatment

Parathyroidectomy to remove three of the four most active or largest parathyroid glands.

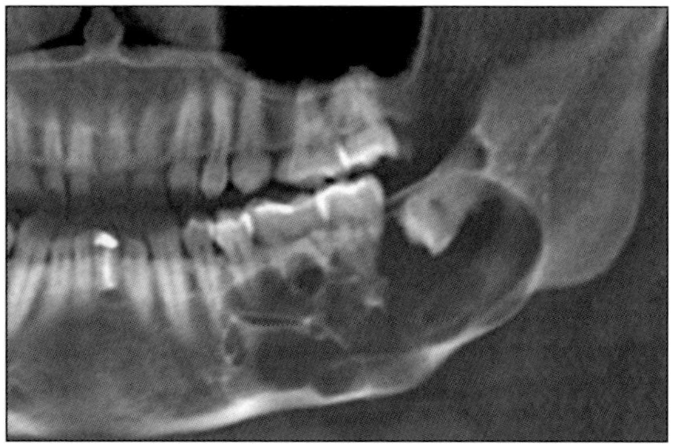

► Large, multilocular odontogenic keratocyst.

Multilocular Radiolucencies

Odontogenic Keratocyst

Nature of disease

Arises from odontogenic epithelium from either dental lamina rests (rests of Serres), the breakup of the Hertwig epithelial root sheath (rests of Malassez), or reduced enamel epithelium after crown development.

Predilections

Slightly more common in the mandibular third molar area. No sex or racial predilection is known. Multiple cysts form in basal cell nevus syndrome.

Clinical features

Most present as a painless expansion in either jaw without objective paresthesia. Rarely they will present with pain and/or trismus if keratin leaks out or if the cyst becomes secondarily infected.

Radiographic presentation

May be multilocular or unilocular. Noted to frequently occur between the premolars. They will displace roots, the sinus floor, the mandibular canal, and adjacent unerupted teeth and may also cause a smooth root resorption. In those arising from reduced enamel epithelium, the associated tooth will be displaced away from the alveolar bone.

Differential diagnosis

If multilocular, one should consider an ameloblastoma, odontogenic myxoma, central giant cell tumor, or a central hemangioma of bone. If between the premolars or between the first premolar and canine, a botryoid odontogenic cyst should be considered. If unilocular and if associated with an unerupted tooth crown, one should consider a dentigerous cyst or an adenomatoid odontogenic cyst if it is in the canine/premolar region. If unilocular and between a first premolar and canine or between premolars, consider a lateral periodontal cyst.

Microscopic features

Epithelial-lined lumen with the specifics of 6 to 10 cells, parakeratin in a corrugated alignment, and a redundant and prominent staining of the basophilic basal cells.

Suggested course of action

Aspiration followed by an incisional biopsy, and/or referral to an oral and maxillofacial surgeon.

Treatment

The mainstay of treatment is a thorough enucleation of the entire cyst. Large unilocular cysts are sometimes marsupialized. Large, destructive cysts or those that have recurred frequently may require a resection.

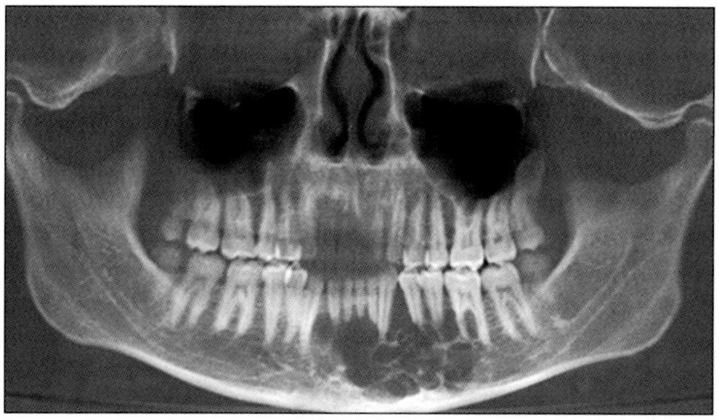

► Multilocular radiolucency from an ameloblastoma.

Ameloblastoma

Nature of disease

A benign neoplasm that can arise from dental lamina rests (rests of Serres), rests from the breakup of the Hertwig epithelial root sheath (rests of Malassez), or epithelium of a dentigerous cyst.

Predilections

Equal male-female distribution, with a slight increase in black individuals with African heritage. Occurs more commonly in young adults (15 to 35 years) but has occurred in nearly every decade of life. The most common site is the mandibular third molar area.

Clinical features

Painless expansion of either jaw without objective paresthesia. Some expansions may be subtle and unnoticed.

Radiographic presentation

Most are multilocular expansions with a thinned cortex. Fewer present as expansile unilocular radiolucencies. The rare desmoplastic ameloblastoma presents as a mixed radiolucent-radiopaque lesion. The mandibular canal outline is usually displaced toward the inferior border when in the mandible. In the maxilla, the tumor often expands into the maxillary sinus and/or the nasal cavity as a soft tissue density. Erupted teeth may be divergent or displaced. Unerupted teeth are usually displaced.

Differential diagnosis

Other lesions that are mostly multilocular radiolucencies are the odontogenic myxoma, central giant cell tumor, odontogenic keratocyst, ameloblastic fibroma, and central hemangioma of bone. Unilocular radiolucencies suggest a dentigerous cyst, a unilocular odontogenic keratocyst, or an adenomatoid odontogenic cyst.

Microscopic features

The follicular pattern has sheets of columnar preameloblasts with their nuclei opposite the basement membrane ("reverse polarization") surrounding an island of stellate reticulum–like cells. Because these stellate reticulum–like cells are ectodermal, they may take on a squamous appearance or a granular cell appearance on occasion. The plexiform pattern has the same preameloblasts pattern, but in this pattern the stellate reticulum–like cells surround the preameloblasts. Both patterns have the same biologic activity and are treated the same. ⟶

Ameloblastoma *(cont)*

Suggested course of action

Aspiration of the lesion to rule out a vascular tumor followed by an incisional biopsy, or referral to an oral and maxillofacial surgeon.

Treatment

Resection of the tumor observing 1.0-cm margins in bone and one uninvolved anatomical barrier such as bone cortex or tissue adjacent to bone (ie, periosteum, adjacent muscle). Reconstructive bone grafting is accomplished either at the time of tumor removal or at a later time and is followed by dental rehabilitation with implant dentistry or a removable appliance. Enucleation and curettage is considered palliative treatment reserved for special cases where resection might not be advised.

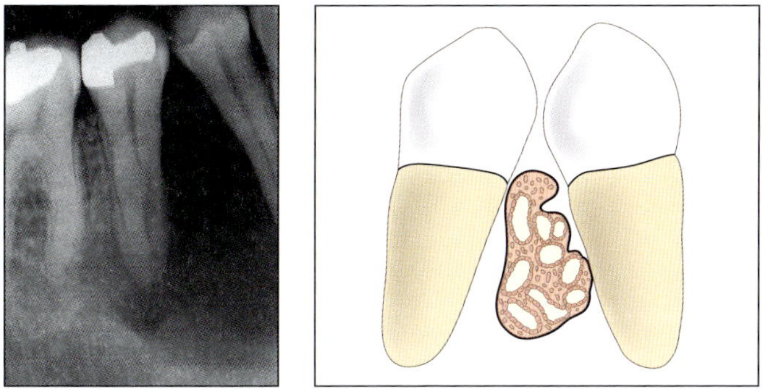

► A multilocular radiolucency between premolar teeth is the usual presentation of a botryoid odontogenic cyst.

Botryoid Odontogenic Cyst

Nature of disease

A thin-walled cyst of multiple compartments that arises from rests of Malassez after the breakup of the Hertwig epithelial root sheath.

Predilections

Rare, with no age, sex, or racial predilection. Occurs mostly between mandibular premolars or between a canine and a first premolar.

Clinical features

A painless expansion between premolars or between a canine and a first premolar with root divergence and an intact gingival mucosa. Some tooth mobility may be present. No paresthesia or objective anesthesia is observed.

Radiographic presentation

Usually a multilocular radiolucency between tooth roots that may cause root divergence.

Differential diagnosis

If the multilocular quality is not readily apparent, a lateral periodontal cyst is to be considered. Otherwise an odontogenic keratocyst, ameloblastoma, central giant cell tumor, and odontogenic myxoma are considerations.

Microscopic features

A multicystic lumen lined by cuboidal or squamous epithelium of only one to three cell layers.

Suggested course of action

Incisional or excisional biopsy, and/or referral to an oral and maxillofacial surgeon for definitive treatment.

Treatment

Complete removal by enucleation and curettage. One should consider orthodontic tooth realignment to correct the root divergence after allowing 6 months for bone regeneration. Larger or recurrent lesions may require moving the associated teeth or accomplishing a peripheral resection.

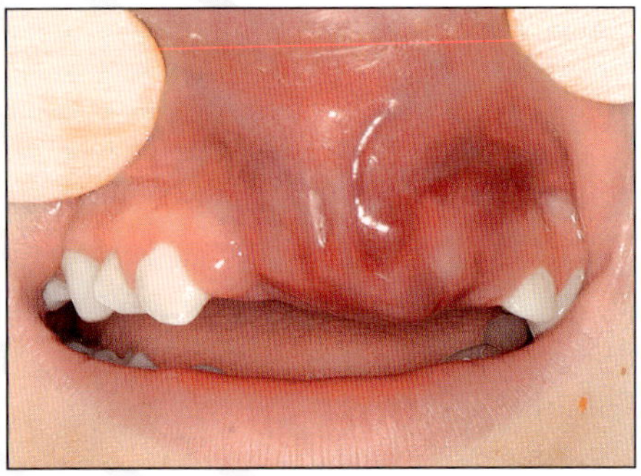

► Central giant cell tumor clinically.

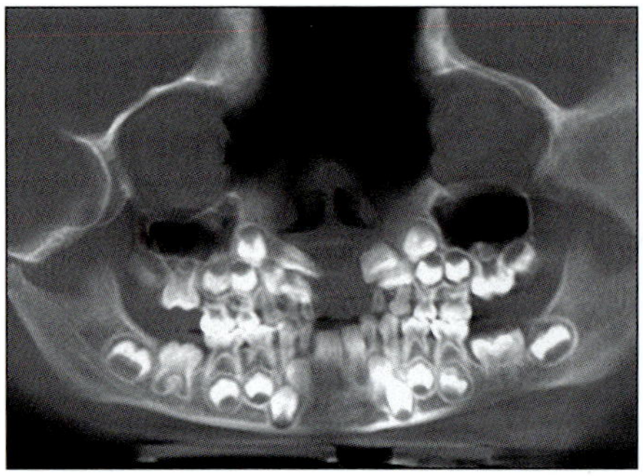

► Radiographic picture of a central giant cell tumor.

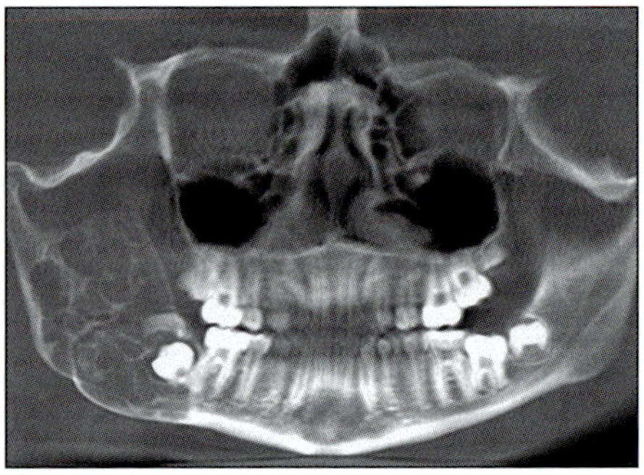

► Large, multilocular radiolucency from a central giant cell tumor.

Central Giant Cell Tumor

Nature of disease

A benign neoplasm of bone marrow osteoclast precursors.

Predilections

Occurs mostly in children, teenagers, and young adults. No sex or racial predilection is known. They occur more frequently in the mandible than in the maxilla.

Clinical features

Expansile mass arising from the mandible or maxilla. They may occur anywhere in the jaws, including the condyle, midline, and across the midline. The overlying mucosa is often thinned, imparting a blue appearance.

Radiographic presentation

Although some are unilocular radiolucencies, most are multilocular. They will often thin out the inferior border or create a cupped-out radiolucency at the inferior border. They will displace teeth, tooth buds, the mandibular canal, and the floor of the sinus.

Differential diagnosis

Ameloblastoma, odontogenic myxoma, ameloblastic fibroma, and odontogenic keratocyst are the important considerations.

Microscopic features

Extravasated red blood cells amid a background of plump fibroblasts with little collagen formation and numerous multinucleated giant cells resembling osteoclasts. Vascular spaces lined by fibroblasts rather than endothelial cells are present.

Suggested course of action

Aspiration and incisional biopsy, and/or referral to an oral and maxillofacial surgeon.

Treatment

Between 30% and 40% of cases will involute in response to intralesional steroid injections of triamcinolone, 10 mg/mL given 1 mL per every 1 cm of lesion once a week for 6 weeks. Enucleation and curettage can also be effective as a primary treatment option or if there is no response to steroid injections. For recurrent lesions or very large destructive lesions, resection observing 1.0-cm margins will be curative. Note: This lesion has had numerous incorrect names, including the following:

- *Central giant cell reparative granuloma*: It is destructive, not reparative, and is not a true granuloma.
- *Central giant cell lesion*: It is not unspecific; it is a benign neoplasm.
- *Aneurysmal bone cyst*: These are central giant cell tumors with larger internal vascular spaces. It is also not a cyst because it does not have an epithelial lining.

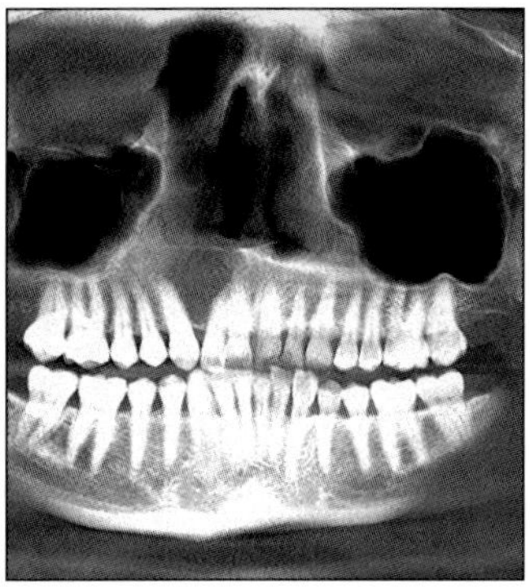

► Glandular odontogenic cyst in the maxilla.

Glandular Odontogenic Cyst

Nature of disease

An uncommon cyst with an epithelial-lined lumen containing mucous cells as a component of the lining. It arises from either prosoplasia of the odontogenic epithelium into mucous cells or entrapment of salivary gland primordia.

Predilections

No age, sex, or racial predilection is known. Most are found in the mandible.

Clinical features

May have no expansion, but more commonly an expansion with an intact overlying mucosa is noted. Larger lesions may displace teeth, prevent their eruption, or cause mobility. Paresthesia or objective anesthesia is absent.

Radiographic presentation

Some are unilocular, but most are multilocular and expansive. Tooth roots may be divergent. The mandibular canal may be displaced toward the inferior border. Teeth may be displaced or embedded by the cyst.

Differential diagnosis

The rarity of this lesion and its presentation make the more common multilocular lesions like ameloblastomas, odontogenic keratocysts, odontogenic myxomas, and central giant cell tumors stronger considerations.

Microscopic features

The lumen is lined by squamous epithelium together with pale-staining cuboidal to columnar cells, some of which show cilia and others of which contain mucin.

Suggested course of action

Incisional biopsy and/or referral to an oral and maxillofacial surgeon for biopsy and definitive treatment.

Treatment

Enucleation and curettage is considered curative. However, recurrences have been noted and identified as either glandular odontogenic tumors or mucoepidermoid carcinomas due to the similarity of the histopathology among these three lesions.

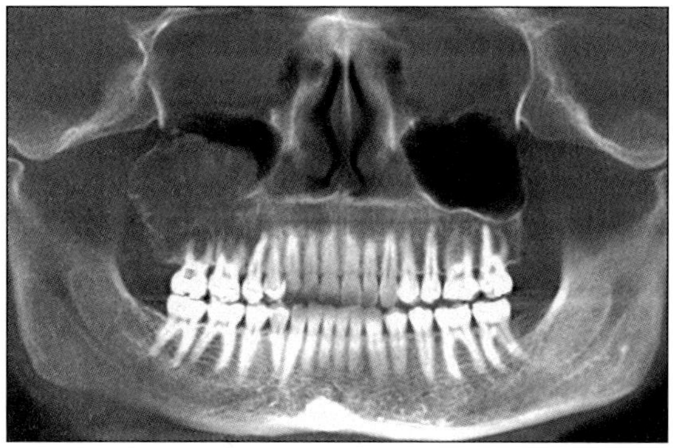

► Odontogenic myxoma of the maxilla.

Odontogenic Myxoma

Nature of disease

A benign neoplasm that arises from odontogenic mesenchyme that originated in the dental papilla of a developing tooth.

Predilections

Occurs mostly in younger individuals age 5 to 30 years, but can occur at any age. Affects the mandible more commonly than the maxilla. No sex or racial predilection is known.

Clinical features

Most are a painless expansion with an intact overlying mucosa, unless it is sufficiently large so as to ulcerate from occlusal trauma. Objective paresthesia is absent.

Radiographic presentation

Most are multilocular radiolucent lesions that often taken on a "soap bubble" appearance. Many will be seen to create thin bony septa arising from the inferior border when in the mandible and from the alveolar crest when in the maxilla. Less commonly, a unilocular radiolucency is seen.

Differential diagnosis

Other similar-appearing radiolucencies with expansion include ameloblastomas, central giant cell tumors, odontogenic keratocysts, central hemangiomas, and in children and teenagers an ameloblastic fibroma.

Microscopic features

Stellate and spindle-shaped fibroblasts loosely arranged within a lightly staining basophilic ground substance and thin immature collagen fibers. Occasionally, odontogenic rests may be seen within this background.

Suggested course of action

Incisional biopsy and/or referral to an oral and maxillofacial surgeon for definitive treatment.

Treatment

Resection with 1.0-cm margins in bone and one tumor-free anatomical barrier of periosteum or adjacent soft tissue. Immediate or delayed bone grafting can also be accomplished.

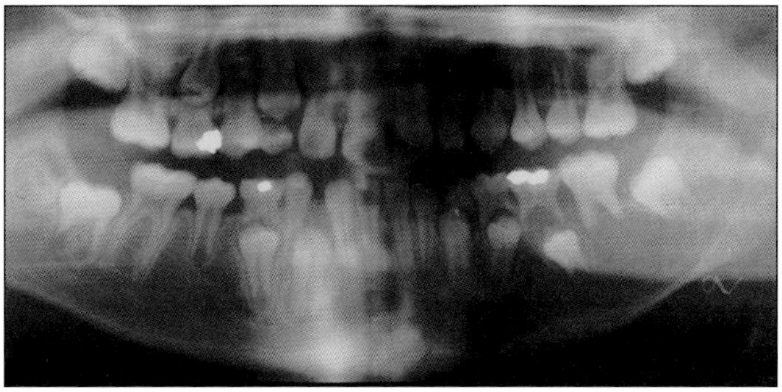

► Arteriovenous hemangioma of the mandible.

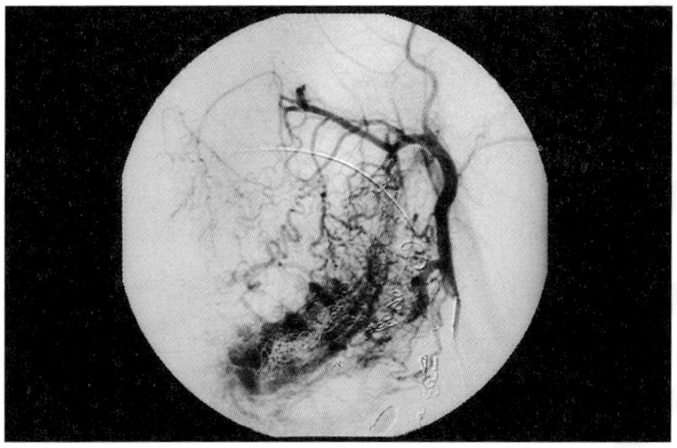

► Angiogram of arteriovenous hemangioma.

Arteriovenous Hemangioma

Nature of disease

A potentially life-threatening bleeding mass from developmental aberrations of arteries and veins. It is caused by the genetic loss of endothelial cell production of platelet-derived growth factors and transforming growth factor beta, which are required to recruit adventitial cells to support blood vessels during vasculogenesis. The result is an expanding vascular mass under arterial pressure as the systemic vascular system matures.

Predilections

Most common in preteen and teenage girls and less common in boys of the same age. No race predilection is known.

Clinical features

Usually an expansile mass that may appear blue. It will have pulsations that may be palpable as well as arterial sounds upon stethoscope or Doppler examination. They are often brought to the attention of health care personnel in the emergency room as a severe bleeding episode.

Radiographic presentation

If the lesion involves bone as well as soft tissue, it will appear as a multilocular radiolucent lesion with mild expansion.

Differential diagnosis

Odontogenic keratocysts, odontogenic myxomas, ameloblastic fibromas, and central giant cell tumors may be considered in this age group.

Microscopic features

Large, dilated, endothelial-lined blood vessels absent of supporting adventitial cells or stroma.

Suggested course of action

Aspiration of the lesion. If blood is returned, avoid biopsy in the office. Refer to an invasive radiology center for an arteriogram and to an oral and maxillofacial surgeon to coordinate treatment.

Treatment

Embolization followed by either debridement and packing of the lesion or resection. Note: Embolization via coils is to be discouraged due to early recanalization of vessels. Use of polyvinyl alcohol beads or cyanoacrylate allows for reduced blood loss surgery 48 to 72 hours later.

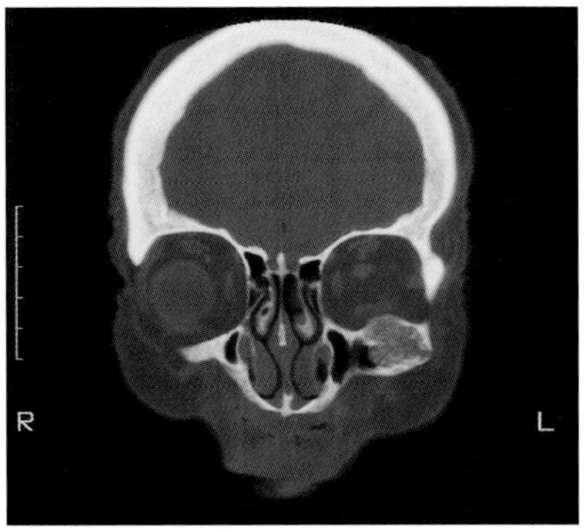

► Central cavernous hemangioma.

Cavernous Hemangioma

Nature of disease

A non-neoplastic proliferation and dilation of veins containing blood under low pressure.

Predilections

Occurs mostly in mature adults. More common in women. There is no racial predilection.

Clinical features

In bone, it will present as a mild expansion without displacement of teeth or the mandibular canal. No paresthesia or objective anesthesia is observed. In soft tissue, it will appear as a painless, blue, lobulated mass. Pulsations are usually not present. Stethoscope and Doppler examination will identify an echoing sound suggestive of venous pressure.

Radiographic presentation

A radiolucency with poorly defined borders, or a trabecular radiopacity due to the stimulation of new bone. Displacement of teeth and/or the mandibular canal is not usually seen.

Differential diagnosis

A radiolucency with ill-defined borders should suggest an idiopathic bone cavity, a metastatic malignancy, a primary malignancy, and an osteomyelitis.

Microscopic features

Large, dilated, endothelial-lined spaces.

Suggested course of action

Aspirate. If blood is returned, refer to an oral and maxillofacial surgeon for workup.

Treatment

If Doppler sounds rule out arterial pressure, a cavernous hemangioma in bone can be curetted without significant blood loss. In soft tissue, sclerosing agents such as sodium morrhuate or sodium tetradecoyl sulfate can fibrose most vessels without surgery, much like the sclerosing varicose veins in the legs. Otherwise, a local excision can be accomplished with minimal bleeding.

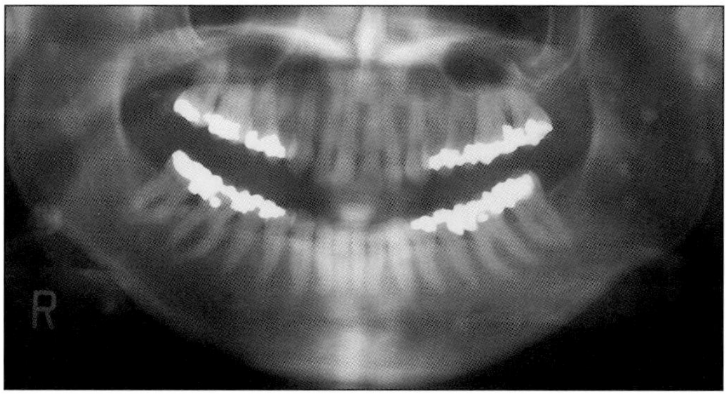

► Multiple bilateral phleboliths from a long-standing bilateral capillary hemangioma.

Capillary Hemangioma

Nature of disease

An overproliferation of capillaries due to overexpression of basic fibroblast growth factor within an embryo.

Predilections

Rare in bone. Most commonly seen in the soft tissues of a newborn or within the first 2 years of life. Some are congenital. These are often termed *juvenile capillary hemangiomas* (see below). Those in bone occur in older individuals.

Clinical features

In bone, most are diagnosed radiographically as the clinical picture is normal. Some will produce a mild, painless expansion.

Radiographic presentation

A multilocular radiolucency with thinned cortices and mild expansion in a new active lesion. Most will be seen with round to oval radiopacities in the soft tissues overlying the mandible, which are phleboliths.

Differential diagnosis

Due to its rarity in bone, lesions such as central giant cell tumors, ameloblastic fibromas, odontogenic myxomas, and odontogenic keratocysts are more realistic considerations.

Microscopic features

Very cellular lesions composed of endothelial cells forming small, tortuous, and poorly canalized lumen.

Suggested course of action

Incisional biopsy and/or referral to an oral and maxillofacial surgeon. Note: Capillary hemangiomas will not return blood upon aspiration.

Treatment

Because capillary hemangiomas in bone are not true neoplasms with continuous growth, they are removed by enucleation and curettage.

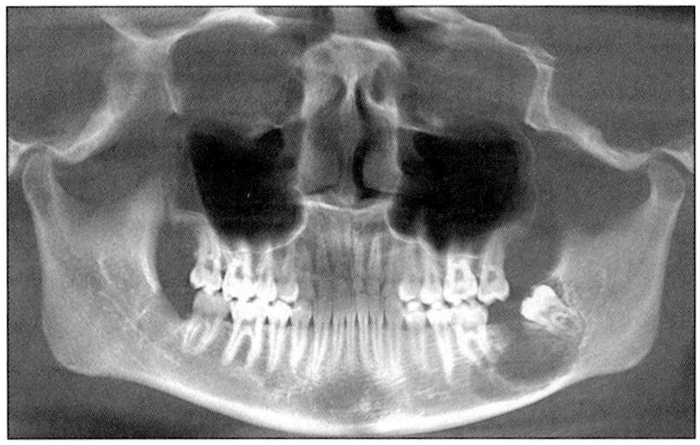

► Central mucoepidermoid carcinoma.

Central Mucoepidermoid Carcinoma

Nature of disease

Central mucoepidermoid carcinomas are low-grade malignancies thought to arise from entrapped salivary gland primordia during embryogenesis.

Predilections

The mandible is affected much more commonly than the maxilla. Occurs only slightly more in the posterior mandible than in the anterior mandible. No obvious age, sex, or racial predilection is known.

Clinical features

Normal or slight bony expansion. The overlying mucosa is intact. Paresthesia or subjective anesthesia may occur.

Radiographic presentation

May be unilocular or multilocular with mild expansion. It may erode tooth roots, displace the mandibular canal, and/or erode bone cortices.

Differential diagnosis

Its presentation will be similar to that of an ameloblastoma, central giant cell tumor, odontogenic myxoma, and an odontogenic keratocyst.

Microscopic features

A mixture of mucus-secreting cells, epidermoid cells, and very small basophilic-staining cells termed *intermediate cells* in cords and lining cystic spaces. Because central mucoepidermoid carcinomas are almost always low grade, there is a preponderance of mucus-secreting cells. To distinguish a central mucoepidermoid carcinoma from a radiographically and microscopically similar glandular odontogenic cyst/tumor, a MAML2 test is used; a positive result indicates mucoepidermoid carcinoma.

Suggested course of action

Incisional biopsy and/or referral to an oral and maxillofacial surgeon.

Treatment

Resection of the affected bone observing 1.5-cm margins. A neck dissection is not required unless there are clinically palpable lymph nodes or lymph nodes identified as suspicious by CT or MRI scan.

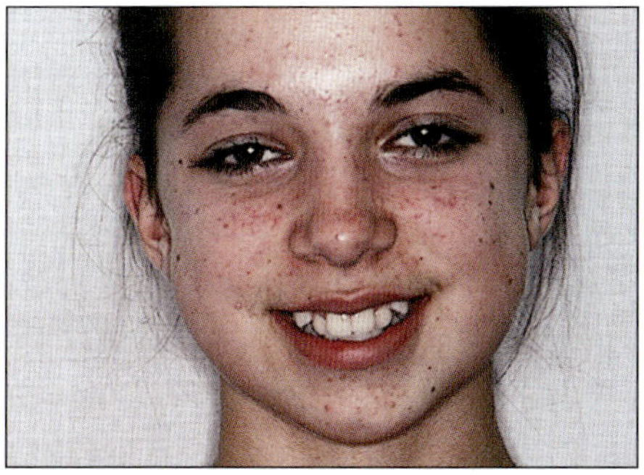

► Type I cherubism.

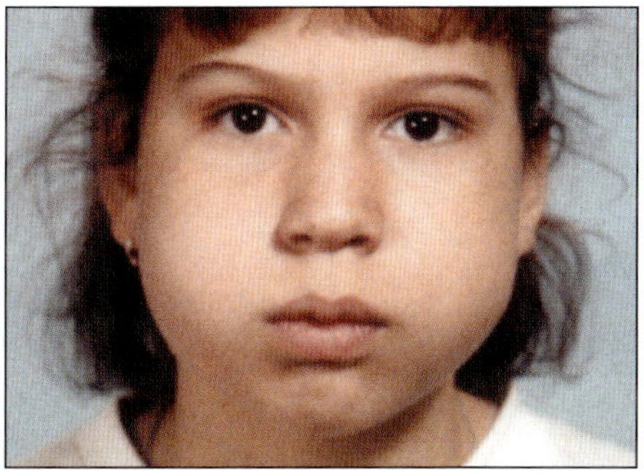

► Type II cherubism.

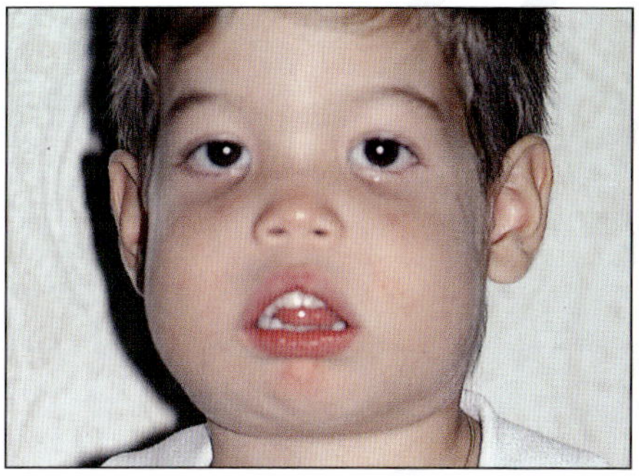

► Type III cherubism.

Cherubism

Nature of disease

An autosomal dominant inherited disease that may also occur as a spontaneous mutation in up to 40% of cases. Affects the embryonic maxilla and mandible. That is, it will also affect the middle turbinate and will spare the condyle.

Predilections

While the genetic defect is present at birth, clinical manifestations are first seen around 3 years of age. There is no sex or racial predilection.

Clinical features

- Type I: A subtle form that may only be apparent radiographically or have a slight expansion of the rami bilaterally.
- Type II: An obvious clinical expansion at the ramus and midbody of the mandible bilaterally as well as the posterior maxilla.
- Type III: Severe bilateral symmetric expansion of the complete clinical mandible and maxilla. The maxillary expansion at the orbital floor may rotate the eyes upward, giving the child a rounded face with the eyes pointed toward heaven, like the depiction of cherubs in Renaissance art (hence the name *cherubism*).

Radiographic presentation

- Type I: Bilateral, slightly expansile multilocular radiolucencies of the rami.
- Type II: Bilateral, multilocular, moderately expansile radiolucencies of the rami extending to the mental foramen.
- Type III: Bilateral, multilocular, severely expansile radiolucencies of the complete maxilla and mandible sparing the condyle.

Differential diagnosis

Cherubism is distinctive by its history, radiographic appearance, and age of the patient. However, Ramon syndrome, Jaffe-Campanacci syndrome, and Noonan syndrome are to be considered as well as an extensive involvement of Langerhans cell histiocytosis.

Microscopic features

A fibrous stroma in which numerous small blood vessels are seen along with scattered giant cells and extravasated red blood cells. →

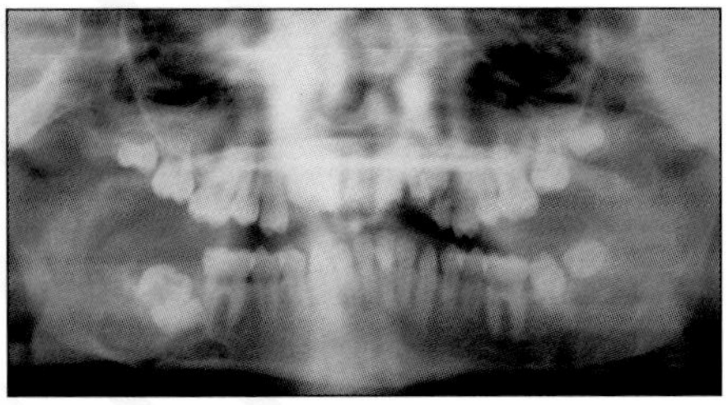

► Type I cherubism.

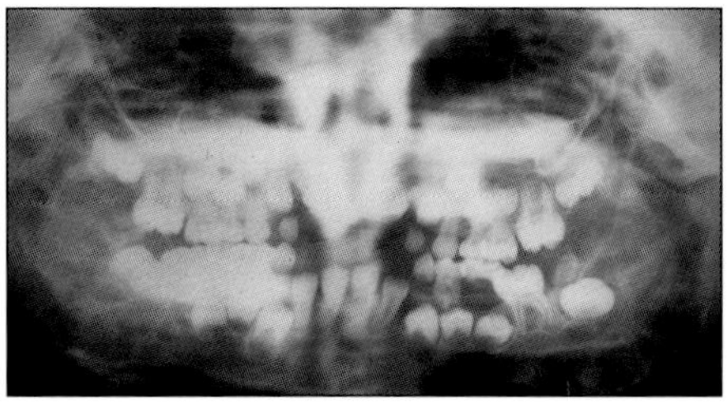

► Type II cherubism.

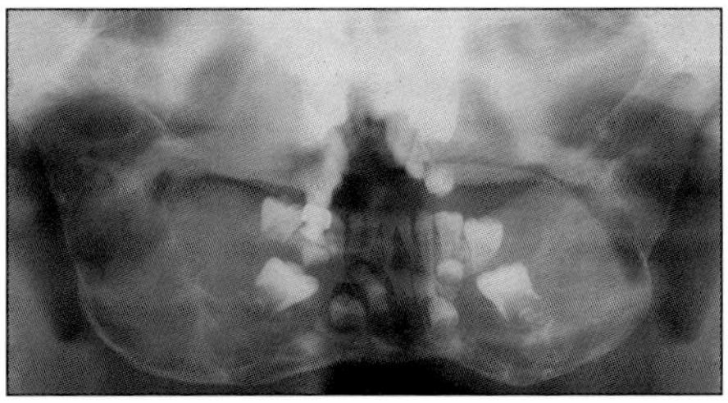

► Type III cherubism.

Cherubism *(cont)*

Suggested course of action

Refer to a geneticist for documentation and counseling. Refer to an oral and maxillofacial surgeon for follow-up.

Treatment

Most cases require no treatment as the expansion begins a self-reducing involution in the mid to late teen years. If residual expansion is present, osseous contouring can be accomplished in the late teens. In adults, missing teeth and impacted teeth are present, which may require removal of impacted teeth, removal of residual cherubic tissue, alveolar grafting, and implant placements.

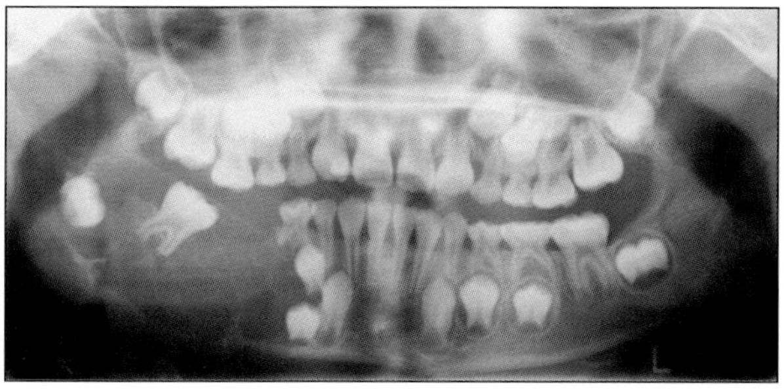

► Ameloblastic fibroma.

Ameloblastic Fibroma

Nature of disease

A hamartomatous proliferation of odontogenic mesenchyme and odontogenic epithelium that arise from the developing tooth germ.

Predilections

Strong predilection for children and teenagers. Note: Identification of a similar histopathology in older individuals should be looked at as suspicious for an ameloblastic fibrosarcoma.

Clinical features

Painless expansion in either the maxilla or mandible with an intact overlying mucosa. A disturbance or delay in the eruption of anticipated teeth may be seen. Objective paresthesia is absent.

Radiographic presentation

May be a unilocular or multilocular radiolucency with expansion. Large multilocular and destructive features should raise a suspicion of ameloblastic fibrosarcoma.

Differential diagnosis

In the child/teenage age range, an odontogenic myxoma, central giant cell tumor, and central hemangioma are the primary considerations. In those somewhat older, ameloblastoma and ameloblastic carcinoma are also to be considered.

Microscopic features

There is a loose arrangement of odontogenic mesenchyme amid a light basophilic ground substance with little or no collagen formation. Within this background are cords of cuboidal or columnar odontogenic epithelium often ending in a bulbous configuration.

Suggested course of action

Incisional biopsy and/or referral to an oral and maxillofacial surgeon for definitive care.

Treatment

For those cases in which an ameloblastic fibrosarcoma has been ruled out or there are no suspicions for it, enucleation and curettage is curative.

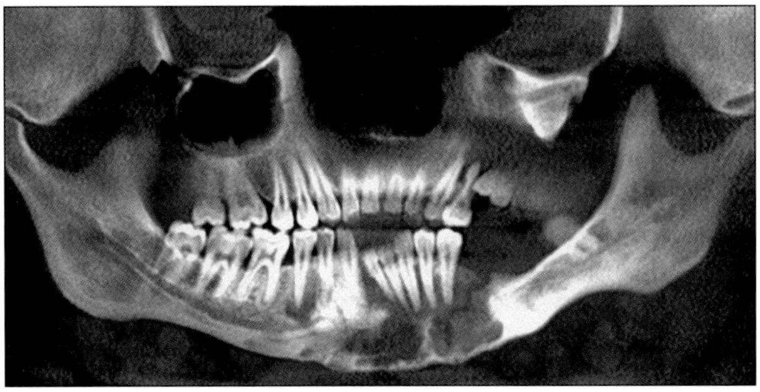

► Multilocular radiolucency of primary hyperparathyroidism.

Primary Hyperparathyroidism

Nature of disease

Primary hyperparathyroidism results mostly from hyperplasia and oversecretion of parathormone from one or more of the four parathyroid glands. Rarely does it result from a benign parathyroid adenoma and rarer still from a parathyroid carcinoma. The oversecretion of parathormone activates osteoclasts, which results in bone-resorption cavities filled with giant cells (osteoclasts), hypercalcemia, hypophosphatemia, and hypercalciuria.

Predilections

More common in women and those over 50 years of age.

Clinical features

Related to the jaws, mildly expansile radiolucencies filled with a red-brown soft tissue called "brown tumors" may be seen. Patients may complain of constipation, fatigue, bone pain, thirst, nausea, and vomiting due to hypercalcemia. Occasionally, tooth mobility unrelated to periodontal disease is observed.

Radiographic presentation

Brown tumors may be unilocular or multilocular. The lamina dura may be absent, and the trabecular bone pattern may be generally ill defined.

Differential diagnosis

The differential diagnosis revolves around radiolucencies with hypercalcemia. Therefore, multiple myeloma, sarcoidosis, small cell carcinoma of the lung, and adrenal insufficiency are considerations.

Microscopic features

A fibroblastic stroma of plump fibroblasts, multinucleated giant cells, and extravasated red blood cells indistinguishable from a central giant cell tumor.

Suggested course of action

Incisional or excisional biopsy that identifies these aforementioned microscopic features. Follow up with serum calcium determination; if above 10.5 mg/dL, refer the patient to a general surgeon for definitive workup and treatment.

Treatment

Parathyroidectomy to remove three of the four most active or largest parathyroid glands.

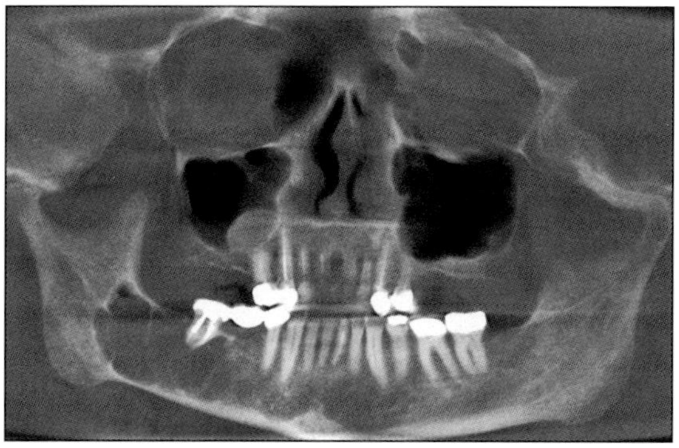

► Glandular odontogenic tumor.

Glandular Odontogenic Tumor

Nature of disease

A very rare odontogenic tumor that is either an aggressive benign or a low-grade malignant tumor thought to arise from prosoplasia of odontogenic rests.

Predilections

Rare but has occurred mostly in the mandible, with a strong adult female predilection.

Clinical features

Expansion and tooth mobility with an intact overlying mucosa. Occasionally pain and/or paresthesia is present.

Radiographic presentation

May be an expansile unilocular or multilocular radiolucency with ill-defined borders.

Differential diagnosis

Mucoepidermoid carcinoma, glandular odontogenic cysts, and renal carcinomas are other clear cell–containing tumors that will bear a resemblance to a glandular odontogenic tumor once the histopathology is obtained. Otherwise, expansile radiolucencies would be consistent with several odontogenic cysts and tumors.

Microscopic features

Clear cells admixed in a fibromyxoid stroma with deeply staining epithelial cells.

Suggested course of action

Incisional biopsy and/or referral to an oral and maxillofacial surgeon for definitive treatment.

Treatment

After a workup to include a CT scan or PET scan, such tumors are treated with resection observing 1.0- to 1.5-cm margins. If the uncommon finding of lymph node involvement is noted, a neck dissection is included.

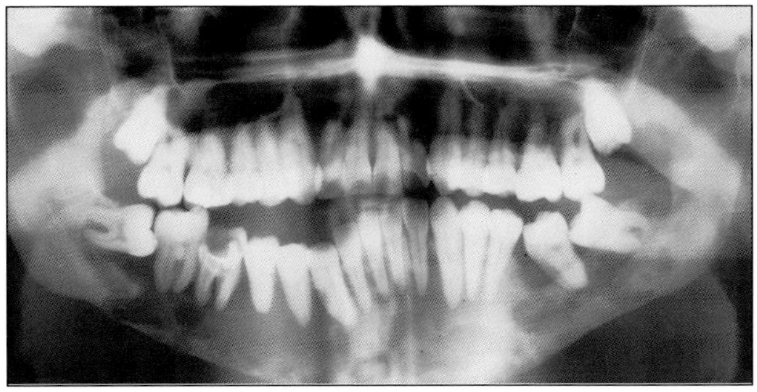

► Extensive bilateral radiolucencies seen in a case of Langerhans cell histiocytosis.

Irregular or Diffuse Radiolucencies

Langerhans Cell Histiocytosis

Nature of disease

A low-grade malignancy from a local or multifocal clonal proliferation of the antigen-presenting cell known as the *Langerhans cell.*

Predilections

Bony lesions are mostly seen in children and young adults. Soft tissue lesions are more common in individuals aged 20 to 40 years.

Clinical features

Mobility of teeth with gingival and bone recession is well known. May also present as a painless jaw expansion.

Radiographic presentation

Alveolar bone loss to the apex of teeth, creating the "floating tooth" appearance, is frequently seen. However, an irregular or multilocular radiolucency with ill-defined borders is also well known.

Differential diagnosis

The radiolucency around teeth that are mobile may also be seen in rapidly progressive juvenile periodontitis, Papillon-Lefèvre syndrome, osteomyelitis, acute lymphocytic leukemia, and other malignancies.

Microscopic features

An inflammatory cell background in which eosinophils may be more numerous than anticipated along with oval cells with a nucleus that has a central groove (Langerhans cells). Electron microscopy will show characteristic Birbeck granules.

Suggested course of action

Remove any mobile teeth, and biopsy what appears to be granulation tissue around teeth. If Langerhans cell histiocytosis is suspected, request a CD1a antigen as a confirmatory test. Or refer the patient to an oral and maxillofacial surgeon for this workup.

Treatment

Unifocal or localized disease is treated with aggressive curettage or a peripheral resection. Recurrent lesions may be treated with 1,800 to 2,400 cGy of radiotherapy. Multifocal disease is treated with chemotherapy (ie, 6-mercaptopurine, vinblastine, etc).

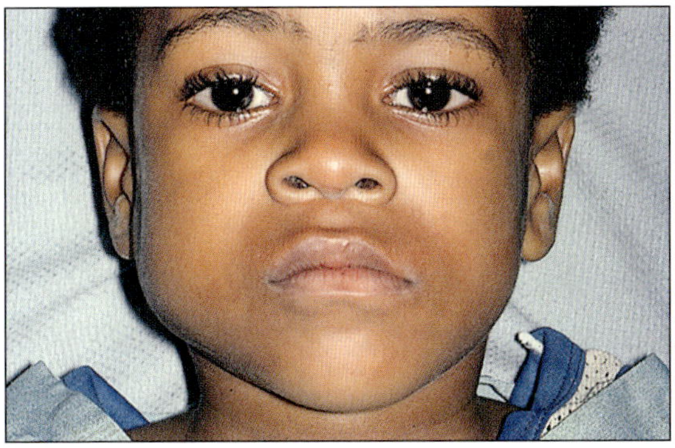

► Ramus expansion due to acute lymphoblastic leukemia.

Leukemias

Nature of disease

All leukemias are bone marrow malignancies that spill malignant white blood cells into the systemic circulation.

Predilections

- Acute lymphoblastic leukemia (ALL): Mostly strikes children in the first decade of life
- Acute myelogenous leukemia (AML): Mostly strikes teenagers and young adults
- Chronic lymphoblastic leukemia (CLL) and chronic myelogenous leukemia (CML): Leukemias affecting adults over age 40 years

Clinical features

Many are asymptomatic with a significantly elevated white blood cell count (≥ 25,000/dL). Some patients will report weakness and fatigue. Cases of leukemic gingival infiltrates causing a puffy, boggy, bleeding gingiva can occur with any leukemia but are very rare. Tooth mobility may be seen, but deep bone pain of long bones is more common. Secondary infections such as pneumonia are frequent, and in AML pericoronitis is often seen.

Radiographic presentation

Most have normal radiographs, but some will show significant irregular alveolar bone resorption or a diffuse radiolucency within the marrow space of the rami.

Differential diagnosis

Those presentations with gingival enlargement, tooth mobility, and alveolar bone loss will be similar to juvenile rapidly progressive periodontitis, Papillon-Lefèvre syndrome, hereditary gingival fibromatosis, and Langerhans cell histiocytosis.

Microscopic features

Peripheral blood smears and bone marrow biopsies will show atypical lymphocytes of a specific type (ie, granulocytes, lymphocytes, monocytes, etc).

Suggested course of action

Suspicious cases should be referred to a hematologist-oncologist.

Treatment

Specific treatments will vary as a function of the cell type and genetic rearrangement of each cell line. Generally, these include type-specific chemotherapy and possible stem cell or bone marrow transplants.

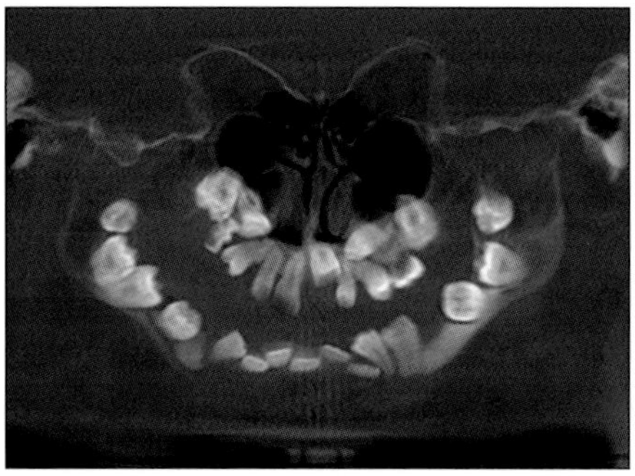

► Gorham-Stout vanishing bone disease affecting the mandible and maxilla.

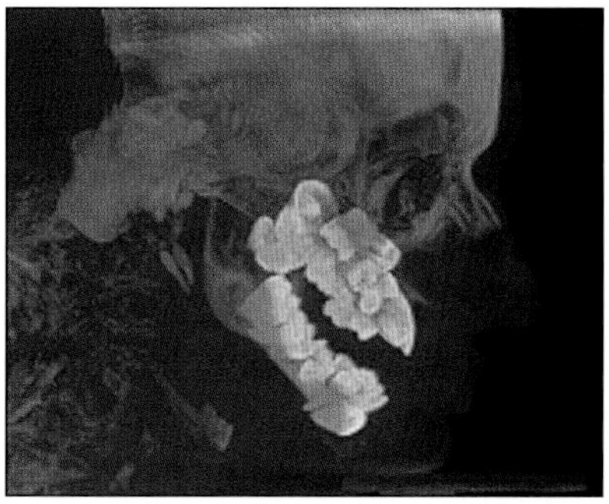

► Gorham-Stout vanishing bone disease affecting the cervical vertebrae.

Gorham-Stout Vanishing Bone Disease

Nature of disease

True Gorham-Stout vanishing bone disease is a diffuse lymphangiomatosis that resorbs bones.

Predilections

A very rare disease in which accurate predilections are unknown. However, most cases are seen in young adults. No sex or racial predilection is known.

Clinical features

Irregular osteolysis in either jaw plus additional bones. Lymphangiomas of skin and/or mucosa should be looked for to confirm a suspected case. Cases involving the jaws will have mobile teeth and often a pathologic fracture with tooth and jaw displacement.

Radiographic presentation

A diffuse and often large area of osteolysis seen in several bones. The mandible, maxilla, zygoma, and vertebrae are most commonly involved.

Differential diagnosis

Many reported cases of Gorham-Stout disease are found to be chronic osteomyelitis cases, which should always be a consideration. Otherwise, multiple myeloma, metastatic cancer, and severe anemias may provide a similar picture.

Microscopic features

Dilated endothelial-lined lymphatic spaces within or adjacent to bone. Bone resorption is not mediated by osteoclasts. Bone appears thin with regular edges.

Suggested course of action

Referral to centers with experience with this rare disease—ie, University of Miami Division of Oral and Maxillofacial Surgery (Miami, Florida), MD Anderson Cancer Center Division of Hematology/Oncology (Houston, Texas), and Memorial Sloan Kettering Cancer Center (New York, New York).

Treatment

There is no known cure. Palliative surgery to relieve pain and titanium plate placements to reinforce weakened bone are often needed. Experimental therapies with bisphosphonates, RANK ligand inhibitors, and alpha-2 interferon may be offered in selected cases.

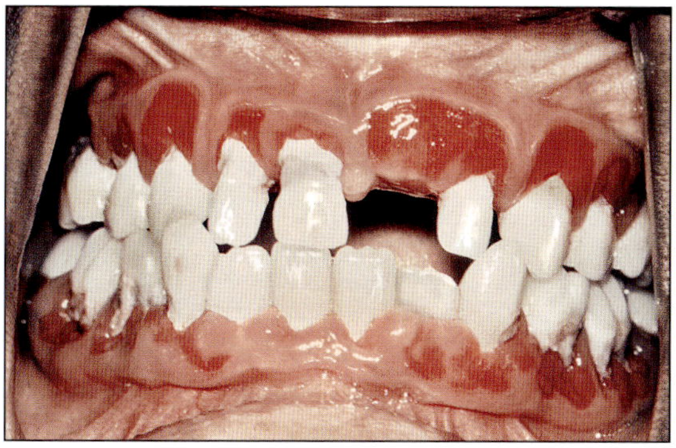

► Juvenile rapidly progressive periodontitis.

Juvenile Rapidly Progressive Periodontitis

Nature of disease

Severe gingival and periodontal inflammation and bone resorption out of proportion to local plaque scores caused by an autosomal recessive leukocyte adherence deficiency. In such cases, macrophages and neutrophils do not respond to chemotactic signals and are not able to bind to and engulf most organisms. Alterations in the cell-surface membrane proteins CD11, CD18, Mac-1, LFA-1, p150, and p95 seem to be the underlying defects.

Predilections

Mostly children and teenagers, but adults up to 30 years old can be affected. There is no known sex or racial predilection.

Clinical features

The localized form involves only incisors and first molars, showing extensive vertical bone loss, mobile teeth, and gingival inflammation that readily bleeds. The generalized form involves all teeth with extensive periodontal pocketing, gingival inflammation with bleeding, and alveolar bone resorption.

Radiographic presentation

Extensive alveolar bone loss corresponding to the area of clinical involvement, creating a floating tooth appearance on periapical and panoramic radiographs.

Differential diagnosis

Subtle or localized cases may seem like common periodontitis from poor plaque control. More severe forms may herald the Papillon-Lefèvre syndrome, of which juvenile rapidly progressive periodontitis is one component. Otherwise, Langerhans cell histiocytosis, acute lymphocytic leukemia in children, and acute myelogenous leukemia in teenagers and young adults should be considered as well as poorly controlled insulin dependence (diabetes).

Microscopic features

Nonspecific but severe chronic inflammation is seen, usually more populated with plasma cells than neutrophils or macrophages. →

Juvenile Rapidly Progressive Periodontitis *(cont)*

Suggested course of action

Suspicious cases should be referred to an advanced periodontal program or to a periodontist with some experience in treating juvenile rapidly progressive periodontitis. Referral to a geneticist to confirm the diagnosis is also advised.

Treatment

Removal of unsalvageable teeth followed by intensive scaling and curettage procedures together with antibiotic therapy of the tetracycline family can contain and control juvenile rapidly progressive periodontitis. A rigid recall schedule is needed. Periodontal flap surgery and bone/soft tissue regenerative surgeries may be accomplished once disease control is obtained and maintained. Dental implant rehabilitation can proceed with caution and must be followed with a rigid recall/surveillance program.

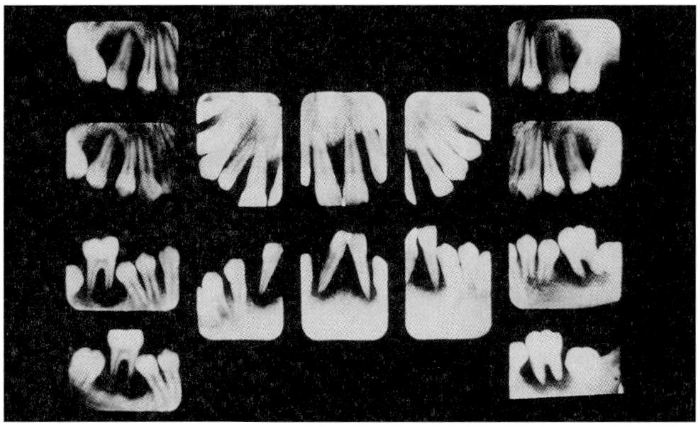

► Bone loss from the rapidly progressive periodontitis component of Papillon-Lefèvre syndrome.

Papillon-Lefèvre Syndrome

Nature of disease

This syndrome is an autosomal recessive trait associated with a leukocyte adherence deficiency similar to that in juvenile rapidly progressive periodontitis. However, this syndrome also results in hyperkeratosis of the palmar and plantar skin surfaces. Like in juvenile rapidly progressive periodontitis, a defect in neutrophil and macrophage membrane surface proteins CD11, CD18, Mac-1, LAF-1, p150, and p95 renders these cells incapable of chemotaxis and engulfing periodontal pathogens.

Predilections

Severe gingival inflammation is usually clinically apparent, and bone loss can be seen on radiographs by age 4 or 5 years. It will involve the primary dentition at this age as well as the permanent dentition that follows. There is no known sex or racial predilection.

Clinical features

The dentition will be seen to have severe and extensive gingival inflammation and recession with tooth root exposures and tooth mobility. The gingiva will readily bleed. Deep periodontal pockets can be probed. The plantar and palmar hyperkeratosis will first appear as a brown "dirty hand" or "dirty foot" with a rough surface texture. As the disease progresses, the hyperkeratosis will appear more hairlike and will be a deeper color of brown, with some black areas. A sour, foul odor is often apparent from the decaying keratin.

Radiographic presentation

Severe generalized alveolar bone loss involving all teeth (to a lesser extent third molars in late teenagers) is seen, creating numerous "floating teeth."

Differential diagnosis

If the palmar and plantar hyperkeratosis is subtle, juvenile rapidly progressive periodontitis becomes the main consideration, followed by Langerhans cell histiocytosis. Otherwise, such bone loss may also be seen in acute lymphocytic leukemia in children and acute myelogenous leukemia in teenagers.

Microscopic features

The gingival lesions will show an intensive nonspecific inflammation with more plasma cells than neutrophils. The palmar and plantar hyperkeratosis is a nonspecific overproduction of orthokeratin. The skin dermis may show a mild nonspecific inflammation as well. →

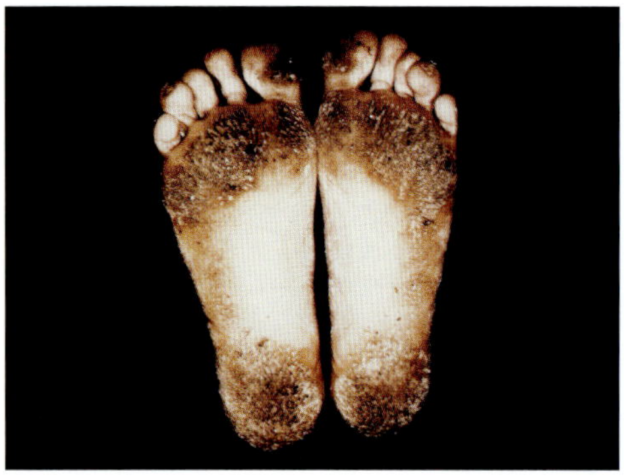

► Hyperkeratosis of the plantar area seen as part of Papillon-Lefèvre syndrome.

Papillon-Lefèvre Syndrome *(cont)*

Suggested course of action

Suspicious cases should be referred to an advanced periodontal program or to a periodontist with some experience in treating periodontitis resulting from an immune deficiency. Referral to a geneticist to confirm the diagnosis is also advised.

Treatment

Unsalvageable teeth are removed followed by intensive scaling and curettage procedures together with long-standing antibiotic therapy of the tetracycline family. If and/or once control is obtained and maintained, soft tissue and bone regenerative techniques can be considered. In selected cases where control is maintained over a period of time, dental implant rehabilitation may be considered. Note that third molars seem to be minimally or not involved. Their retention is often valuable in later oral reconstructive efforts. Excessive keratin may be removed with 6% salicylic acid water soaks. A reduction in keratin production can be obtained with systemic isotretinoin (Accutane, Roche) 0.5 to 2.0 mg/kg twice daily.

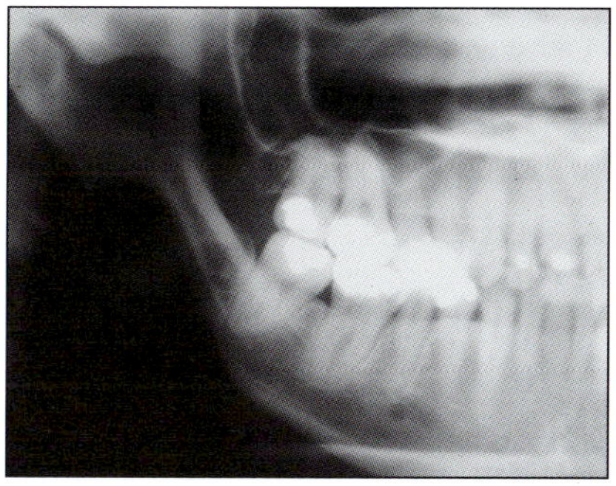

► Ramus resorption in diffuse progressive systemic sclerosis.

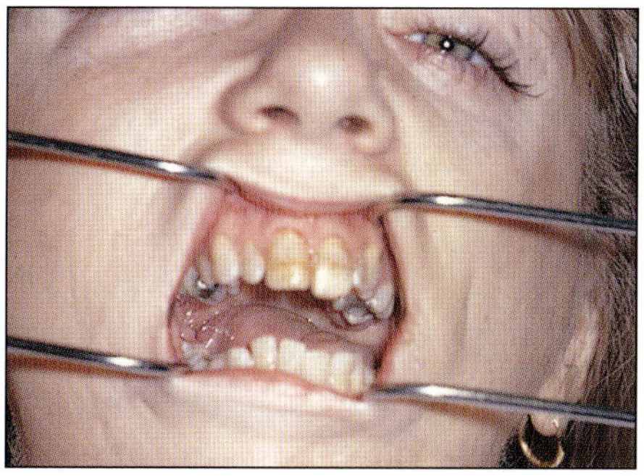

► Limited mouth opening in progressive systemic sclerosis.

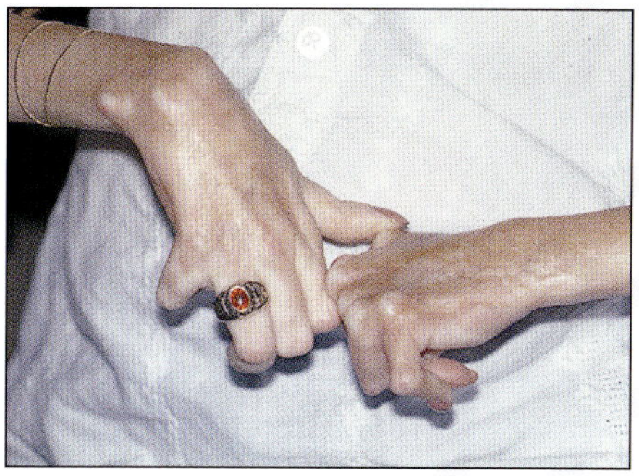

► Flexion contraction seen in diffuse progressive systemic sclerosis.

Progressive Systemic Sclerosis (Scleroderma)

Nature of disease

Progressive systemic sclerosis is an autoimmune disease whereby antibodies to several ribonucleic proteins (ie, Scl-70, topoisomerase, etc) develop. Variable extents of this autoimmune disease result in three possible clinical presentations:

1. Linear scleroderma (Parry-Romberg syndrome)
2. CREST syndrome
3. Diffuse progressive systemic sclerosis

In all three types, normal cellular elements are lost and are replaced by collagen.

Predilections

In all types, women are affected much more often than men (4:1). No racial predilection is known.

Clinical features

1. Linear scleroderma (Parry-Romberg syndrome) begins in the early teens and runs a 3-year course. On one side of the face, arrested development and atrophy create significant asymmetry. The subcutaneous fat layer and facial muscle decrease in size, followed by the underlying bone in severe cases or those that begin before the teenage years. If the scalp on one side is involved with atrophy and alopecia, it gives the appearance of a sword injury and is known as the *coup de sabre deformity*.
2. CREST syndrome is an acronym representing **C**alcinosis of the joints and fascia; **R**aynaud phenomenon whereby fingers turn blue, red, or white due to vasospasm from cold temperatures; **E**sophageal hypomotility from weakness in the throat and esophagus muscles; **S**clerodactyly from tightness of the skin around the fingers; and **T**elangiectasia from dilated capillaries most prominently seen on the fingers and labial mucosa.
3. Diffuse progressive systemic sclerosis has the features most associated with the older term *scleroderma*: tight oral commissures, hyperflexed hands and wrists with prominent sclerodactyly, alopecia, hyperpigmented skin, and skin fixed to underlying bone and internal organ involvement.

Radiographic presentation

1. Linear scleroderma will show an even thinning of any involved bone while retaining its general shape.
2. In CREST syndrome, irregular, fluffy-appearing calcified masses may be seen in joints or within tendons or muscles.
3. Diffuse progressive systemic sclerosis will often show widening of the periodontal ligament space and resorption of the angle of the mandible. Other radiographs may show deformities and dislocations at the wrist, ankles, or metacarpophalangeal joints. →

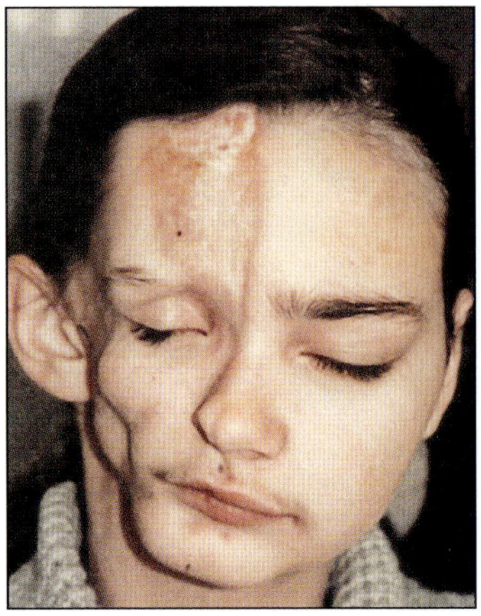

► Coup de sabre deformity in Parry-Romberg linear scleroderma.

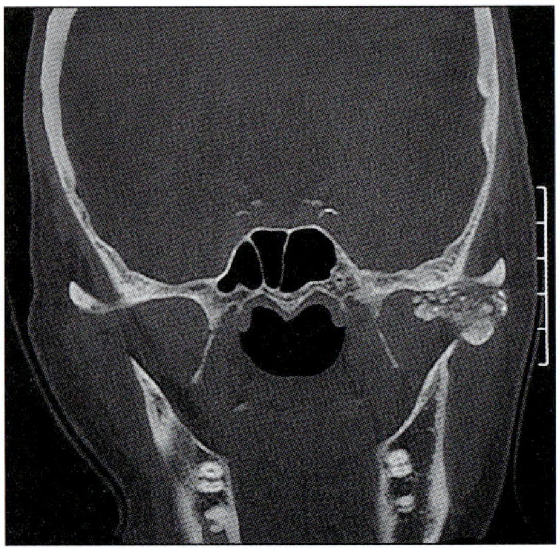

► The calcinosis in CREST syndrome.

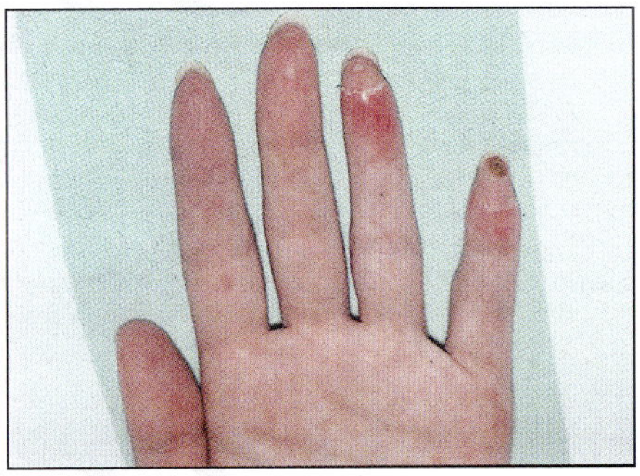

► The Raynaud phenomenon in CREST syndrome.

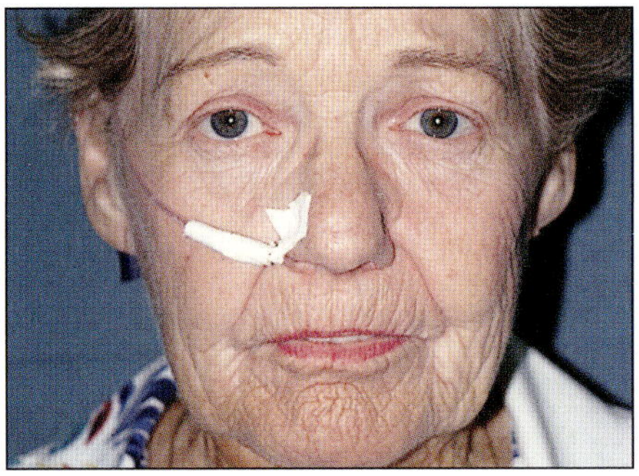

► Nasal feeding tube required due to the esophageal hypomotility in CREST syndrome.

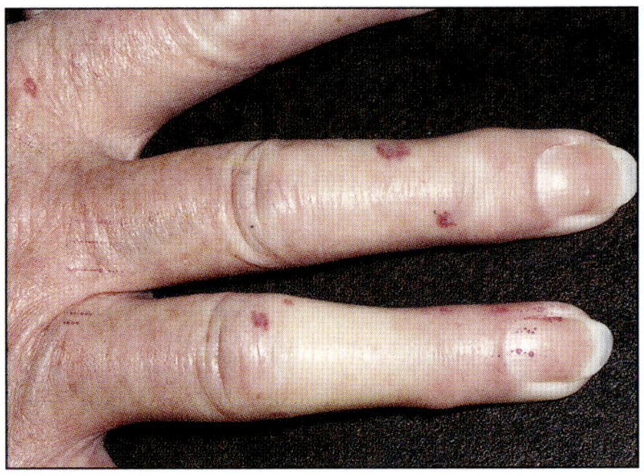

► The sclerodactyly and telangiectasia in CREST syndrome.

Progressive Systemic Sclerosis (Scleroderma) *(cont)*

Differential diagnosis

Each of the fully developed variants of progressive systemic sclerosis is a straightforward diagnosis. However, in its early stages it may resemble systemic lupus erythematosus, mixed connective tissue disease, and Sjögren syndrome as well as nonspecific muscle aches and weakness.

Microscopic features

Tissue specimens will show an excessive deposition of collagen. Surface epithelium will be thin, with sparse skin appendages and sparse minor salivary glands of the oral mucosa.

Suggested course of action

Refer to a rheumatologist for evaluation and workup. Restorative dental work is safe to perform provided the jaw opening is sufficient. If microstomia inhibits access to dental care or the patient desires facial contour improvement, refer to an oral and maxillofacial surgeon for evaluation. Note: Be sure to include questions about medication in the medical history specific to bisphosphonates and RANK ligand inhibitors because many of these patients are prescribed these drugs for steroid-induced osteoporosis.

Treatment

Rheumatologists treat these patients with prednisone and a variety of other immune-suppressive drugs (ie, mycophenolate, azathioprine, methotrexate) in an attempt to slow it down and/or control its progression. Oral commissurotomies are often done to increase access for oral hygiene and dental care. Facial fat grafts, onlays, and sometimes microvascular flaps are used to restore facial symmetry.

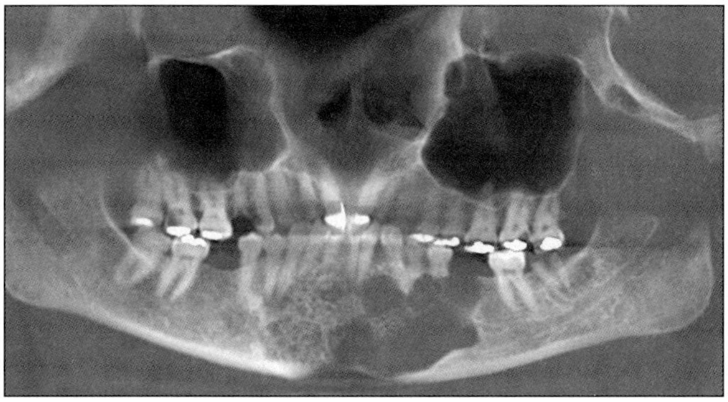

► Primary intraosseous carcinoma.

Primary Intraosseous Carcinoma

Nature of disease

Malignant transformation of primordial epithelial cells in the jaws from tooth development (rests) or from entrapped epithelium during embryogenesis.

Predilections

Very rare but seen mostly in adults over 40 years old. No sex or racial predilection is known.

Clinical features

Often an asymptomatic radiographic finding. Otherwise may present with a painful or painless bony expansion. Paresthesias are common, and in the absence of previous trauma, malignancy should be expected.

Radiographic presentation

A mildly expansile or sometimes nonexpansile irregular radiolucency. The cortex may be thinned or eroded.

Differential diagnosis

Intraosseous carcinomas are unanticipated findings. Considerations would be an osteosarcoma, osteomyelitis, and metastatic cancer.

Microscopic features

Atypical epithelial cells consistent with squamous cell carcinoma. Depending on the differentiation, keratin pearls may be seen.

Suggested course of action

Intrabony exploration and biopsy, and/or referral to an oral and maxillofacial surgeon.

Treatment

Intraosseous carcinomas are considered stage IV due to their location. A complete workup of a PET scan and other imaging is required. Treatment involves resection of the involved bone observing 1.5- to 2.0-cm margins, with consideration for postoperative radiotherapy and/or chemotherapy as per the results of the workup.

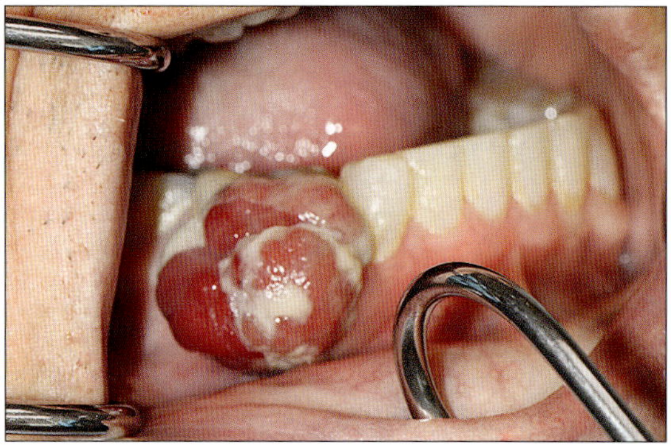

► Breast cancer metastasis to the mandible.

Metastatic Carcinoma

Nature of disease

A proliferation of malignant cells that spread to the jaws mostly via the venous routes and less so via arteries and lymphatics. The route from those primary sites above the diaphragm is via local veins or arteries to the jaws. Those from below the diaphragm are via the paravertebral veins of Batson.

Predilections

The most common primary sites are the breast (31%), lung (27%), kidney (14%), bone (10%), thyroid (6%), and others (<5%).

Clinical features

May be an incidental finding of a radiolucency in the jaw. More commonly, it is seen as a soft tissue gingival mass or mass arising from bone around a tooth or from a recent extraction socket. Paresthesia or overt anesthesia of a nerve distribution is common.

Radiographic presentation

Most will show a poorly demarcated radiolucency and mild expansion. Others may appear normal, and some (such as in metastatic breast cancer) will have some radiopacities.

Differential diagnosis

Primary carcinomas, peripheral giant cell proliferations, pyogenic granulomas, and some cases of osteomyelitis are considerations.

Microscopic features

A malignant cell population appearing as cells from the distant primary site. Note: Special stains are often needed to determine the cell type and origin of the metastasis. Occasionally, the primary site has not yet been identified.

Suggested course of action

Incisional biopsy and/or referral to an oral and maxillofacial surgeon.

Treatment

Metastasis portends a poor prognosis. The primary site and metastatic sites may be treated with surgery, focal radiotherapy, and/or chemotherapy for disease and pain control. Cure is unlikely.

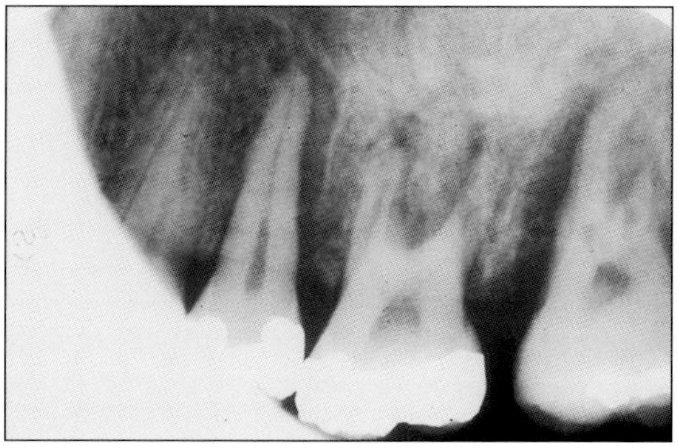

► Supraerupted molar, widened periodontal ligament, open contact, and a diffuse radiopacity in an osteosarcoma.

Osteosarcoma

Nature of disease

A proliferation of malignant mesenchymal stem cells/osteoprogenitor cells that forms neoplastic bone.

Predilections

May occur at any age but mostly seen in young adults. In the jaws, it is well known to occur 10 to 15 years later than those in long bones. No sex or racial predilection is known.

Clinical features

A bony, hard to fleshy mass arising from and expanding the involved area. The surface mucosa may be ulcerated and friable. Paresthesia or complete anesthesia of a nerve distribution is common. Pain may be present but is uncommon. Teeth in the area are often mobile and/or displaced.

Radiographic presentation

Most are seen as a combined osteolytic radiopaque mass with irregular outlines. Early osteosarcomas may first be noted by a widening of the periodontal ligament space known as a *Garrington sign* and an opening of tooth-to-tooth contact. Extracortical neoplastic bone is frequently seen arising from a disrupted cortex at right angles and is referred to as a "sunray appearance."

Differential diagnosis

Paget disease, fibrous dysplasia, chronic sclerosing osteomyelitis, suppurative osteomyelitis, osteoblastomas, and some ossifying fibromas can produce a similar clinical and radiographic appearance.

Microscopic features

A neoplastic spindle-cell stroma with deep-staining pleomorphic nuclei is seen to produce immature tumor bone and even mature-appearing bone.

Suggested course of action

Incisional biopsy and/or referral to an oral and maxillofacial surgeon or medical oncologist.

Treatment

Combined chemotherapy and surgery. Surgery requires 3.0-cm margins in bone and 2.0-cm margins in soft tissue, often necessitating flap reconstruction as well. Radiotherapy is used only in selected cases.

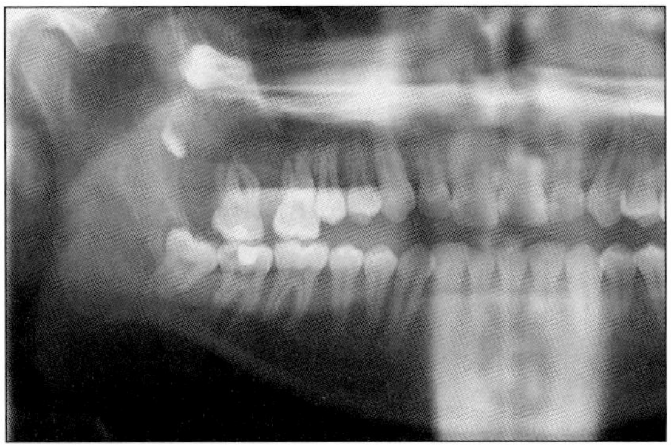

► Chondrosarcoma of the maxilla.

Chondrosarcoma of the Jaws

Nature of disease

A malignant proliferation of mesenchymal stem cells/progenitor cells with a partial differentiation into chondroblasts without any differentiation into bone.

Predilections

Mostly seen in young adults but can occur at any age. No sex or racial predilection is known.

Clinical features

A firm, expansile mass arising from bone and often growing out of bone. Paresthesia and overt anesthesia may be present. Tooth mobility and tooth displacement are common. Pain may be present but is uncommon.

Radiographic presentation

An outline of a soft tissue mass is noted in a resorbed area of the jaws with indistinct borders. Some striae of ossifications may be seen due to periosteal reactive bone, but chondrosarcomas are otherwise radiolucent.

Differential diagnosis

Osteosarcomas, fibrosarcomas, pleomorphic sarcomas, and osteomyelitis may have similar presentations.

Microscopic features

A pleomorphic cellular stroma of atypical mesenchymal cells, some of which may develop large chondrocytic lacunae often with multiple nuclei.

Suggested course of action

Exploration and incisional biopsy from the center of the mass, and/or referral to an oral and maxillofacial surgeon.

Treatment

Most cases are treated with surgical resection observing 2.0-cm margins. Uncommonly, chemotherapy is used as an adjunct.

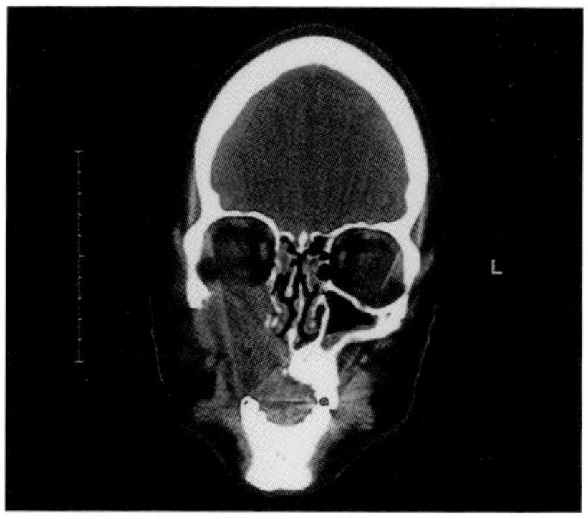

► Extensive destruction and orbital invasion from a pleomorphic sarcoma of the maxilla.

Pleomorphic Sarcoma of the Jaws

Nature of disease

A highly aggressive proliferation of primordial stem cells that show a slight fibroblastic differentiation or histiocytic differentiation. Note: Previously known as *malignant fibrous histiocytoma*.

Predilections

Adults, with no known sex or racial predilection.

Clinical features

A very destructive soft tissue mass growing out of and resorbing bone. Paresthesia and overt anesthesia are common. Pain is sometimes present. Tooth mobility and displacement are common.

Radiographic presentation

A soft tissue mass is seen to replace bone via resorption. Tooth roots are often resorbed. Tooth displacement is common.

Differential diagnosis

Other high-grade malignancies such as some osteosarcomas, squamous cell carcinomas, fibrosarcomas, metastatic carcinoma, and even a suppurative osteomyelitis may be considered.

Microscopic features

A cellular proliferation of pleomorphic fibroblast-appearing cells with clear cytoplasm resembling a histiocyte often in a swirled pattern of darker-staining cells around a center of lighter-staining cells, referred to as the *storiform pattern*.

Suggested course of action

Incisional biopsy and/or referral to an oral and maxillofacial surgeon.

Treatment

Resection of the tumor observing 3.0-cm margins followed by postoperative chemotherapy and radiation therapy.

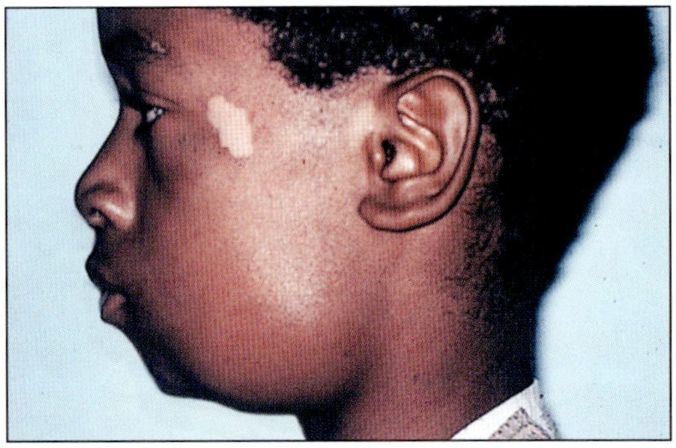

► Clinical picture of Burkitt lymphoma African type.

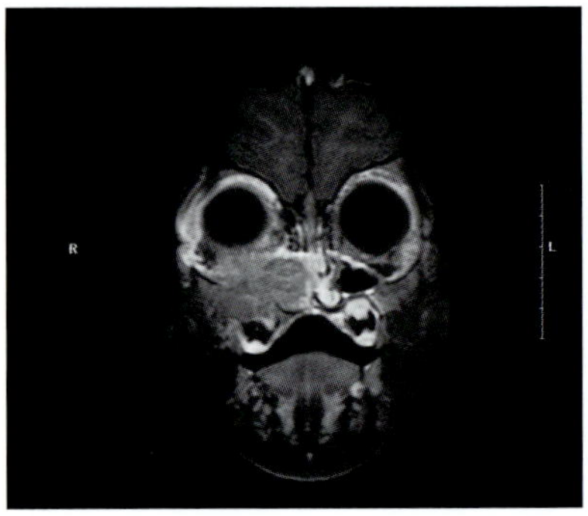

► CT scan of a Burkitt lymphoma African type in the maxilla.

Burkitt Lymphoma

Nature of disease

A rare and very aggressive B-cell lymphoma of two types: *(1)* the African type, which mostly affects the jaws, and *(2)* the American type, which mostly affects the contents of the abdomen. Although an association with the Epstein-Barr virus is often discussed, only 30% are associated with it, while the *c-MYC* proto-oncogene undergoes deregulation in most cases.

Predilections

Children and early teenagers are mostly affected; 75% of cases occur before age 14 years. The African type is common in equatorial Africa but very uncommon elsewhere. The maxilla is involved twice as often as the mandible. The American type is uncommon everywhere.

Clinical features

1. African type: The African type will present as a destructive, poorly demarcated expansile mass arising from either the maxilla or mandible. Paresthesia is common.
2. American type: An abdominal mass is not usually palpable until late in its staging, and symptoms of pain, nausea, constipation, and vomiting have occurred. Jaw tumors can occur but are rare.

Radiographic presentation

Panoramic radiographs will show an expansile, irregular radiolucency and destruction of surrounding bone. CT scans will show an infiltrating mass growing into soft tissues and adjacent anatomical spaces.

Differential diagnosis

The aggressive African type will resemble a rhabdomyosarcoma, Ewing sarcoma, and osteosarcoma.

Microscopic features

The classic description of a Burkitt lymphoma is that of the "starry sky" appearance. This is caused by dark-staining neoplastic B cells often with mitotic figures coalesced together but separated by light-staining and almost clear macrophages, giving it the appearance of bright stars against a black night sky.

Suggested course of action

Masses in the jaws of such a destructive nature require a biopsy. If feasible, accomplish an incisional biopsy. If not, refer to an oral and maxillofacial surgeon for a biopsy and further workup.

Treatment

Despite the aggressive behavior of Burkitt lymphomas, this childhood malignancy is curable. Surgery is not usually indicated. Instead, multidrug chemotherapy using rituximab, etoposide, and oncovin as the cornerstone drugs has been effective.

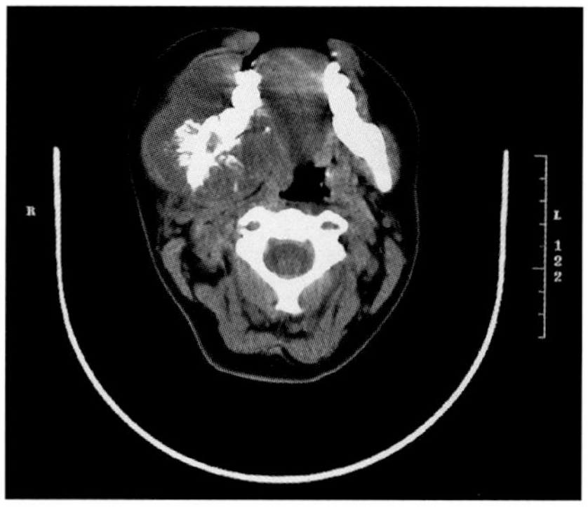

► Ewing sarcoma of the mandible.

Ewing Sarcoma

Nature of disease

A rare and aggressive, genetically and histologically distinct round cell sarcoma of bone. It arises from a specific reciprocal translocation of chromosomes 11 and 22 in bone marrow stem cells referred to as *primitive neuroectodermal tumors* (PNETs).

Predilections

Eighty percent occur before age 20 years. It is rare to almost nonexistent in black individuals of African heritage. There is also a slight predilection for boys.

Clinical features

Ewing sarcoma will present as a fast-growing, destructive bony lesion with mobile teeth and soft tissue necrosis. It is often accompanied by pain, paresthesia, and fever.

Radiographic presentation

Ewing sarcoma will be seen as a significantly osteolytic destructive radiolucency that may resorb tooth roots and produce a sunray-type of extracortical bone. It should be noted that older textbooks often describe an "onionskin" pattern of extracortical bone such as that seen in Garré sclerosing osteomyelitis; however, this is rarely if ever seen in true cases of Ewing sarcoma. Instead, the aggressive destruction produces irregular sequestra and more of the sunray pattern.

Differential diagnosis

The aggressive bony destruction seen in Ewing sarcoma in young individuals may also be seen in Burkitt lymphoma, rhabdomyosarcoma, osteosarcoma, and fibrosarcoma.

Microscopic features

Ewing sarcoma will have uniform round cells densely packed together with little stroma. The nuclei are seen to be round to oval, with a distinct nuclear membrane and finely granular chromatin. Areas of necrosis are common.

Suggested course of action

Refer to a cancer center or hematologist/oncologist for workup and treatment. If a biopsy is required, refer to an oral and maxillofacial surgeon.

Treatment

Ewing sarcomas are treated with multimodal therapy, usually starting with extirpative surgery followed by chemotherapy (commonly etoposide and ifosfamide for 6 to 12 months) and then radiation therapy of 5,000 to 6,000 cGy.

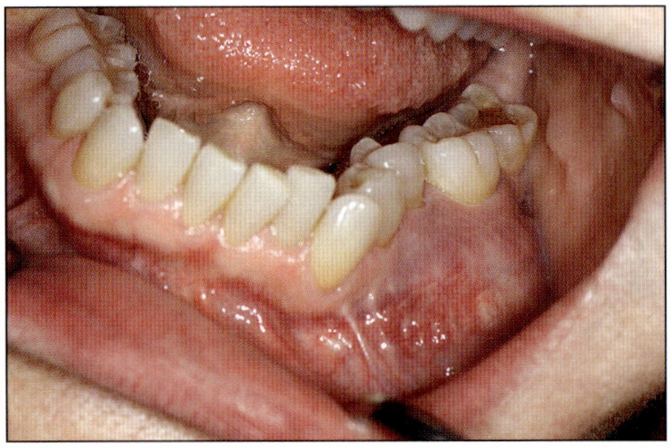

► Neurosarcoma of the mandible.

Neurosarcoma

Nature of disease

A rare malignancy of peripheral nerve sheath cells (ie, Schwann cells and neurofibroblasts) associated with mutations on chromosomes that affect the production and function of the p53 tumor suppressor protein. A rare variant that has rhabdomyoblast features and is even more highly malignant is known as the "triton tumor" because it is known to grow in the Triton salamander.

Predilections

Some occur in the normal population, but most occur as a transformation of a benign neurofibroma in hereditary neurofibromatosis type 1. In those with hereditary neurofibromatosis type I who also have the 17p mutation, it is inherited as an autosomal dominant trait. There is no known sex or racial predilection. The tumor itself is more common in the extremities.

Clinical features

In the jaws and head and neck, it will present as either an expansile and destructive mass within and emerging from bone or a similar soft tissue mass fixed to surrounding tissues.

Radiographic presentation

Those arising from bone will be seen as a diffuse irregular radiolucency with the ability to displace teeth and resorb roots on panoramic radiographs. CT scans will identify infiltration into adjacent areas of either soft tissue or bone.

Differential diagnosis

Neurosarcomas are sufficiently rare so that they are not included on a differential list. Other more common malignancies such as osteosarcomas, fibrosarcomas, rhabdomyosarcomas, and even oral squamous cell carcinoma are to be considered.

Microscopic features

Neurosarcomas will be seen as spindle-cell neoplasms infiltrating normal tissues. Mitotic figures will be numerous. Occasionally, a palisading pattern may be seen reminiscent of a benign schwannoma.

Suggested course of action

Refer to an oral and maxillofacial surgeon for a biopsy and workup or to a regional cancer center.

Treatment

Resection of the tumor observing 3.0-cm margins in bone and/or soft tissue. Immediate reconstruction is often provided, and adjunctive radiation therapy is considered.

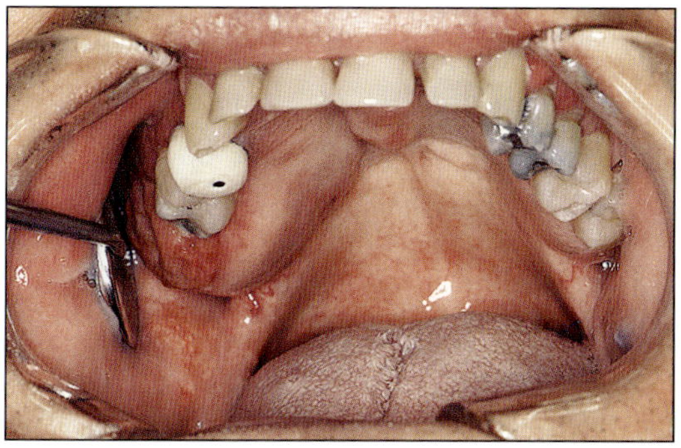

► Clinical view of a fibrosarcoma.

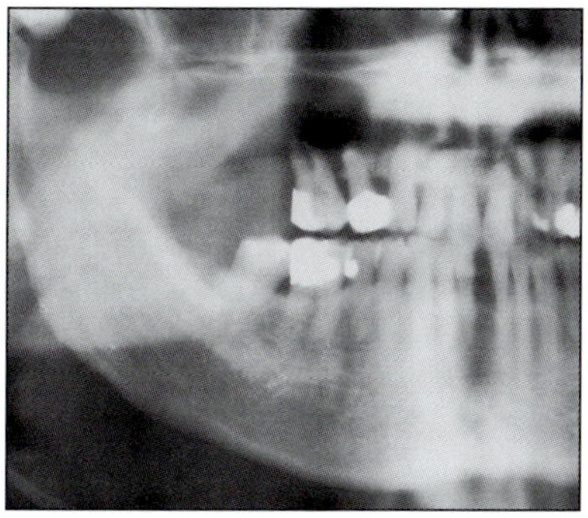

► Extensive osteolysis from a grade 3 fibrosarcoma.

Fibrosarcoma

Nature of disease

A malignant proliferation of mesenchymal stem cells and/or fibroblast precursors that partially differentiate into still-immature fibroblasts.

Predilections

A slight predilection for young adults. No sex or racial predilection is known.

Clinical features

Fibrosarcomas will present as fleshy to firm soft tissue masses adherent to and intertwined with adjacent tissues. If the tumor invades into bone or arises as a central fibrosarcoma, tooth mobility is likely. The mass is not painful unless biting trauma or secondary infection from ulcerations occurs.

Radiographic presentation

If the fibrosarcoma is limited to soft tissue, no radiographic features will be seen. If it invades into bone from thc soft tissue or arises centrally from bone, an irregular osteolysis will be seen with a variable extent, up to a pathologic fracture in some cases.

Differential diagnosis

Aggressive fibromatosis and nodular fasciitis are considerations in children, teenagers, and young adults, as are osteosarcomas and Ewing sarcoma. In older adults, squamous cell carcinoma and a metastatic deposit to the jaws should be considered.

Microscopic features

Fibrosarcomas are spindle cell neoplasms; depending on their grade, they may show a small amount of collagen production or none at all. Well-differentiated tumors will often show a herringbone pattern and will have only a few mitotic figures. Less-differentiated tumors have less collagen (and sometimes none) and a greater number of mitotic figures.

Suggested course of action

Referral to an oral and maxillofacial surgeon or a cancer center for biopsy, workup, and treatment.

Treatment

Fibrosarcomas are treated with soft tissue and bony resection if bone is involved, observing 2.0-cm margins controlled by frozen sections (for soft tissue). Neck dissection is not usually required.

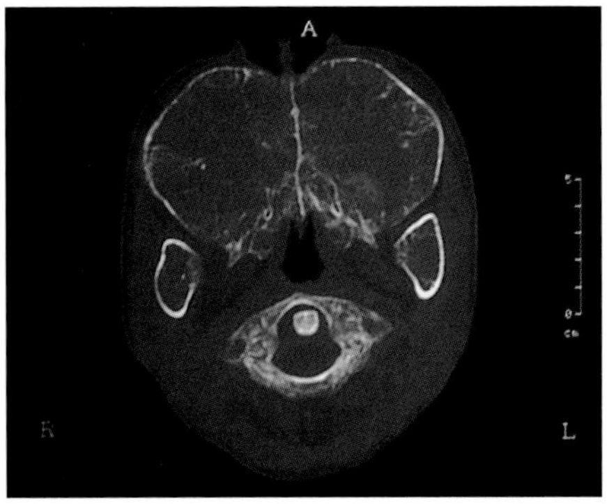

► Extreme expansion of the maxilla due to active hematopoiesis in beta thalassemia intermedia.

Beta Thalassemia Intermedia or Major

Nature of disease

A point mutation in the beta globin chain of hemoglobin A resulting in misshapen red blood cells with fragile cell membranes. The red blood cells are thus prone to rupture and loss of hemoglobin (hemolysis).

Predilections

Clinical signs begin early in life, around age 2 to 5 years. Males and females are affected equally, with no racial predilection.

Clinical features

The individual will present to the dental team with a generally short stature and symmetric expansion of the maxilla and mandible. Hepatosplenomegaly will be apparent. The teeth may be mobile and displaced, corresponding to the expanded bone. These features are caused by extramedullary hematopoiesis as the body uses other marrow spaces and organs to keep pace with the continual loss of red blood cells.

Laboratory values will show a severe microcytic, hypochromic anemia with hemoglobins in the range of 6 to 10 mg/dL and depressed Wintrobe indices. The patient's urine will be tea-colored due to hemoglobinuria.

Radiographic presentation

Panoramic radiographs will show symmetric jaw expansion of both jaws with a diffuse ground-glass picture. A chest radiograph will reveal cardiomegaly. CT scans will confirm a symmetric jaw expansion but will also identify a severely thinned cortex with very fine trabeculations in the marrow space. CT scans will also show involvement of all the bones in the volume scanned, noting a thickening and foggy pattern. In the calvarium, fine trabeculations involving the outer table will provide a "hair on end" pattern.

Differential diagnosis

Similar jaw expansions of a significant degree can be seen in cherubism, fibrous dysplasia, and Ramon syndrome. The radiographic pattern can also be seen in other severe anemias such as homozygous sickle cell anemia and hereditary spherocytosis.

Microscopic features

Blood smears will show deformed and ruptured red blood cells. ⟶

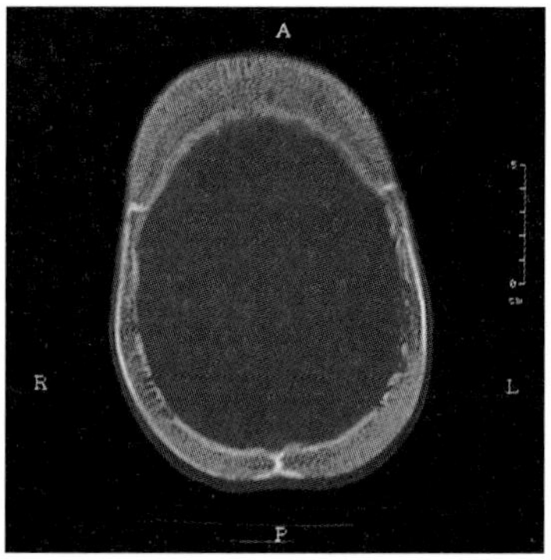

► Cranial expansion and "hair on end" effect from beta thalassemia intermedia.

Suggested course of action

Suspected cases should be referred to a hematologist. Restorative dentistry can be accomplished once the thalassemia is reasonably controlled. However, invasive procedures such as periodontal surgeries and oral surgery are best accomplished in a hospital setting.

Treatment

Patients with beta thalassemia require regular blood transfusions (one to three units per month). They also must have the extra iron that is spilled out from the ruptured red blood cells eliminated; this requires chelation with deferoxamine (Desferal, Novartis).

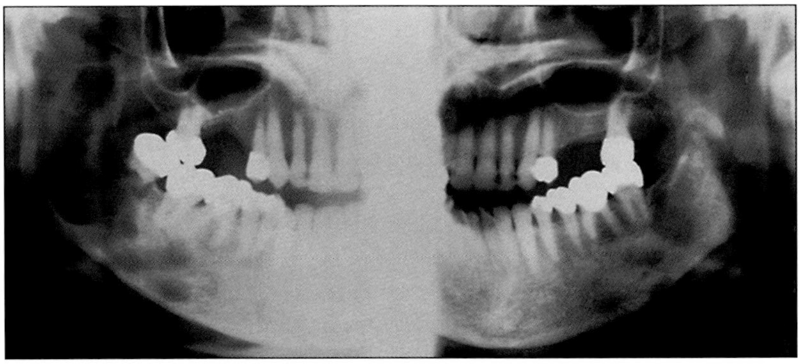

► Multiple radiolucencies in the mandible from multiple myeloma.

Multiple Myeloma and Plasma Cell Dyscrasias

Nature of disease

A monoclonal neoplastic proliferation of plasma cells that involves multiple bone marrow sites. Occasionally, extraskeletal sites are involved or only a single bone is involved, in which case it is termed a *plasmacytoma*. The specific oncogene seems to result from a translocation of chromosomes t(11:14).

Predilections

Men are slightly more affected than women, and 90% of cases develop after 40 years of age. Black individuals are slightly more affected than white individuals.

Clinical features

Otherwise healthy patients may have abnormal laboratory studies leading to the diagnosis. Others may express weakness or fatigue from secondary anemia, hypercalcemia, or bone pain from multiple lytic lesions. There is an accepted tetrad of possible clinical and laboratory findings that lead to a diagnosis of multiple myeloma:

1. Multifocal osteolytic lesions
2. Proliferation of atypical plasma cells in these osteolytic lesions
3. Serum studies identifying a specific immunoglobulin (Ig) increase (IgM, IgA, IgE, or IgG) termed a *monoclonal gammopathy.*
4. Polymerase chain reaction identifying gene rearrangement

Note: Plasmacytomas will not have all four of these systemic features. Instead, they will present as a large soft tissue mass protruding from bone. The lesion itself will contain neoplastic plasma cells and have gene rearrangement, but it will not secrete an Ig component or be multifocal.

Radiographic presentation

Classic "punched out" osteolytic lesions can be found in any skeletal site. The skull, ribs, pelvis, and vertebrae are common locations. In the jaws, the rami and posterior body of the mandible are often involved. The rare plasmacytoma will appear as a large (2- to 6-cm), unilocular, expansile radiolucency.

Differential diagnosis

The main differential diagnosis centers around the specific myeloma protein (ie, IgG, IgA, IgM, or IgE). However, other diseases that are known to produce osteolytic lesions in multiple bony sites include primary hyperparathyroidism, metastatic small cell lung cancer, and Langerhans cell histiocytosis.

⟶

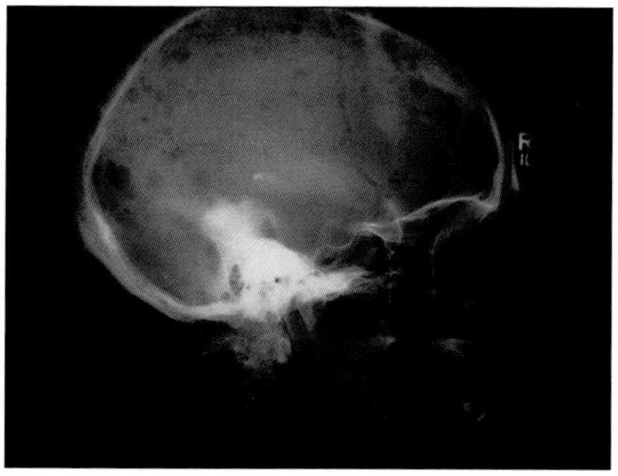

► Classic "punched out" radiolucencies in the skull from multiple myeloma.

Microscopic features

Light microscopic slides will show a monotony of identical-appearing plasma cells with almost no stroma.

Suggested course of action

Suspicious cases are best referred to a hematologist/oncologist for workup and treatment. If a biopsy of jaw lesions is required, refer to an oral and maxillofacial surgeon.

Treatment

Multiple myeloma today is treated with a variety of chemotherapy agents, such as bortezomib and lenalidomide, as well as stem cell transplants from filtering peripheral blood and bone marrow transplants. The dental practitioner needs to begin a preventive dental program of prophylaxis, caries control, and periodontal maintenance and needs to be aware that prednisone and/or zoledronate is often used together with these regimens, placing the patient at risk for drug-induced osteonecrosis of the jaws.

Sickle Cell Anemia

Nature of disease

Sickle cell anemia is an autosomal recessive trait that causes a point mutation in a single position on the beta hemoglobin chain. The mutation substitutes the amino acid valine for the normal glutamine in the sixth position on the chain. Therefore, affected patients have abnormal hemoglobin commonly called *hemoglobin S*. This causes a misshapen and fragile red blood cell that results in a chronic anemia and episodes of crisis triggered by hypoxemia, which creates sludging, intravascular clots, and therefore tissue ischemia and necrosis.

Predilections

Almost exclusive to black individuals of African heritage. The *hemoglobin S* gene is thought to be present in 81% of black people. No sex predilection is known.

Clinical features

Heterozygous individuals are clinically normal but can progress into a crisis mode during strenuous periods, causing hypoxemia. Homozygous individuals will be of short stature, weak, and will often need walking aids or wheelchairs due to bleeding into their joints, with later fibrosis or ischemic bone necrosis. Tooth eruption is often delayed, and the teeth may be dysplastic or underdeveloped. Temporomandibular joint (TMJ) ankylosis causing an open bite deformity may also be present.

Radiographic presentation

Heterozygous individuals will have normal radiographs. Homozygous individuals may show a destroyed TMJ or areas of osteolysis with bony sequestra. Unerupted teeth and teeth with short roots are often noted. CT scans will show vertical extracortical bone formation and a thickened calvarium, creating the "hair on end" appearance. Other bones will show a thickened cortex and some sclerosis.

Differential diagnosis

Homozygous sickle cell anemia is distinctive by the many signs, symptoms, and laboratory values. However, clinically, the initial presentation may suggest beta thalassemia or either acute lymphocytic leukemia or acute myelogenous leukemia.

Microscopic features

Blood smears will show misshapen red blood cells of various sizes (anisocytosis). →

Suggested course of action

Heterozygous individuals (sickle cell trait) can be treated as any other patient in regard to their dental needs. The availability of supplemental oxygen is advised but rarely needed. Procedures involving intravenous sedation should have ongoing supplemental oxygen available and should be fully monitored. Homozygous individuals require shorter procedure appointments, preventive dental and hygiene care, and restorative dentistry. Extractions and other oral surgery procedures are best referred to an oral and maxillofacial surgeon and are usually accomplished in a hospital setting.

Treatment

There is no cure for homozygous sickle cell anemia. Supportive care is needed in the form of blood transfusions, folate and vitamin B12 supplements, and avoidance of hypoxic conditions. The pneumococcal vaccine is highly recommended for these individuals.

7

Radiopaque and Mixed Radiolucent-Radiopaque Lesions

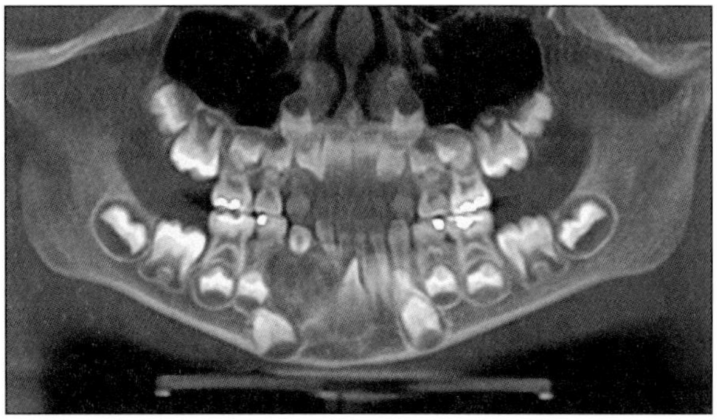

► Ossifying fibroma.

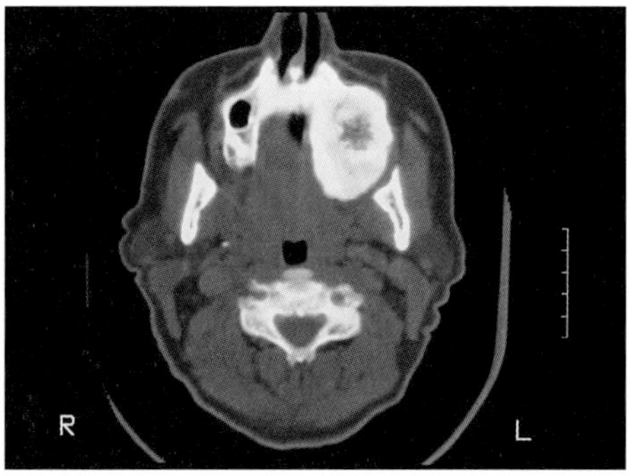

► Ossifying fibroma appearance on a CT scan.

Ossifying Fibroma

Nature of disease

A benign neoplasm of primitive fibroblasts that shows both fibroblastic and osteoblastic differentiation, producing both collagen and bone.

Predilections

Occurs in all bones but is much more common in the jaws due to the presence of teeth and the cementum-bone interaction, giving rise to the term *cemento-ossifying fibroma* when it occurs in the tooth-bearing areas of the jaws. Moderate predilection for children and young adults but can occur at any age. There is no sex or racial predilection. Note that it is known to develop from another bony disease such as fibrous dysplasia or cemento-osseous dysplasia.

Clinical features

A firm to hard expansion of bone with an intact overlying mucosa. Paresthesia or anesthesia is absent. Unerupted teeth and erupted teeth are often displaced.

Radiographic presentation

A round to oval mixed radiolucent-radiopaque mass with distinct borders and a thinned but identifiable cortex. There is no formation of extracortical bone. In early cases, the lesion may be totally radiolucent. Note: Ossifying fibromas are often confused with or misdiagnosed as fibrous dysplasia. These radiographic features should distinguish ossifying fibromas from fibrous dysplasia.

Differential diagnosis

Oval partially radiopaque masses are seen with osteoblastomas, ameloblastic fibro-odontomas, developing odontomas, and osteosarcoma.

Microscopic features

A benign but neoplastic fibroblastic stroma with deep basophilic staining together with islands of bone with regular and blunted edges. Scattered to rare osteoclasts may also be seen. If the biopsy included soft tissue, a capsule will be noted; otherwise, the neoplastic cells and bone are seen to interdigitate into normal bone without a capsule.

Suggested course of action

Incisional biopsy and/or referral to an oral and maxillofacial surgeon.

Treatment

Resection observing 0.5-cm margins in bone and a pericapsular dissection in soft tissues.

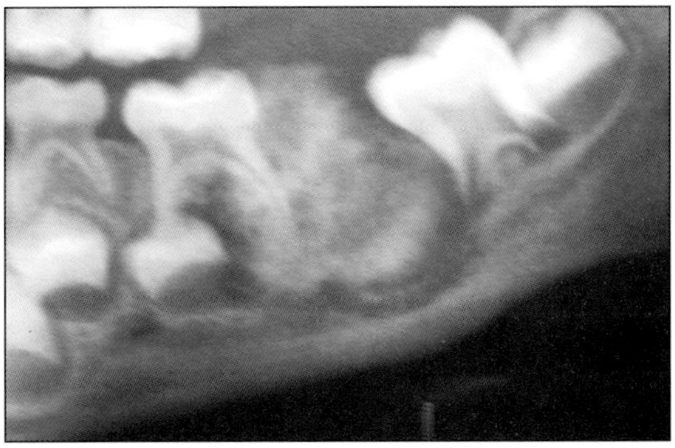

► Osteoblastoma.

Osteoblastoma/Osteoid Osteomas

Nature of disease

These two names describe the same disease, which is a benign neoplastic proliferation of osteoblasts.

Predilections

Strong predilection for teenagers and young adults. Most common in males. No racial predilection is known.

Clinical features

A firm to hard expansion of the involved area frequently associated with a dull but deep pain. The overlying mucosa is intact. Teeth may be mobile and/or displaced. Paresthesia or anesthesia is not reported.

Radiographic presentation

Depending on their duration and size, osteoblastomas may be seen as well-delineated mixed radiolucent-radiopaque lesions or may be completely radiopaque. The mandibular canal may be displaced. Teeth may also be displaced and roots partially resorbed.

Differential diagnosis

Ossifying fibromas are the main lesion to be considered. Others include a developing odontoma, an ameloblastic fibroma, and a calcifying odontogenic cyst.

Microscopic features

Irregular trabecular bone is seen to arise from plump, dark-staining osteoblasts rimming its surface. The stroma is composed of loosely arranged collagen with numerous small blood vessels. A fibrous capsule is variably present.

Suggested course of action

Exploration and bone biopsy and/or referral to an oral and maxillofacial surgeon.

Treatment

Peripheral resection observing 0.5-cm margins.

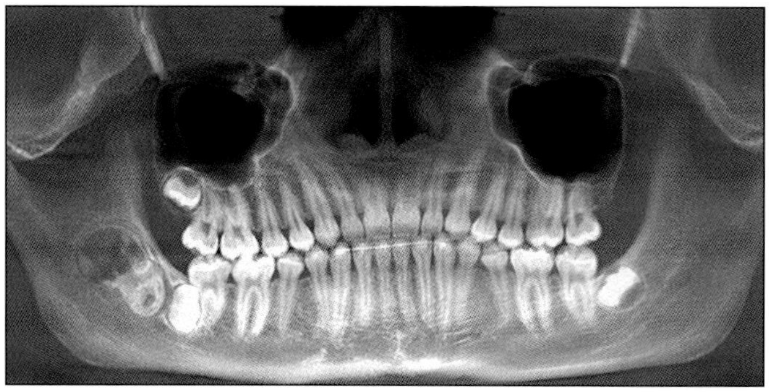

► Ameloblastic fibro-odontoma as seen on a panoramic radiograph.

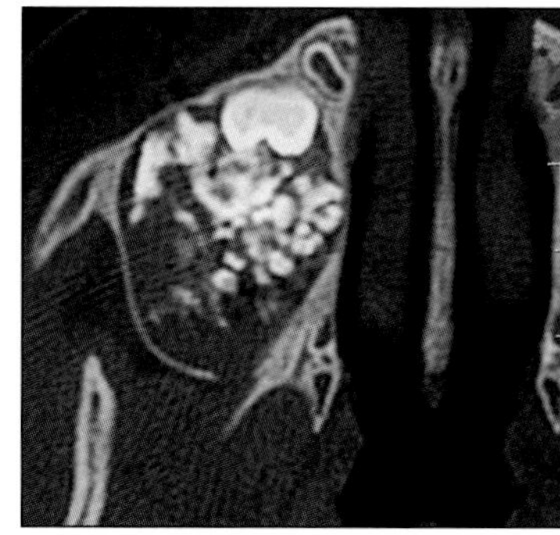

► Large ameloblastic fibro-odontoma as seen on a CT scan.

Ameloblastic Fibro-odontoma

Nature of disease

An aborted attempt at tooth formation representing a hamartomatous proliferation of ameloblasts, stellate reticulum, and incompletely formed dentin.

Predilections

Mostly seen in children and teenagers. No sex or racial predilection is known.

Clinical features

Most are an asymptomatic incidental radiographic finding. A fewer number present as a painless, hard bony expansion. An anticipated tooth is often clinically absent.

Radiographic presentation

A mixed radiolucent but mostly radiopaque mass is seen within the alveolar bone. The mass is of greater density than the surrounding bone and is well delineated from the bone. The adjacent cortices may be expanded and thin.

Differential diagnosis

The density of the dentin within an ameloblastic fibro-odontoma as seen on radiographs will strongly suggest a complex odontoma. Other considerations may include mature and well-mineralized osteoblastomas, ossifying fibromas, or calcifying odontogenic cysts.

Microscopic features

Part of the lesion will identify cords and islands of ameloblasts with a center of stellate reticulum within a very loose arrangement of gray- to blue-staining odontogenic mesenchyme absent of any eosinophilic collagen. This portion is identical to an ameloblastic fibroma. However, within and around this soft tissue component will be dense areas of eosinophil-stained dentin in which columnar odontoblasts and dentinal tubules may be discerned.

Suggested course of action

Exploration and enucleation of the mass or referral to an oral and maxillofacial surgeon.

Treatment

Exploration and enucleation of the mass, which will be readily separated from bone.

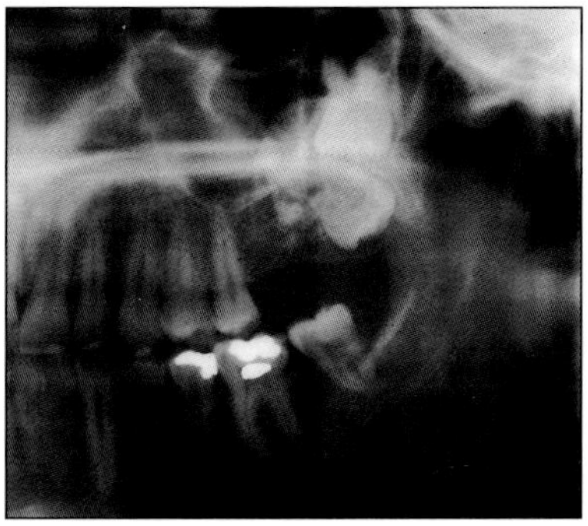

► Complex odontoma.

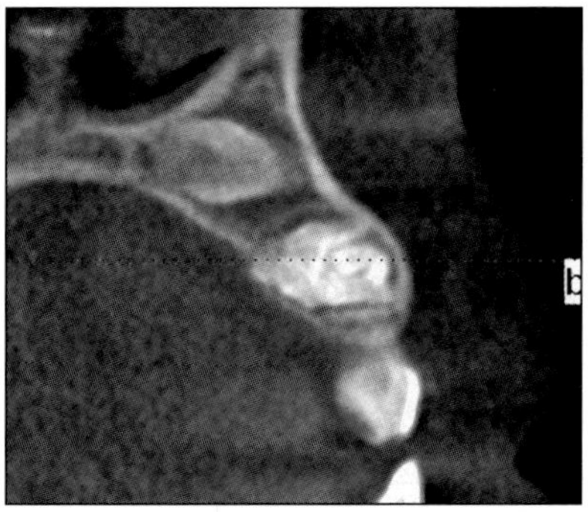

► Compound odontoma.

Odontomas

Nature of disease

A *complex odontoma* is an aborted attempt at tooth formation representing a hamartomatous overproduction of dentin. A *compound odontoma* is a dysregulated attempt at tooth formation in which multiple smaller or incomplete teeth are formed in place of an anticipated tooth or as an extra focus of odontogenesis.

Predilections

Mostly seen in teenagers and young adults, with a slight male predilection. There is no racial predilection.

Clinical features

Most are asymptomatic incidental radiographic findings. Less commonly, a slight bony expansion with an intact overlying mucosa is observed. Some are associated with the absence of an anticipated tooth.

Radiographic presentation

- A complex odontoma will appear as an irregular, dense, poorly delineated mass within the alveolar bone. Large ones may extend into the maxillary sinus or into the basilar bone of the mandible. The relative density will be much greater than that of the surrounding bone.
- Compound odontomas will appear to have more than one and oftentimes multiple small teeth with a single root resembling the morphology of a premolar. The mass will be well delineated from the surrounding bone.

Differential diagnosis

- A complex odontoma will appear similar to an osteoblastoma or a very heavily mineralized ossifying fibroma. A cementoblastoma and focal cemento-osseous dysplasia may also be considered.
- Compound odontomas are radiographically distinct.

Microscopic features

- Complex odontomas will be almost entirely comprised of dentin with dentinal tubules and rare odontoblasts.
- Compound odontomas will be seen as complete, albeit small, teeth with enamel, dentin, and pulp.

Suggested course of action

Exploration and enucleation or referral to an oral and maxillofacial surgeon.

Treatment

Exploration and enucleation of the mass. Compound odontomas will readily separate from a crypt with bone. Complex odontomas also readily separate from surrounding bone but may be undercut by adjacent bone, impairing the delivery of the hard mass.

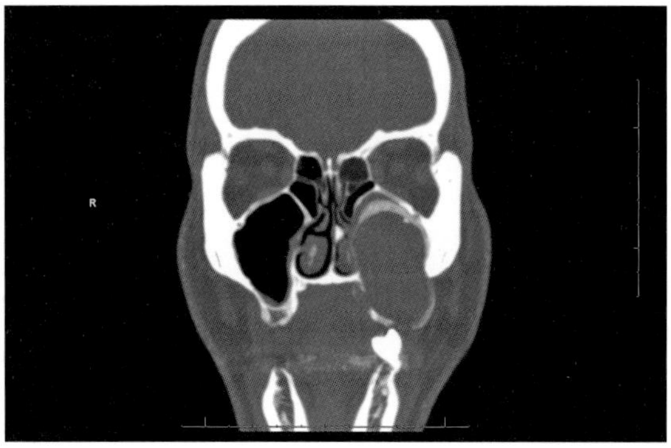

► Calcifying odontogenic cyst.

Calcifying Odontogenic Cyst

Nature of disease

A pathologic cavity lined by epithelium that uniquely produces calcifications and keratinizations within the lining.

Predilections

No age, sex, or racial predilection is known. Occurs more commonly in the premolar regions.

Clinical features

Usually an asymptomatic expansile lesion with an intact overlying mucosa. Many will present as an incidental radiographic finding. Paresthesias and anesthesia are absent. In some cases, tooth displacement and/or tooth mobility will be present.

Radiographic presentation

While some will be a completely radiolucent unilocular lesion, most will show calcifications best seen on a cone beam CT scan in one of two general patterns. The most common pattern is a ring or crescent moon–shaped layer of calcification at the periphery of the radiolucency. The other pattern is one of scattered flecks of calcifications. Almost all are primordial cysts unassociated with an unerupted tooth but will displace other unerupted teeth as well as erupted teeth.

Differential diagnosis

Other unilocular radiolucencies known to be seen with calcifications include the adenomatoid odontogenic cyst, the desmoplastic ameloblastoma, ossifying fibroma, and some osteoblastomas and calcifying epithelial odontogenic tumors.

Microscopic features

This cyst has a unique lining beginning with the basal cell layer, which is cuboidal to columnar and exhibits reverse polarization (ie, nuclei at a distance from the basement membrane) similar to that of an ameloblastoma. The squamous epithelium protrudes into the lumen and contains large, pale vacuolated cells (ghost cells) and focal areas of keratinization. Throughout this layer, focal areas of eosinophil-stained calcifications are seen as well. The connective tissue cyst wall is usually thicker than those of dentigerous cysts.

Suggested course of action

Aspiration, exploration, and incisional biopsy and/or referral to an oral and maxillofacial surgeon.

Treatment

Enucleation and curettage.

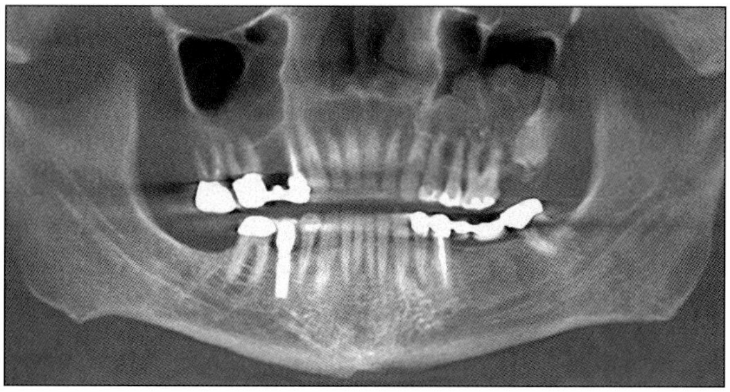

► Calcifying epithelial odontogenic tumor.

Calcifying Epithelial Odontogenic Tumor

Nature of disease

A true but slowly growing odontogenic neoplasm thought to arise from cells of the stellate reticulum.

Predilections

Mostly adults. There is no known sex or racial predilection.

Clinical features

An asymptomatic expansile mass. Paresthesia and anesthesia are absent. The mucosa is intact, but erupted teeth may be displaced or absent.

Radiographic presentation

Although most will present as a multilocular mixed radiolucent-radiopaque lesion, some (usually smaller ones) will be unilocular. Tooth displacement, root resorption, and absence of anticipated teeth may be present.

Differential diagnosis

The less common unilocular presentation of a calcifying epithelial odontogenic tumor will be similar to a calcifying odontogenic cyst, an adenomatoid odontogenic cyst, and an ossifying fibroma. The more common multilocular ones will be similar to a desmoplastic ameloblastoma and some osteosarcomas.

Microscopic features

This tumor consists of sheets, cords, and nests of cells with prominent nuclear pleomorphism, suggesting that it is more aggressive or that it is a more dedifferentiated tumor than is noted clinically. There may also be sheets of clear-staining cells. The eosinophilic calcifications seen throughout are in concentric rings like those seen in trees and are referred to as *Liesegang rings*. Deposits of amyloid are seen throughout and can be highlighted by congo red–staining or thioflavin T fluorescence.

Suggested course of action

Exploration and incisional biopsy and/or referral to an oral and maxillofacial surgeon.

Treatment

Resection observing 1.0- to 1.5-cm margins.

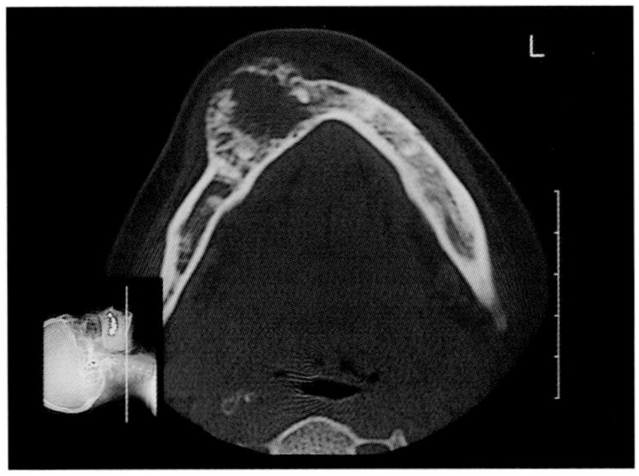

► Desmoplastic ameloblastoma.

Desmoplastic Ameloblastoma

Nature of disease

An uncommon and unique variant of an ameloblastoma that induces a dense deposition of collagen, which undergoes dystrophic calcifications in scattered areas.

Predilections

Mostly adults. There is no known sex or racial predilection.

Clinical features

An asymptomatic expansile mass with an intact overlying mucosa. Tooth displacement and the absence of anticipated teeth are common. Paresthesia or anesthesia is not observed.

Radiographic presentation

A mixed radiolucent-radiopaque expansile mass with irregular borders is common. The calcifications are indistinct and provide a somewhat uniform hazy appearance. Teeth and the mandibular canal may be displaced as well as the floor of the maxillary sinus when it occurs in the maxilla. Root resorption may also be seen.

Differential diagnosis

The diffuse radiopacity and indistinct borders are similar to a calcifying epithelial odontogenic tumor or even fibrous dysplasia. Other considerations include ossifying fibromas, osteoblastomas, and even an osteosarcoma.

Microscopic features

This tumor will be mostly composed of dense acellular collagen in which cords and nests of odontogenic cuboidal and low columnar cells with reverse polarization will be noted.

Suggested course of action

Exploration and incisional biopsy and/or referral to an oral and maxillofacial surgeon.

Treatment

Resection observing 1.0- to 1.5-cm margins.

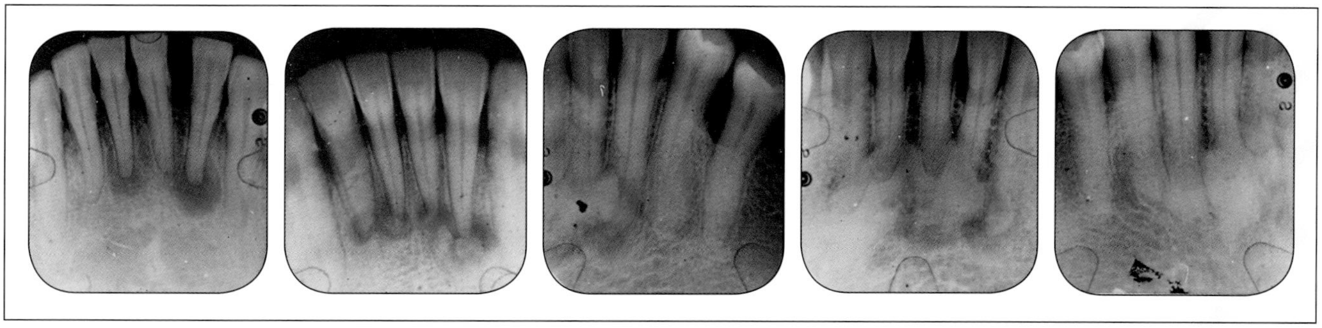

► The progression of periapical cemental dysplasia.

Periapical Cemental Dysplasia

Nature of disease

A genetically driven dysmorphogenesis of the cementum–periodontal ligament–lamina dura complex.

Predilections

Almost all occur in adult women of black African heritage. Known to occur in the mandibular anterior incisor-canine area.

Clinical features

Mostly an asymptomatic incidental radiographic finding. Uncommon cases may report dull pain or a slight expansion in the anterior mandibular vestibule. Teeth will be vital to pulp testing unless nonvital from an unrelated cause.

Radiographic presentation

Periapical cemental dysplasia is limited to the mandibular anterior six teeth and known to develop in three phases—phase I: an apical radiolucency; phase II: an apical mixed radiolucent-radiopaque lesion; phase III: a predominantly radiopaque apical lesion. However, many are seen with different anterior teeth in various stages of this maturity.

Differential diagnosis

In the radiolucent phase, these lesions may closely resemble apical periodontitis or an apical cyst. As they mature, florid cemento-osseous dysplasia and periapical hypercementosis may be considered, as well as condensing osteitis.

Microscopic features

Few are biopsied. However, the lesion is seen to have cells resembling cementoblasts/osteoblasts forming and rimming a dense irregular bone (or perhaps cementum) island.

Suggested course of action

Pulp test the associated teeth. Document the findings and preserve the radiographs. Follow the patient with serial radiographs.

Treatment

No treatment. A concerted effort should be made to avoid unnecessary root canal treatments or extractions.

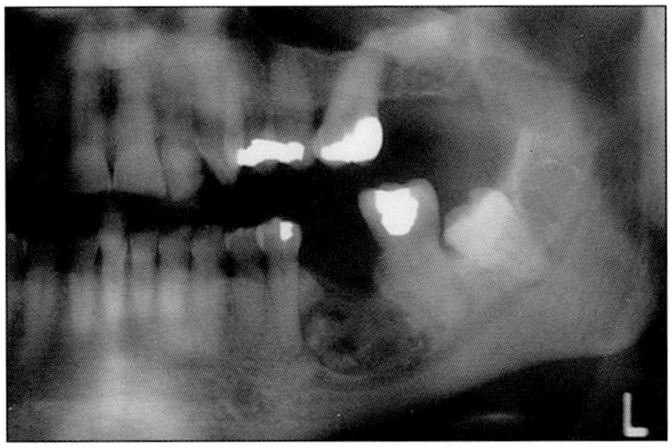

► Focal cemento-osseous dysplasia.

Focal Cemento-osseous Dysplasia

Nature of disease

A genetically driven dysmorphogenesis of the cementum–periodontal ligament–lamina dura complex.

Predilections

Seen almost exclusively in adult women of black African heritage. Associated with mandibular premolar and molar teeth.

Clinical features

Most are asymptomatic incidental radiographic findings. Less commonly, dull tooth or bone pain is reported or there is a slight expansion in the vestibule around the involved area.

Radiographic presentation

As with periapical cemental dysplasia, an apical lesion develops that progresses through three phases—phase I: an apical radiolucency; phase II: a mixed radiolucent-radiopaque apical lesion; phase III: a predominantly radiopaque apical lesion. In focal cemento-osseous dysplasia, only one or at most two teeth are involved, usually premolar or molar teeth.

Differential diagnosis

Depending on the stage of maturity, cemento-osseous dysplasia may resemble different lesions. In the radiolucent phase, apical periodontitis and various cysts such as odontogenic keratocysts and lateral periodontal cysts may be considered. However, in its phase II and phase III presentations, calcifying odontogenic cysts, ossifying fibromas, cementoblastomas, odontomas, and osteoblastomas are considerations.

Microscopic features

Plump cells with dark-staining nuclei are seen in sheets and lining islands of dense bone (or perhaps cementum). In some cases, inflammatory cells may be seen with the lesion.

Suggested course of action

Pulp test the associated tooth/teeth. Perform an exploration and remove the lesion to rule out the more serious pathologies on the differential diagnosis, and/or refer to an oral and maxillofacial surgeon.

Treatment

Removal of the lesion via curettage to establish a diagnosis and rule out more concerning pathologies.

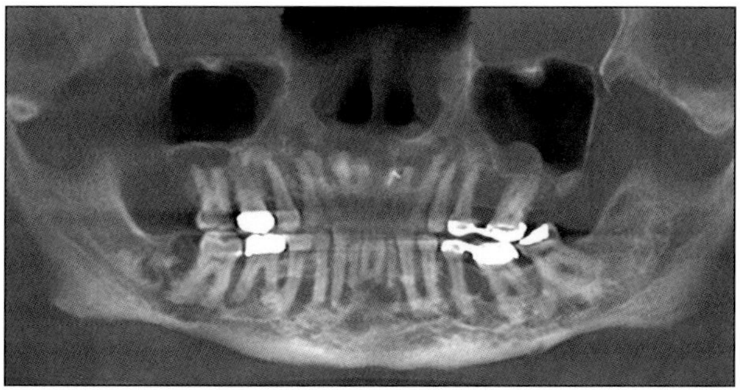

► Florid cemento-osseous dysplasia in a dentate individual.

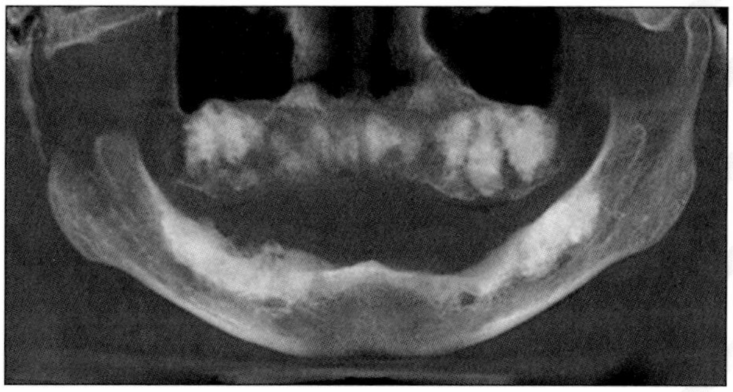

► Florid cemento-osseous dysplasia in an edentulous patient.

Florid Cemento-osseous Dysplasia

Nature of disease

A genetically driven dysmorphogenesis of the cementum–periodontal ligament–lamina dura complex.

Predilections

Almost exclusively involves adult women of black African heritage. Very rare cases may involve men.

Clinical features

Most present as an asymptomatic incidental radiographic finding. However, others may present with expansion and dull pain. Still others may present with exposed alveolar bone from a recent extraction. In those patients who report pain, either the lesion is in its initial radiolucent active phase, or secondary infection has resulted via either a pulpal route, a periodontal route, or exposed bone from an extraction.

Radiographic presentation

Like periapical cemental dysplasia and focal cemento-osseous dysplasia, florid cemento-osseous dysplasia may be seen in any of three phases from radiolucent to mixed radiolucent-radiopaque to nearly completely radiopaque. All four quadrants are involved in each phase, more overtly in the mandible than in the maxilla. The involvement is usually limited to the alveolar bone but on occasion may be seen to extend to the inferior border or the maxillary sinus if secondarily infected. On rare occasions, a large, round radiopaque mass is seen to grow out of an existing florid cemento-osseous dysplasia. This is usually an ossifying fibroma/cemento-ossifying fibroma.

Differential diagnosis

Florid cemento-osseous dysplasia is radiographically and racially distinct so that few pathologies other than periapical cemental dysplasia, focal cemento-osseous dysplasia, and Paget disease may be considered.

Microscopic features

Dense acellular bone is prominent. In some cases, inflammatory cells are also seen as well as rare plump cells suggestive of osteoblasts (perhaps cementoblasts).

Suggested course of action

Accomplish comprehensive preventive and restorative dentistry so as to avoid extraction of teeth, which frequently creates a nonhealing extraction socket and secondary infection.

Treatment

Elective dentoalveolar surgery risks bone exposure and secondary infection and is therefore avoided if possible. In those cases of pain and/or secondary infection, surgical removal of the involved bone is necessary. Note: Bone that regenerates in such defects is normal bone. Grafts in these defects also regenerate normal bone.

Odontoameloblastoma

Nature of disease

An extremely rare simultaneous occurrence of an odontoma and an ameloblastoma sometimes referred to as a "collision tumor."

Predilections

Occurs mostly in teenagers and younger adults. There is no sex or racial predilection.

Clinical features

A painless expansile mass with an intact overlying mucosa. Displacement of erupted or unerupted teeth may be seen as well as the absence of an anticipated tooth.

Radiographic presentation

A radiodense mass with the density of dentin, as in a complex odontoma, or a radiodense mass with small teeth representing a compound odontoma will be seen adjacent to a multilocular radiolucent lesion. The radiolucent component may be seen to displace erupted or unerupted teeth and resorb roots.

Differential diagnosis

The odontoma portion will be radiographically distinct. The radiolucent portion may represent other odontogenic neoplasms or cysts such as an odontogenic myxoma or an odontogenic keratocyst. If the radiolucent component is seen to envelop the odontoma component, a calcifying epithelial odontogenic tumor may also be considered.

Microscopic features

The odontoma component of a complex odontoma will be predominantly dentin with identifiable dentinal tubules. If a compound odontoma is instead present, complete teeth with enamel, dentin, cementum, and pulp will be seen. These components will be mostly separate from the ameloblastoma component but may also be within it. The ameloblastoma will likely be a follicular pattern showing cuboidal to columnar odontogenic epithelial cells with reverse polarization (ie, their nuclei are away from the basement membrane) surrounding islands of stellate reticulum. If the ameloblastoma is of a plexiform pattern, these same odontogenic epithelial cells will be themselves surrounded by stellate reticulum.

Suggested course of action

Exploration and incisional biopsy and/or referral to an oral and maxillofacial surgeon.

Treatment

Odontoameloblastomas are treated as per the neoplastic biology of the ameloblastoma component—that is, a resection observing 1.0- to 1.5-cm margins.

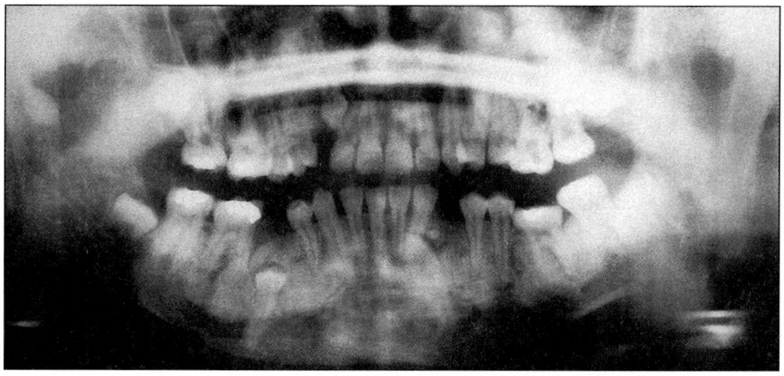

► Osteoma from the condyle and multiple exostoses in Gardner syndrome.

Gardner Syndrome

Nature of disease

An autosomal dominant trait from a mutation in the *adenomatous polyposis coli (APC)* gene on chromosome 5 that causes numerous polyps in mostly the colon, with a very high cancerous transformation along with other manifestations such as osteomas of the jaws and skull, epidermoid cysts, desmoid tumors, and supernumerary teeth.

Predilections

No sex or racial predilection is known. Most cases develop sufficient signs and/or symptoms to be diagnosed in the preteen or early teenage years.

Clinical features

Intestinal polyposis may be asymptomatic. However, cramping, bloody stools, and diarrhea may occur. Osteomas are common and are usually noticed at the inferior border of the mandible as a hard mass or similarly on the skull. Facial, scalp, or extremity epidermoid cysts may be seen as distended skin expansions. Desmoid tumors will be seen as a firm fibrotic mass arising from an aponeurosis or from periosteum.

Radiographic presentation

The common osteomas will be readily apparent on plain radiographs. Osteomas on the mandible will be seen as a teardrop-shaped bony mass attached to a pole of the condyle or hanging from the inferior border. Desmoid tumors are best seen on a CT scan as a soft tissue density arising from a bony surface and creating a resorption of the cortex. Endosteomas in the jaws along with supernumerary teeth are noted on a panoramic radiograph. The intestinal polyps are best seen with CT scans or an MRI scan as broad-based masses arising from the intestinal wall and growing out into the colonic lumen.

Differential diagnosis

A fully expressed Gardner syndrome will be similar to other syndromes associated with colon or small intestinal polyps. Therefore, familial adenomatous polyposis, attenuated adenomatous polyposis, Turcot syndrome, Cowden syndrome, and even Peutz-Jeghers syndrome may be considered. If osteomas are seen by the dental provider without symptoms or knowledge of intestinal polyposis, one may consider florid osseous dysplasia and periapical cemental dysplasia in black women or cleidocranial dysostosis or even tori superimposed on the radiograph in others. →

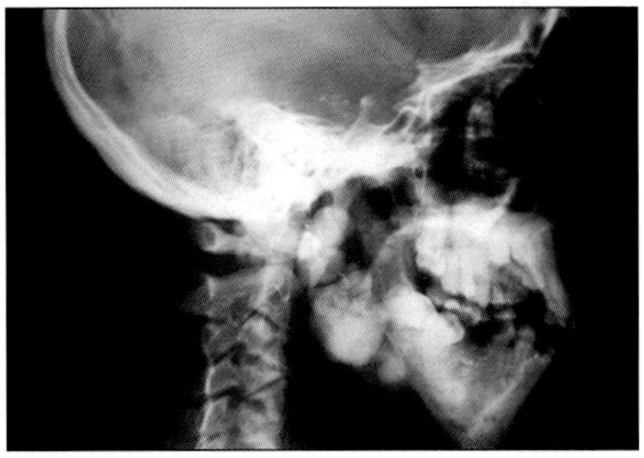

► Osteomas from the inferior border of the mandible in Gardner syndrome.

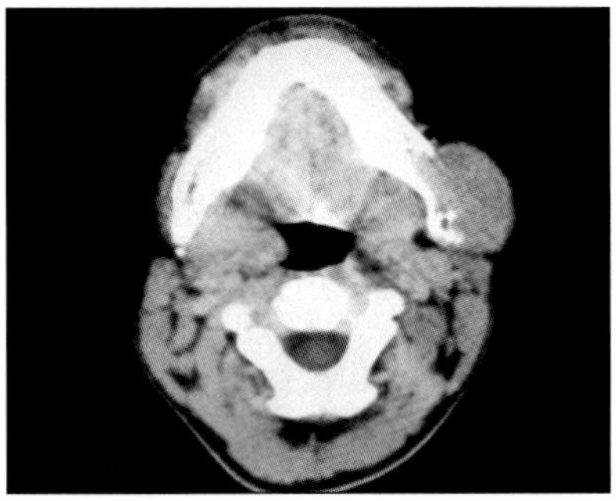

► Desmoid tumor in Gardner syndrome.

Gardner Syndrome *(cont)*

Microscopic features

Intestinal polyps will be villous proliferations of multiple branches into the gut lumen. The common malignant transformation will show atypical mucin-secreting glandular cells invading into the intestinal wall. Epidermoid cysts will show a squamous lined cavity that may be filled with keratin or a sebaceous secretion. Desmoid tumors will show spindle-shaped cells growing between muscle fibers in cords and fascicles. Osteomas will be seen as round to teardrop-shaped collections of mature bone with lamellar architecture and Haversian systems.

Suggested course of action

Any patient in whom a dental practitioner identifies a true osteoma (ie, one at the inferior border or off the condyle) should be referred to a gastroenterologist.

Treatment

A confirmed Gardner syndrome patient will be treated with a prophylactic colectomy due to the nearly 100% malignant transformation rate of their colonic polyps. Once that is accomplished, symptomatic epidermoid cysts and desmoid tumors can be removed. Osteomas may remain but may also be removed if they interfere with function or cause a cosmetic deformity.

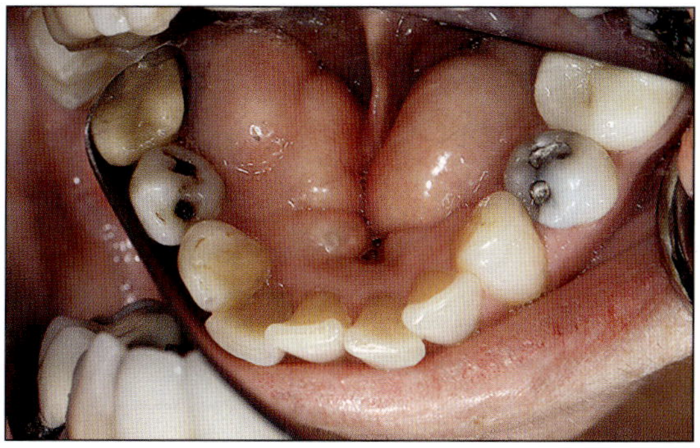

► Multiple large tori in the mandible.

Mandibular and Maxillary Tori/Exostoses

Nature of disease

A benign overgrowth of normal, compact cortical bone arising from a bony surface of the jaws.

Predilections

Adults. No sex or racial predilection is known. Most occur on the lingual surface of the mandible or on the palate. Those less common ones that occur on the buccal surfaces of the mandible or maxilla may be referred to as *exostoses*.

Clinical features

A nontender bony hard expansion covered with a thin overlying mucosa.

Radiographic presentation

Most appear as a radiodense shadowing on panoramic and periapical radiographs. A cone beam CT scan will more clearly identify a broad base of dense bone with an outgrowth and a well-delineated outline.

Differential diagnosis

Tori are usually clinically apparent and distinctive. However, an ossifying fibroma, an osteoblastoma, and a cementoblastoma may appear in a similar manner.

Microscopic features

Dense compact bone with Haversian systems and lamellar architecture lacking a defined cortex and marrow space.

Suggested course of action

Reassure the patient that these growths are a variation of normal bone requiring no treatment unless removal is required to make room for a prosthesis or its large size interferes with function. Note: The surface of tori remodel somewhat rapidly, which makes them a vulnerable site for drug-induced osteonecrosis of the jaws.

Treatment

None required except to facilitate a prosthodontic treatment plan or to remove an encumbrance to function.

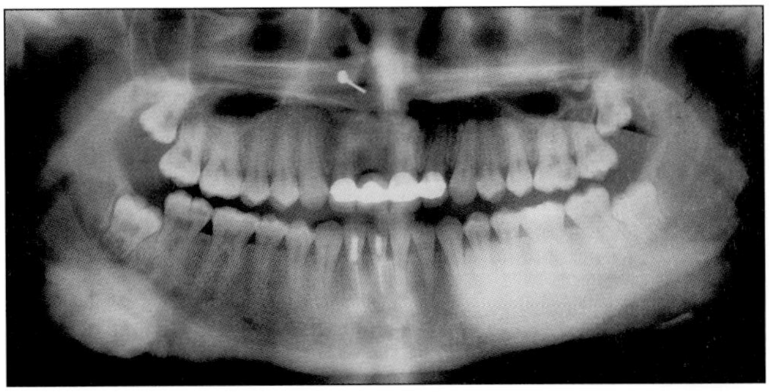

► Osteosarcoma of the mandible as seen on a panoramic radiograph.

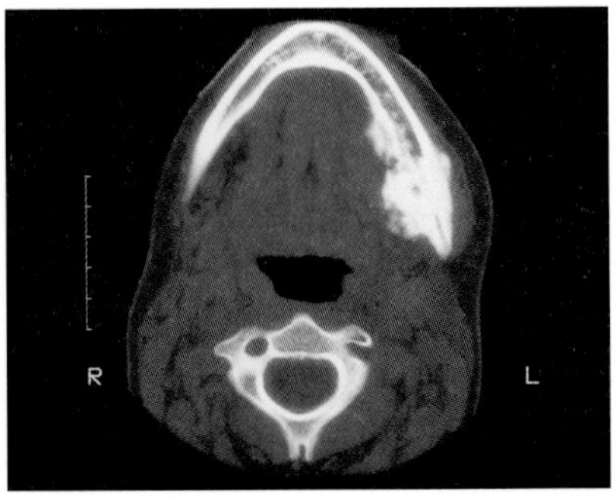

► Osteosarcoma of the mandible with irregular cortex and jagged extracortical bone production perpendicular to the cortex.

Osteosarcoma of the Jaws

Nature of disease

A malignant proliferation of mesenchymal stem cells/progenitor cells into a partial osseous differentiation.

Predilections

May occur at any age, but most in the jaws are seen between the ages of 15 and 40 years. No sex or racial predilection is known.

Clinical features

A firm to bony hard expansile mass arising in and often growing out of bone. Paresthesia and overt anesthesia may be present. Pain is an occasional symptom but is uncommon. Tooth separation and mobility are common.

Radiographic presentation

A mixed radiolucent-radiopaque expansile mass will be seen. A destroyed cortex with extracortical bone arising from the mass at right angles, referred to as the "sunray appearance," is common. Widening of the periodontal ligament space, recently opened contacts of teeth, and supraeruption of teeth may be seen as early findings.

Differential diagnosis

Chondrosarcomas, fibrosarcomas, Paget disease, osteoblastomas, and some fibrosarcomas will be very similar in their presentation.

Microscopic features

A pleomorphic cellular stroma of atypical spindle-shaped mesenchymal cells producing immature "tumor" bone.

Suggested course of action

Exploration and biopsy of the central portion of the mass. (Note: A superficial biopsy may show only misleading benign reactive bone.) Referral to an oral and maxillofacial surgeon for either the biopsy or workup and definitive treatment.

Treatment

Upfront chemotherapy (usually three cycles) followed by resection observing 3-cm margins in bone and 2-cm margins in soft tissue, as well as one or two cycles of postsurgical chemotherapy. In cases of a larger tumor interfering with function or those rapidly growing, surgery is accomplished first, followed by three to five cycles of chemotherapy. Radiation therapy is only used in select cases.

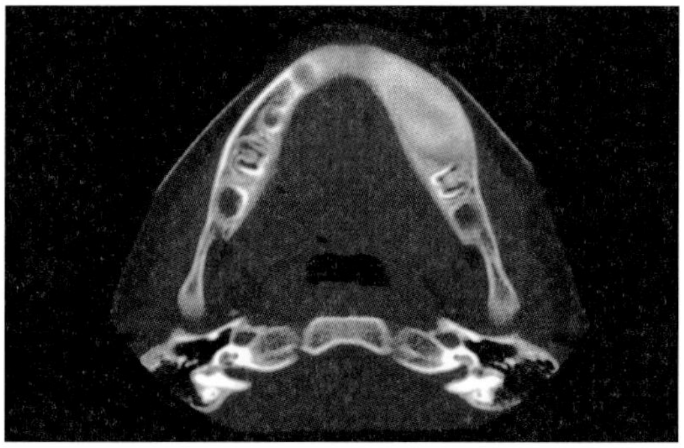

► Monostotic fibrous dysplasia.

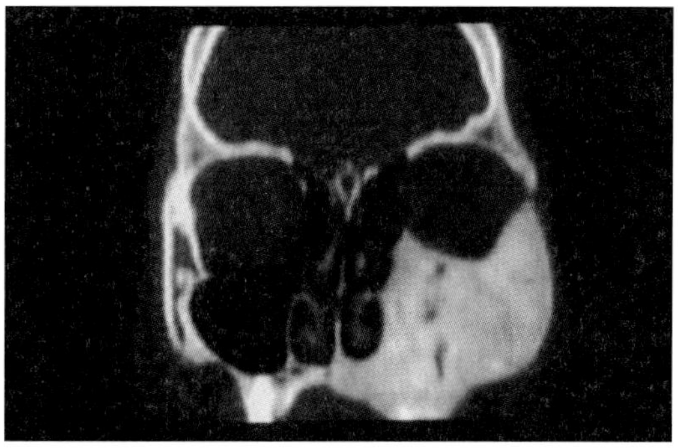

► Craniofacial fibrous dysplasia.

Fibrous Dysplasia

Nature of disease

A noninherited genetic mutation during embryologic development that affects bone remodeling/maturation and may also affect endocrine function. This mistake during embryologic development is in the *GNAS-1* gene (guanine nucleotide-binding protein alpha stimulating activity polypeptide-1) and, depending on the stage of development of the embryo, may result in any one of the four known clinical expressions.

Predilections

Clinical manifestations become apparent in the later part of the first decade of life or early teenage years. All clinical manifestations are present before the age of 20 years. There is no sex or racial predilection known.

Clinical features

There are four clinical expressions of fibrous dysplasia:

1. Monostotic type: A single bone is involved with usually a fusiform painless expansion that has an intact overlying mucosa.
2. Craniofacial type: Several adjacent (contiguous) bones of the skull or facial skeleton are involved, usually in a unilateral fashion. More rarely, a bilateral expression occurs. The expansions are bony, hard, painless, and will have intact mucosa and skin.
3. Polyostotic type without precocious puberty (Jaffe-Lichtenstein type): Multiple noncontiguous bones are involved together with either the monostotic jaw type or the craniofacial type, usually the femur, metacarpals, and metatarsals.
4. Polyostotic type with precocious puberty (McCune-Albright type): Multiple noncontiguous bones such as the femur, ribs, metacarpals, and metatarsals are involved together with either the monostotic jaw type or the craniofacial type along with early signs (age 5 to 10 years) of genital development, voice changes, and breast enlargement and menarche in girls, etc.

Radiographic presentation

Plain radiographs and CT scans will show a fusiform expansion of bone with a foggy appearance referred to as the "ground-glass" appearance. Notably, the cortex will be remodeled with this type of bone so that no distinctive cortex is seen on right-angle radiographs. Also, extracortical bone as may be seen in Garré osteomyelitis, other osteomyelitises, or osteosarcoma is not seen in fibrous dysplasia. PET scans and technetium bone scans will show a distinct increased uptake in areas of fibrous dysplasia.

Differential diagnosis

Garré osteomyelitis, chronic sclerosing osteomyelitis, and ossifying fibromas are frequently confused with fibrous dysplasia and need to be ruled out. Osteosarcoma and the rare Ewing sarcoma may also be considered. →

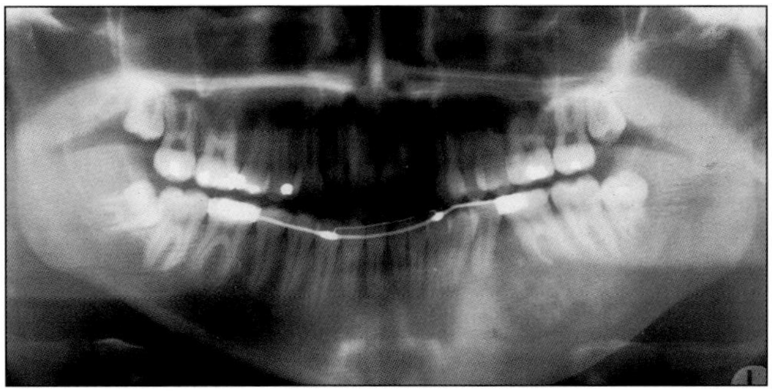

► Fibrous dysplasia as seen on a panoramic radiograph.

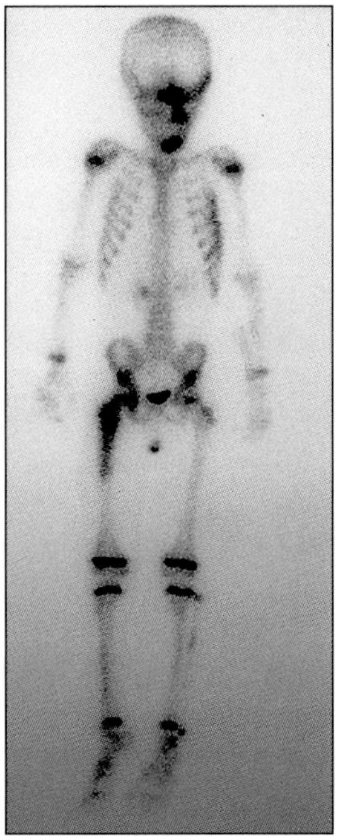

► Polyostotic fibrous dysplasia.

Fibrous Dysplasia *(cont)*

Microscopic features

The classic appearance is that of irregular bone trabeculae emerging from a benign but hyperplastic fibrous stroma. Osteoblastic rimming of the trabeculae is sparse or absent. In long-standing cases of fibrous dysplasia, a few more areas with osteoblastic rimming are seen and are often coalesced to a more mature bone with lamellar architecture.

Suggested course of action

Suspicious cases require good imaging and a workup. At the minimum, a panoramic radiograph is required. Either order a head and neck CT scan and a total body PET scan to assess the type of fibrous dysplasia, or refer the patient to his or her primary care physician or to an oral and maxillofacial surgeon for this workup.

Treatment

Genetic counseling is advised to assure individuals that it is not an inherited trait. Surgical sculpting is often required and is best done during a documented period of quiescence. Sculpting before the cessation of growth will likely require a resculpting procedure later. Even into mid-adulthood (30 to 50 years old), some patients may experience a spontaneous regrowth requiring a resculpting procedure.

Special notes:

- Biopsies do not accelerate regrowth.
- Surgical sculpting does not accelerate regrowth.
- Surgical sculpting does not stimulate a transformation to a malignancy.
- Radiation therapy *does* stimulate a transformation to malignancy and is contraindicated.
- Diagnostic radiographs have not been known to stimulate a transformation to malignancy.

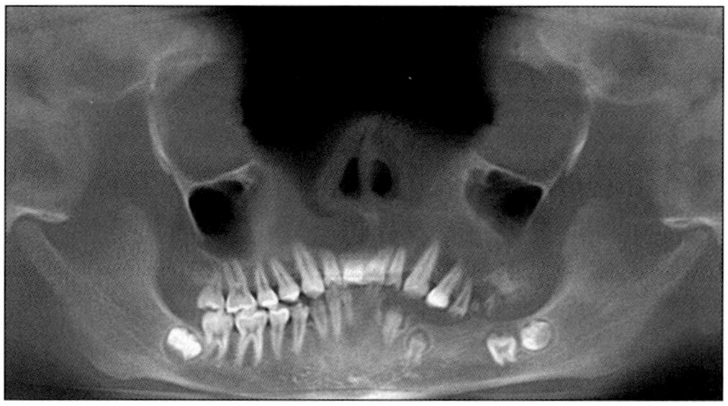

► Segmental odontomaxillary dysplasia.

Segmental Odontomaxillary/Odontomandibular Dysplasia

Nature of disease

A very rare, noninherited defect in a localized area of either jaw (usually the maxilla) whereby the bone and overlying soft tissues are expanded. There is no identified cause known at this time.

Predilections

Most common in the premolar region of the maxilla. Males are affected 2:1 over females. Clinical manifestations are usually noted at or just before puberty. No racial predilections are known.

Clinical features

The involved bone will be expanded, and local teeth will be displaced with the expansion or may be hypoplastic. The expansion is painless. The gingiva may show some hypertrophy and be thicker than normal but with no ulceration or granulation tissue.

Radiographic presentation

A foggy, diffuse, ground-glass appearance similar to that of fibrous dysplasia is seen. There will be no definitive line of demarcation to that of uninvolved bone.

Differential diagnosis

The localized area of bony expansion will suggest a monostotic fibrous dysplasia or an incomplete hemifacial hypertrophy. Additionally, a focal cemento-osseous dysplasia or a chronic sclerosing osteomyelitis may also be considered.

Microscopic features

Normal-appearing immature trabecular bone with osteoblasts rimming remodeling osteoclasts and abundant normal capillaries are seen in the rare specimens taken.

Suggested course of action

Good-quality images are important. Request a CT scan and a total body PET scan to assess the areas of involvement. An office panoramic view to begin is recommended. Refer to an orthodontist or an oral and maxillofacial surgeon for further workup and definitive treatment.

Treatment

Each case is unique and will require an individualized treatment plan that will include orthodontic tooth alignment and surgical bone contouring. Frequently, extraction of teeth is necessary, requiring provisional restorations until somatic growth slows down and dental implants can be placed.

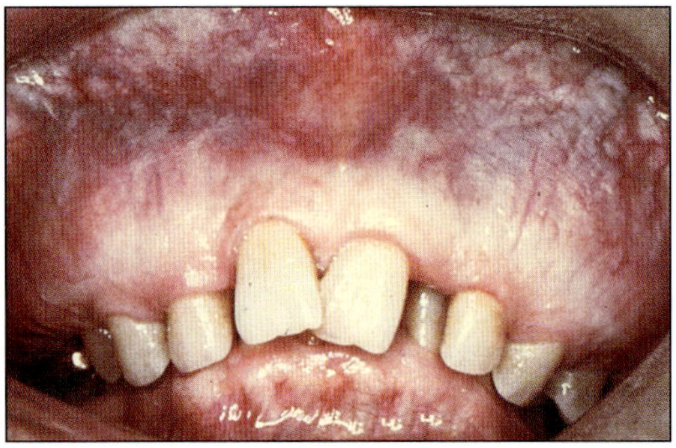

► Expansion of the maxilla seen in Paget disease.

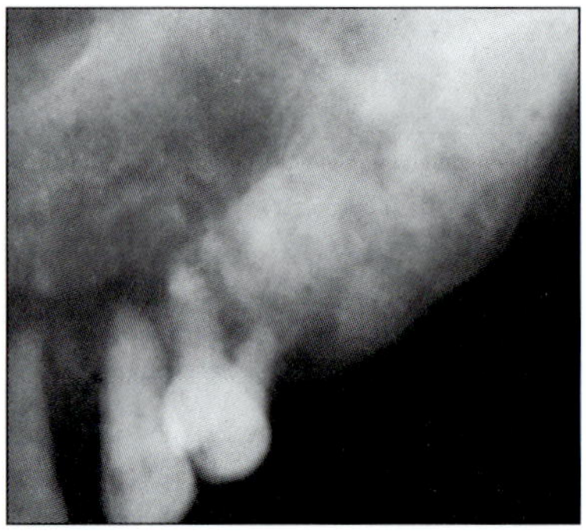

► "Cotton wool" appearance of bone in Paget disease.

Paget Disease

Nature of disease

A focal area or multifocal areas of accelerated bone turnover resulting in expansion of the involved area(s). An unproven viral etiology has been suspected.

Predilections

Occurs exclusively in adults, with an increase in incidence with advancing age. No sex or racial predilection is known.

Clinical features

In the jaws, Paget disease presents as a diffuse expansion of bone. The bone is well vascularized, causing a warmth to the touch and an appearance of localized dilated veins. Teeth will be evenly displaced, creating diastemas and crossbites or a scissor bite. Laboratory tests will show a very large, increased alkaline phosphatase value with high normal calcium and low normal phosphate values. These values relate that bone deposition and resorption are somewhat balanced, although there is a net gain in bone mass.

Radiographic presentation

An expansile, mostly radiopaque enlargement of the involved bone or bone area. The bone will appear mottled with irregular contours. The margins will be ill defined.

Differential diagnosis

Osteosarcomas, chronic sclerosing osteomyelitis, fibrous dysplasia, osteoblastomas, and some ossifying fibromas may present in a similar fashion.

Microscopic features

Areas of dense bone rimmed with plump, deeply staining osteoblasts together with numerous osteoclasts actively resorbing bone.

Suggested course of action

Suspected cases should be referred to a rheumatologist for workup, diagnosis, and treatment.

Treatment

Non-nitrogen–containing bisphosphonates such as tiludronate are the standard drugs used. Note: *(1)* Paget disease has been declining in incidence since the 1980s due to unknown factors. *(2)* Paget disease has a known 1% to 3% spontaneous transformation rate into osteosarcoma, and it is well known to transform into osteosarcoma should it be treated with radiation therapy.

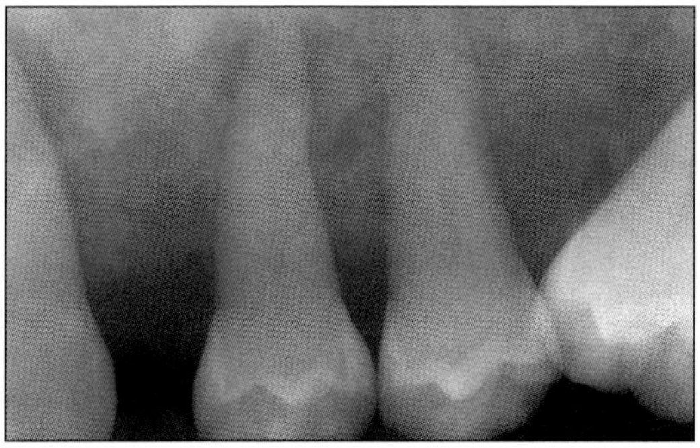

► Loss of lamina dura and ground-glass appearance of bone in secondary hyperparathyroidism.

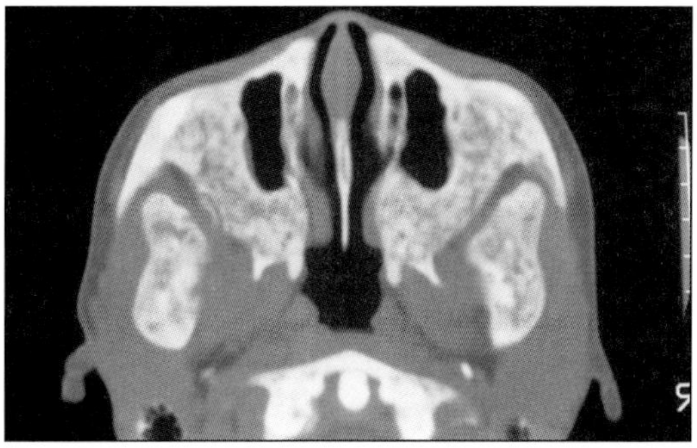

► In secondary hyperparathyroidism, all bones have a mottled appearance.

Secondary Hyperparathyroidism

Nature of disease

This form of hyperparathyroidism is secondary to renal failure with loss of calcium through the urine (hypercalciuria), which results in hypocalcemia. This hypocalcemia triggers the normal parathyroid gland to oversecrete parathormone in a vain attempt to return serum calcium levels to normal. The effect of activating osteoclasts with increased levels of parathormone is what causes the bony changes seen clinically.

Predilections

Can occur in anyone with renal failure. Most patients are adults and may have polycystic kidney disease or lupus nephritis or may already be on dialysis.

Clinical features

In many cases, no clinical signs or symptoms are apparent. In some cases, mobile teeth or jaw expansions are noted. Others may have various bone pains, lethargy, muscle cramps, twitches, carpopedal spasms, or, if severe, tetany.

Radiographic presentation

A generalized loss of the lamina dura and a diffuse mottling of the bony jaws as well as the skull and all other bones may be noted. This is often referred to as *osteitis deformans* or *Von Recklinghausen disease of bone*. In some cases, an ill-defined radiolucency representing a "brown tumor" may also be present.

Differential diagnosis

The clinical and radiographic presentation may resemble Paget disease, thalassemia intermedia, and craniofacial fibrous dysplasia.

Microscopic features

Bone specimens will show normal trabecular bone with thicker trabeculae that are more mineralized. The radiolucent areas will be composed of a plump fibroblastic stroma with little collagen and numerous multinucleated cells appearing identical to an osteoclast.

Suggested course of action

Take good periapical and panoramic radiographs. Suspected cases should be referred to an endocrinologist.

Treatment

Dialysis or kidney transplant.

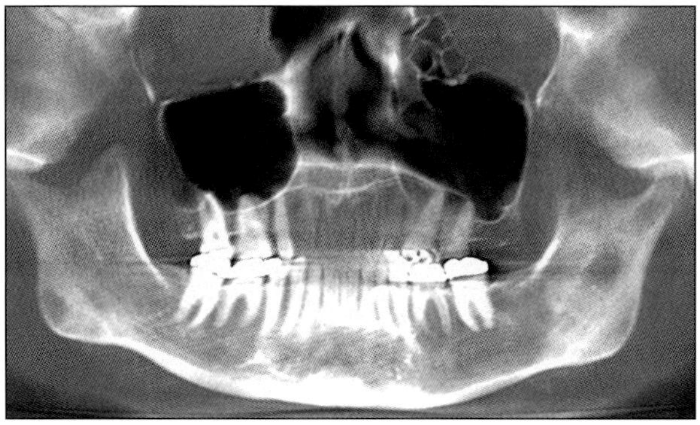

► Metastatic breast cancer to the mandibular rami.

Metastatic Carcinoma

Nature of disease

A proliferation of malignant cells that spread to the jaws mostly via the venous routes and less so via arteries and lymphatics. The route from those primary sites above the diaphragm is via local veins or arteries to the jaws. Those from below the diaphragm are via the paravertebral veins of Batson.

Predilections

The most common primary sites are the breast (31%), lung (27%), kidney (14%), bone (10%), thyroid (6%), and others (<5%).

Clinical features

May be an incidental finding of a radiolucency in the jaw. More commonly, it is seen as a soft tissue gingival mass or mass arising from bone around a tooth or from a recent extraction socket. Paresthesia or overt anesthesia of a nerve distribution is common.

Radiographic presentation

Most will show a poorly demarcated radiolucency and mild expansion. Others may appear normal, and some (such as in metastatic breast cancer) will have some radiopacities.

Differential diagnosis

Primary carcinomas, peripheral giant cell proliferations, pyogenic granulomas, and some cases of osteomyelitis are considerations.

Microscopic features

A malignant cell population appearing as cells from the distant primary site. Note: Special stains are often needed to determine the cell type and origin of the metastasis. Occasionally, the primary site has not yet been identified.

Suggested course of action

Incisional biopsy and/or referral to an oral and maxillofacial surgeon.

Treatment

Metastasis portends a poor prognosis. The primary site and metastatic sites may be treated with surgery, focal radiotherapy, and/or chemotherapy for disease and pain control. Cure is unlikely.

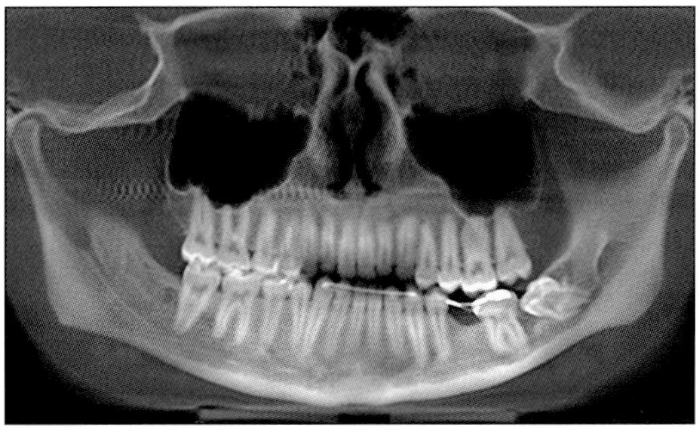

► Garré osteomyelitis in a teenager related to the eruption of a third molar.

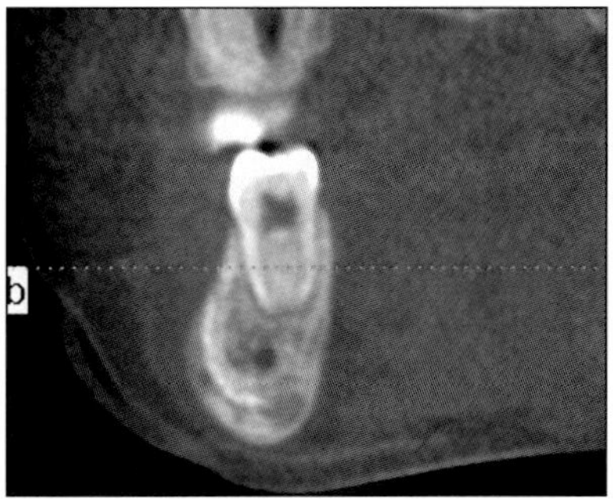

► Extracortical bone formation from inflamed periosteum.

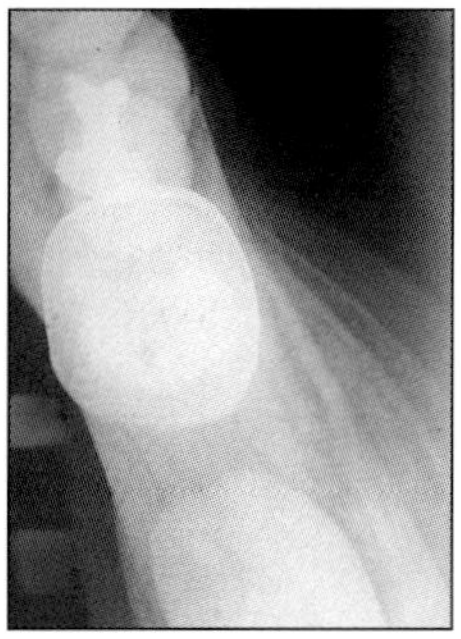

► Occlusal view of a Garré osteomyelitis often shows an onionskin effect.

Garré Osteomyelitis

Nature of disease

A limited and localized infection due to a low-virulence bacteria in an immune-competent host with an adequate blood supply, which will stimulate the periosteum to lay down extracortical bone.

Predilections

Most common in children and teenagers and rare over the age of 25 years. No sex or racial predilection is known. It occurs mostly in the mandible and is extremely rare in the maxilla, but it has occurred in long bones.

Clinical features

Most present as an asymptomatic expansion. Rare cases may have dull pain. The expansion is hard with no erythema or pus. Most occur associated with an abscessed tooth. Rare cases may be secondary to trauma, causing a stimulation of periosteum via a subperiosteal hematoma.

Radiographic presentation

Layers of extracortical bone best seen on occlusal radiographs or axial CT scans are often noted. The extracortical bone will arise from an intact cortex and have a ground-glass or onionskin appearance. If an abscessed tooth is the etiology, a radiolucency may be seen around that tooth.

Differential diagnosis

The diseases on a differential diagnosis representing a similar presentation are much more concerning than Garré osteomyelitis. These include osteosarcoma, Ewing sarcoma, chronic sclerosing osteomyelitis, and fibrous dysplasia.

Microscopic features

A normal-appearing cortex will be seen to have parallel layers of bone 25 to 100 microns thick outside the cortex. These layers may be connected by trabecular struts of a similar thickness. An outer layer of periosteum with inflammatory cells will rim the outer layer of bone.

Suggested course of action

Obtain right-angle occlusal radiographs or CT scans. Examine for a source of infection. Refer to an oral and maxillofacial surgeon for confirmation or a second opinion.

Treatment

Removal of any identifiable source of infection and antibiotics such as phenoxymethylpenicillin or doxycycline.

8

Radiopaque Lesions in Soft Tissue

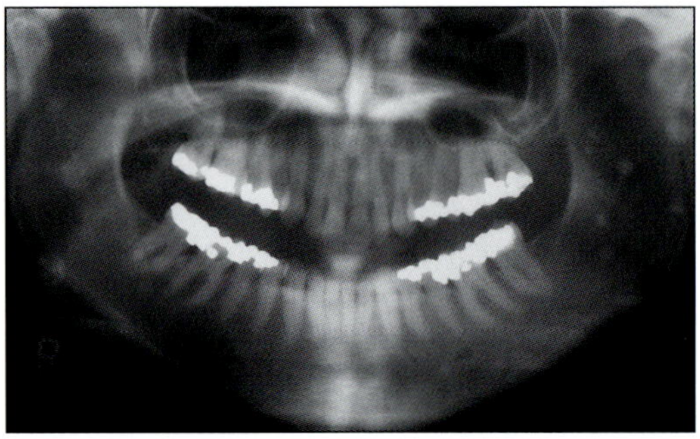

► Phleboliths in parotid hemangiomas superimposed over each ramus.

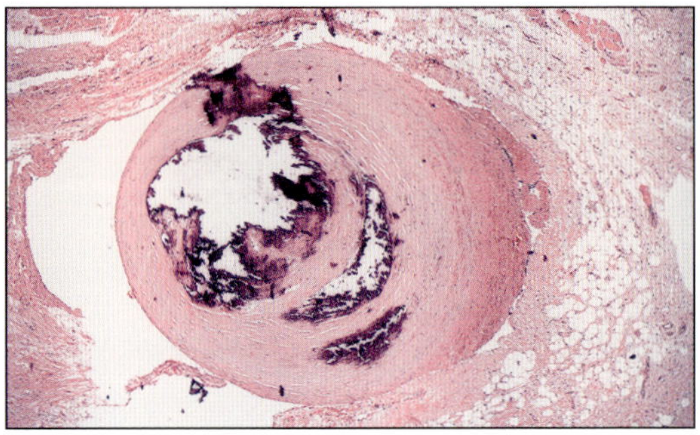

► Phlebolith with concentric rings of dystrophic calcifications around the nidus of a blood clot.

Phleboliths

Nature of disease

Calcium carbonate stones that form in the lumen of veins. Most form due to blood stasis in the lumen of veins of a hemangioma that has atrophied. Others may form from chronic inflammation in a vein, known as *phlebitis*.

Predilections

Most are first recognized in young adults or mature adults from childhood hemangiomas. No sex or racial predilection is known. Most occur in the parotid region.

Clinical features

Most are asymptomatic radiographic findings. Uncommon ones will have a diffuse fullness of the soft tissue in the area and/or remnants of the original hemangioma.

Radiographic presentation

Multiple round to oval radiodense structures with smooth outlines measuring 2 to 10 mm are seen within the involved soft tissues. Because most occur in the parotid region, these radiodense structures will be seen superimposed over the ramus and adjacent areas.

Differential diagnosis

Most cases are radiographically distinctive. Multiple tonsilloliths, sialoliths, antroliths, and a calcification of the carotid bifurcation can provide a somewhat similar picture.

Microscopic features

Concentric layers of mineral, mostly calcium carbonate, around a nidus of the remnants of an old blood clot will be seen.

Suggested course of action

Obtain a CT scan to pinpoint the number and location of the phleboliths. Refer to an oral and maxillofacial surgeon for opinion and confirmation.

Treatment

None required unless the phlebolith is infected or symptomatic. Then removal may be necessary.

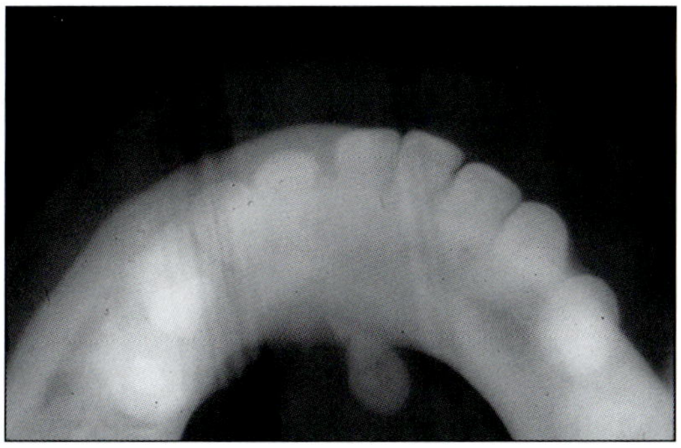

► Sialolith at the opening of the submandibular duct.

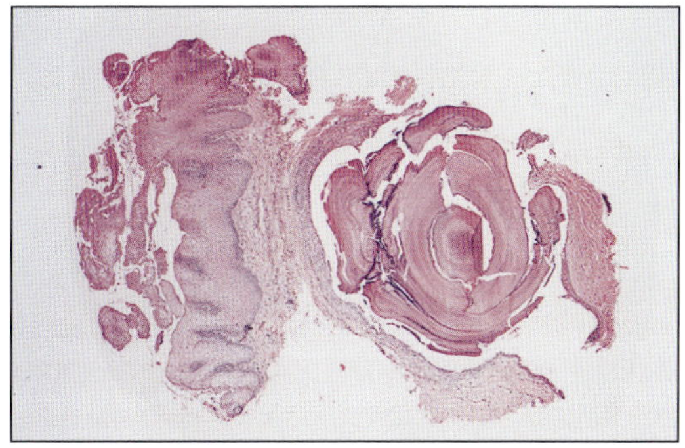

► Sialolith with concentric rings around a central nidus.

Sialoliths

Nature of disease

The formation of calcium carbonate or, rarely, calcium oxalate stones in the duct or parenchyma of a salivary gland. Most are due to inflammation and salivary stasis resulting from infection, which creates a nidus upon which calcium concretions develop. Less commonly, a salivary gland tumor may create a blockage of salivary flow. The stasis that is created then results in a stone.

Predilections

Occurs mostly in the submandibular gland system and rarely in the parotid or sublingual gland systems. Adults are mostly affected. No sex or racial predilection is known.

Clinical features

The most common presentation is that of a firm to hard mass in the submandibular triangle. Those in which there is an active infection will be painful, while others will not be. If the stone is in the submandibular duct, there may be swelling and erythema in the floor of the mouth on that side.

Radiographic presentation

Small stones may be subtle and superimposed over the mandible on a panoramic radiograph. Occlusal radiographs are best to show stones in the floor of the mouth. Medical CT scans are best to show stones in other areas and confirm that they are in the gland parenchyma.

Differential diagnosis

Phleboliths and significant calcifications in the carotid bifurcation should be considered. A calcified lymph node representing a dystrophic calcification from a resolved lymphadenitis, particularly a tuberculous or actinomycosis lymphadenitis, may also present with a similar radiographic appearance.

Microscopic and gross specimen features

The sialolith itself will be a chalky, yellow-colored stone that breaks apart easily. Sometimes a layered effect of concentric rings around the center will be noted. The surrounding gland will be seen to have a chronic inflammatory infiltrate with loss of acini.

Suggested course of action

Obtain an occlusal radiograph to either confirm or rule out the position of the stone in the floor of the mouth. Order a CT scan with axial and coronal cuts to document that the calcification is in the submandibular gland rather than a lymph node, phlebolith, or part of the carotid bifurcation.

Treatment

Symptomatic glands require excision. Asymptomatic glands may be observed provided a CT scan or MRI has shown no suspicion of a concomitant tumor. Sialoliths within the ductal system are removed and the duct sutured open into the floor of the mouth (sialodochoplasty).

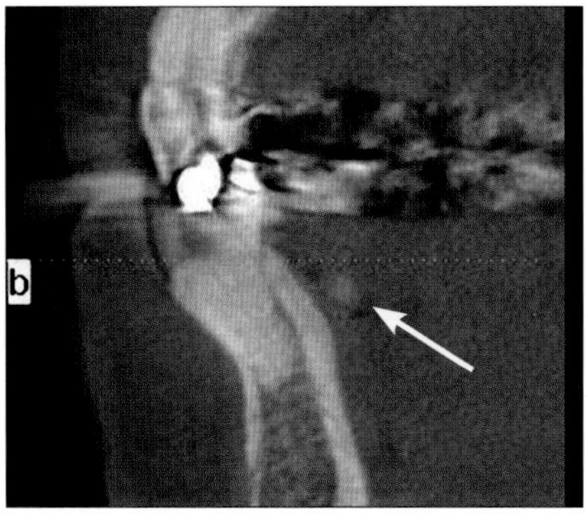

► Bone density calcification in the soft tissues of the floor of the mouth from an osseous choristoma.

Osseous Choristomas

Nature of disease

A very rare phenomenon whereby multipotent stem cells in soft tissue (most commonly the tongue or floor of the mouth) differentiate into osteoblasts and form normal bone.

Predilections

No age, sex, or racial predilection is known.

Clinical features

Most present as an asymptomatic mass in either the tongue or floor of the mouth. The mass is hard and nontender to palpation. The mass may be fixed within the tissue or freely movable. The overlying mucosa is intact.

Radiographic presentation

A round to oval mass of bony density is seen within the muscle bundles of the tongue or within the submucosa in the floor of the mouth.

Differential diagnosis

Foreign bodies in these same locations, a sialolith, or a torus are the most serious considerations. Phleboliths and calcified lymph nodes may also be considered.

Microscopic features

The bone is normal-appearing compact bone with Haversian systems and lamellar architecture similar to a torus.

Suggested course of action

Obtain occlusal radiographs to define its location. Order a CT scan to rule out other considerations on the differential diagnosis. Refer to an oral and maxillofacial surgeon for treatment.

Treatment

Excision via either a pericapsular dissection or with 1- to 2-mm margins of surrounding soft tissue.

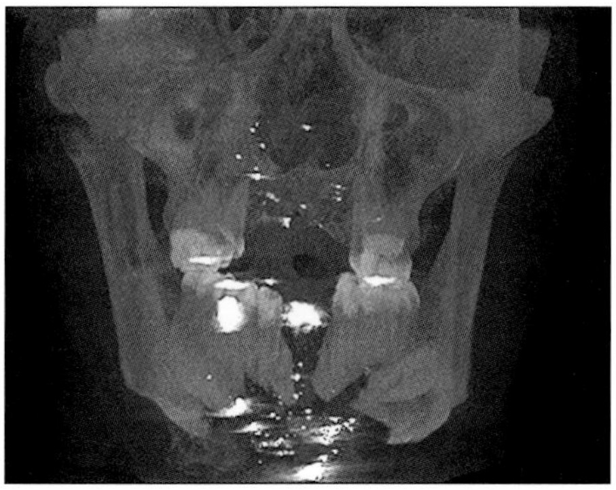

► Multiple bullet fragment foreign bodies from a gunshot wound.

Foreign Bodies

Nature of disease

Nonhuman materials embedded into soft tissue from previous accidents or surgeries or by patient intention.

Predilections

There is no age, sex, or racial predilection.

Clinical features

Many are incidental radiographic findings. Others are known to be present and are asymptomatic. Less commonly, the foreign body can be palpated or causes pain.

Radiographic presentation

Metallic foreign bodies such as bullet fragments, titanium screws, plates, and wires will appear bright white. Items such as buttons and acrylic beads will appear opaque. Items such as silicone implants, hyaluronic acid, and some other cosmetic fillers may appear radiolucent.

Differential diagnosis

Metallic foreign bodies are identifiable as metal even though the specific object may not be recognized. Opaque foreign bodies may simulate sialoliths, phleboliths, and calcified lymph nodes. Items with a density less than that of the surrounding soft tissue may appear as an abscess, a lipoma, or a lymphangioma.

Microscopic features

None pertinent.

Suggested course of action

Obtain radiographs and/or CT scans to identify the location of the foreign body and assess for any local tissue reaction. Refer symptomatic cases to an oral and maxillofacial surgeon.

Treatment

Observation and follow-up of asymptomatic foreign bodies. Surgical removal for those that are symptomatic.

Calcified Lymph Nodes

Nature of disease

Chronic infection and necrosis within a lymph node that settles out calcium salts known as *dystrophic calcifications.*

Predilections

There is no age, sex, or racial predilection. In the cervical chains, most are secondary to tuberculosis lymphadenopathy or actinomycosis.

Clinical features

Most are asymptomatic incidental radiographic findings. Occasionally, the lymph node calcifications may occur while the lymph node remains inflamed, thereby causing pain. Larger ones may be palpable. Note: Calcified lymph nodes are more common in the lungs, known as a *Ghon focus.*

Radiographic presentation

A round to oval radiopaque mass will appear on panoramic radiographs, cone beam CT scans, and medical CT scans. The medical CT scan will rule out sialoliths, phleboliths, and calcifications of the carotid bifurcation and identify the mass to be in the submandibular or jugulodigastric lymph node chains.

Differential diagnosis

Submandibular gland sialoliths, phleboliths, and calcifications in the carotid bifurcation should be considered.

Microscopic features

There is usually little left of the lymph node. That remnant may show chronic inflammatory cells and some fibrosis. The majority of the lymph node will be replaced by an eosinophilic dense calcium deposit seen only on uncalcified specimens.

Suggested course of action

For cases discovered on panoramic radiographs or cone beam CT scans, order a medical CT scan to confirm its location and rule out the other entities on the differential diagnosis.

Treatment

Usually none is required. Symptomatic cases require an exploration and removal for biopsy and culture.

Calcification of the Carotid Bifurcation

Nature of disease

Dystrophic calcifications within the tunica intima and tunica media at the carotid bifurcation.

Predilections

Adults with risk factors such as poorly controlled hypertension, cigarette smoking, and hypercholesterolemia, and those with a history of radiation to the neck. No sex or racial predilection is known.

Clinical features

An asymptomatic radiographic finding.

Radiographic presentation

A panoramic radiograph or cone beam CT scan will identify a radiopaque mass often in a concentric half-moon shape in the soft tissue of the upper neck. A medical CT will pinpoint and confirm the calcification to be in the carotid bifurcation and will more often show the half-moon shape.

Differential diagnosis

Calcified submandibular or jugulodigastric lymph nodes as well as submandibular gland sialoliths and phleboliths will present a similar radiographic finding to a calcification of the carotid bifurcation.

Microscopic features

Autopsy specimens are the only source of specimens. The gross examination shows white to yellow plaques on the intimal wall that are fragile and may split off fragments with compression, which may also occur during palpation and may produce a stroke. Microscopic calcified ground specimens show an eosinophilic dystrophic calcification in the intima often extending into the tunica media.

Suggested course of action

Send a note to the patient's physician identifying the finding and alerting him or her to its relationship to hypertension, cigarette smoking, hypercholesterolemia, etc.

Treatment

Reduce the risk factors: smoking cessation, control of hypertension, diet modifications, and possible statin medications.

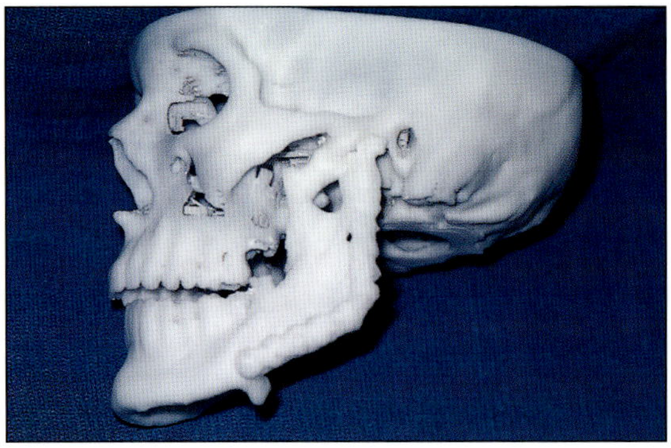

► Bone formation in the temporalis muscle/coronoid process after a surgery.

Traumatic Myositis Ossificans

Nature of disease

A crush injury where bone-forming cells (ie, periosteal cells) are implanted into muscle or muscle precursors retaining the ability to differentiate into bone-forming cells and are stimulated to do so by the environment created by the crush injury.

Predilections

Mostly children and young adults. No sex or racial predilection is known.

Clinical features

Most present with a limited jaw motion or a palpably hard muscle with reduced functional ability.

Radiographic presentation

Most cases produce a mechanical limitation of opening seen as radiodense bone connecting the temporal bone and zygomatic arch to the mandible via either the masseter, medial pterygoid, or temporalis muscle and sometimes via the sphenomandibular ligament. More rarely, the buccinators will be involved with radiodense bone.

Differential diagnosis

Aberrant bone formation in soft tissue should register a concern for osteosarcoma and even chondrosarcoma or Ewing sarcoma via reactive bone. Less likely is an arteriovenous hemangioma that has multiple phleboliths.

Microscopic features

Specimens are seen to be composed of mature, dense bone with lamellar architecture and Haversian systems. Occasionally, inflammatory cells accompany the bone.

Suggested course of action

Refer to an oral and maxillofacial surgeon for workup and treatment.

Treatment

Improvement in motion is gained by a surgical excision of the aberrant bone followed by aggressive physical therapy.

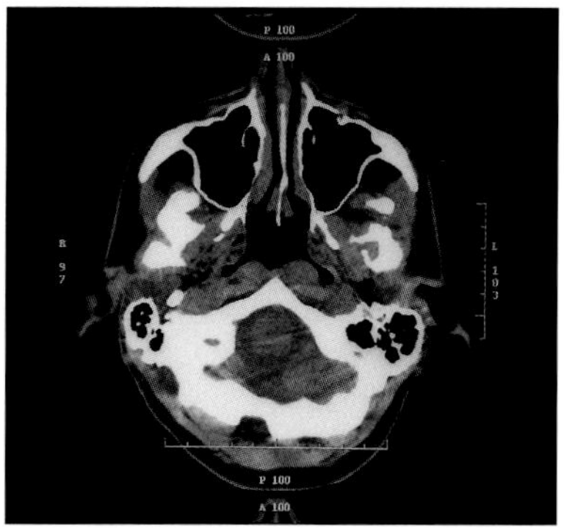

► Multiple areas of bone formation within the muscles of mastication seen in an individual with myositis ossificans progressiva.

Myositis Ossificans Progressiva

Nature of disease

Also termed *fibrodysplasia ossificans progressiva*, this disease is an autosomal dominant inherited trait whereby tendons and aponeuroses as well as muscle fascia progress through stages of fibrous proliferations to endochondral immature bone formation and finally into mature lamellar bone.

Predilections

Clinical manifestations develop in the preteen and teenage years. No sex or racial predilection is known.

Clinical features

Dental practitioners will note a limited jaw movement of 10 mm or less in a teenager or young adult and may also appreciate a bony hard mass in one of the muscles of mastication or buccinators. Other outward signs that may be noted are a stiff gait, shortened metatarsals and phalanges, limited arm motion, and stiff neck.

Radiographic presentation

In the jaws, bony replacement of muscles often joining the skull base (ie, temporal and sphenoid bones) to the ramus of the mandible is common and extensive. Replacement of the buccinators with radiodense bone may also be seen. Panoramic and cone beam CT scans will also identify fusion of the cervical vertebrae in many cases.

Differential diagnosis

Myositis ossificans progressiva is characteristic by its presentation and extent. In mild cases, traumatic myositis ossificans or osteosarcoma may be considered. In fully developed cases, the clinical picture may resemble the rare Murray Puretic-Drescher syndrome, another inherited autosomal dominant trait that manifests with similarly hyaline fibrotic lesions but without bone.

Microscopic features

Specimens will show mature bone with lamellar architecture and Haversian systems.

Suggested course of action

In cases suspicious for myositis ossificans progressiva, resist any intention of biopsy because surgery will incite further ossifications. Instead, refer to a major medical center with a strong rheumatology and/or orthopedic program.

Treatment

There is no effective treatment for this genetically driven disease. Treatments aimed at its progression include 13-cis-retinoic acid, slow administration of corticosteroids, etidronate disodium, and low-dose radiation therapy or 800 to 2,000 cGy to selective sites.

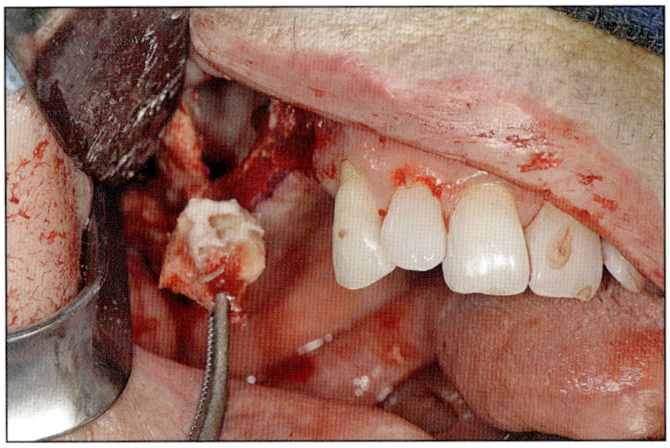

► An antrolith removed from the right maxillary sinus.

Antroliths

Nature of disease

Antroliths are dystrophic calcifications that develop in the maxillary sinus cavity as a result of chronic infection.

Predilections

Mostly adults. No sex or racial predilection is known.

Clinical features

Usually, an asymptomatic radiographic finding. Pain and swelling may also be present as some result from chronic sinusitis.

Radiographic presentation

Antroliths will appear as irregular radiopaque masses within the maxillary sinus cavity. Most are located within the soft tissue outline representing a swollen sinus membrane. If an active sinus infection is present, there may be an air-fluid level as well.

Differential diagnosis

On a panoramic radiograph, phleboliths and tonsilloliths may be superimposed over the sinus. Additionally, a condensing osteitis, a cementoblastoma, and an odontoma associated with the maxillary premolars or molars may mimic an antrolith.

Microscopic and gross specimen features

The gross specimen will be a hard white or yellow friable mass that may crumble. Microscopically, the calcification is lost in routine decalcification procedures.

Suggested course of action

Obtain a cone beam CT scan or medical CT scan to confirm its position in the sinus, then refer to an otorhinolaryngologist or an oral and maxillofacial surgeon.

Treatment

Transnasal endoscopic exploration and removal of the antrolith with cultures and sinus washing. In some cases, an open transoral Caldwell-Luc approach may be used. This is followed by a 10-day course of antibiotics and nasal decongestants.

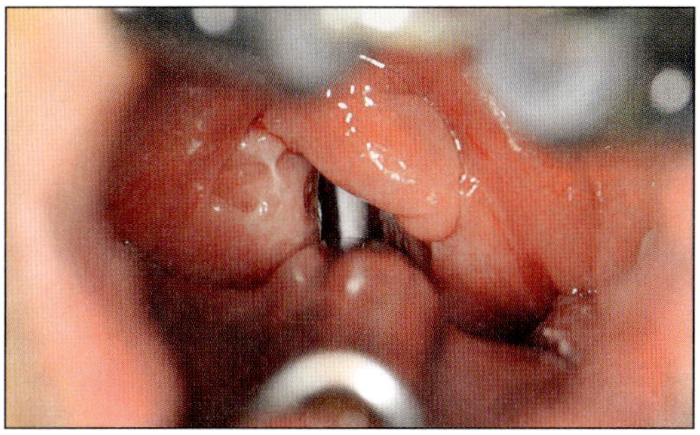

► Tonsillolith seen in the lower part of the left tonsil during tonsillectomy.

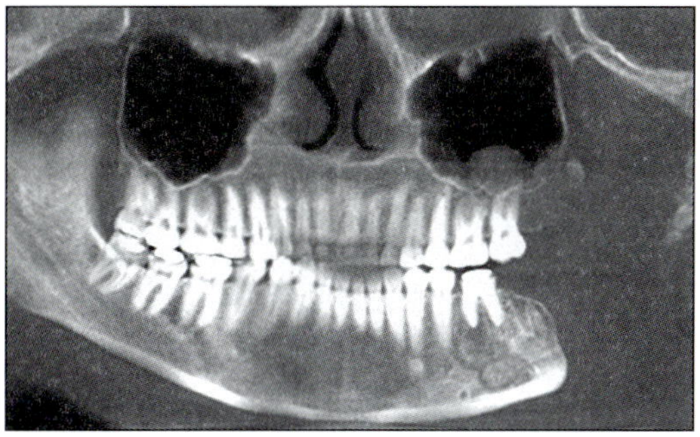

► Tonsillolith superimposed over the posterior maxilla.

Tonsilloliths

Nature of disease

Dystrophic calcifications that develop in the crypts of the pharyngeal tonsils as a result of chronic tonsillitis, most often from *Actinomyces* infections.

Predilections

No age, sex, or racial predilection is known.

Clinical features

Most are asymptomatic yellow masses noted within the crypts of enlarged tonsils. Others will be seen with active tonsillitis, which will have the symptoms of erythema and edema of the tonsil. Some will also have a slight purulent drainage. The patient will then complain of pain and dysphagia.

Radiographic presentation

A tonsillolith is usually incompletely calcified and will therefore either go unnoticed or present as a subtle radiopaque mass superimposed over the ramus on a panoramic radiograph. Cone beam CT scans and medical CT scans are better suited to identify a tonsillolith, which will appear as an irregular radiopaque mass within the soft tissues medial to the ramus.

Differential diagnosis

Clinically, tonsilloliths are somewhat distinctive. However, a foreign body in the tonsil may appear in a similar fashion. Radiographically, phleboliths and antroliths may be considered.

Microscopic features

A decalcified specimen will not show the tonsillolith but may show colonies of *Actinomyces* organisms and undecalcified surrounding neutrophils termed a *sulfur granule*. Undecalcified specimens will show an eosinophilic concretion often times together with *Actinomyces* organisms.

Suggested course of action

Obtain a medical CT scan to confirm the location of the tonsillolith and assess the contralateral tonsil. Refer to an otorhinolaryngologist.

Treatment

In asymptomatic tonsils, removal of the tonsillolith and irrigation of the crypts are often all that is necessary. In chronically inflamed tonsils with tonsilloliths, tonsillectomy is preferred.

9

Pigmented Lesions of Mucosa and Facial Skin

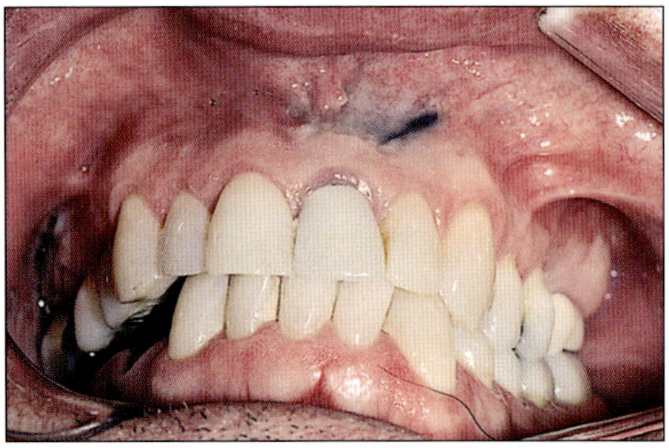

► Amalgam tattoo.

Amalgam Tattoo

Nature of disease

Small silver/mercury amalgam particles from dental restorations implanted into the mucosa beneath the basement membrane by the high-speed handpiece removal of amalgam restorations or from an apicoectomy with an amalgam retrofill.

Predilections

There is no sex or racial predilection. Seen mostly in adults due to the replacement of preexisting restorations with either newer materials or crowns.

Clinical features

Amalgam tattoos will appear as an asymptomatic blue to black discoloration usually in the mucosa apical to the attached gingiva. On rare occasions, mild inflammation causing discomfort can occur.

Radiographic presentation

Most amalgam tattoos are composed of particles too fine to appear on periapical or panoramic radiographs. Coarser particles will appear as an irregular-shaped metal object with rough edges.

Differential diagnosis

The innocuous amalgam tattoo will be very similar to an oral melanoma. Otherwise, lesions with a brown/blue/black color include melanotic macules, mucoceles/mucous cysts, low-grade mucoepidermoid carcinomas, and hemangiomas/lymphangiomas.

Microscopic features

Basophilic-stained metal particles randomly positioned in the connective tissue or in a concentration around the walls of blood vessels will be seen.

Suggested course of action

Thoroughly review the history of removing a previous amalgam restoration. If the area presents with an induration or nodular presentation, or if you are unsure whether the lesion represents an amalgam tattoo, accomplish an incisional biopsy or refer to an oral and maxillofacial surgeon for a biopsy.

Treatment

Rule out other more concerning pathologies. Otherwise, no specific treatment is required.

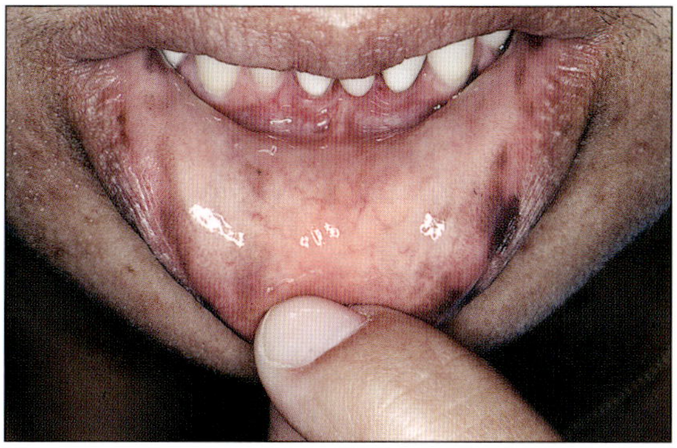

► Melanotic macules.

Melanotic Macules

Nature of disease

An increased production of melanin by the normal melanocytes in the area, with the melanin being taken up by the basal cells along the basement membrane and macrophages in the lamina propria beneath the basement membrane.

Predilections

Seen in patients with Peutz-Jeghers syndrome, Addison disease, hereditary neurofibromatosis type 1, and polyostotic fibrous dysplasia, but most are random in the general population, with no age, sex, or racial predilection.

Clinical features

Melanotic macules are flat, brown-black, asymptomatic areas seen on the oral mucosa similar to those seen on the skin as freckles. They are usually less than 1.5 cm in diameter and may be multiple.

Radiographic presentation

None.

Differential diagnosis

The most important disease to distinguish from a melanotic macule is a melanoma. Otherwise, Peutz-Jeghers syndrome, Addison disease, smoker's melanosis, hereditary neurofibromatosis type 1, and polyostotic fibrous dysplasia should be considered.

Microscopic features

The basal cells will show a brown intracellular pigmentation in a linear band. Some melanin may also be seen within the cytoplasm of macrophages just beneath the basement membrane.

Suggested course of action

Examine the area closely to rule out induration, nodularity, and pain, which would be suspicious for melanoma. If unsure about the clinical diagnosis of a melanotic macule, accomplish an incisional biopsy or refer to an oral and maxillofacial surgeon for a second opinion and/or biopsy.

Treatment

None required.

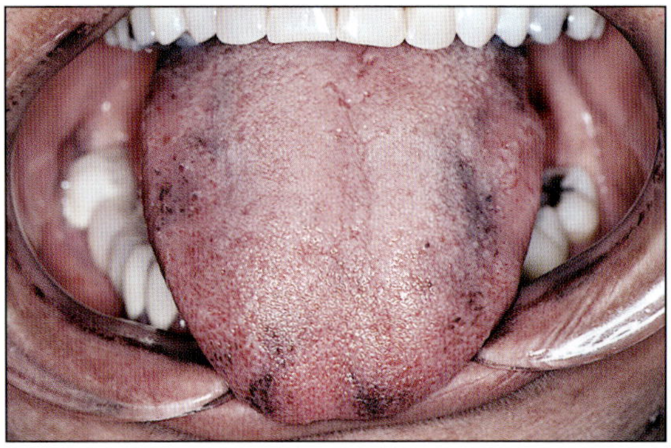

► Melanotic macules in Peutz-Jeghers syndrome.

Peutz-Jeghers Syndrome

Nature of disease

An autosomal dominant trait that results in melanotic macules on the oral mucosa and skin together with polyps of the intestines. The syndrome is the result of a mutation in the *STK11* (serine/threonine kinase 11) gene on chromosome 19p.

Predilections

Most individuals are young (less than 30 years) at the time of diagnosis. Most polyps are benign and develop in the small intestines; however, up to 30% occur in the colon, and 30% become malignant over time in any of their locations.

Clinical features

The dental practitioner may notice numerous brown macules on the lips, palate, labial and buccal mucosa, and tongue. Various melanotic macules can also be noted on the skin, particularly on the fingers.

Radiographic presentation

There are no radiographic features in the jaws. CT scans and dye studies of the gastrointestinal tract will show the polyps arising from the intestinal lining projecting into the lumen.

Differential diagnosis

The clinician should distinguish the melanotic macules from a melanoma with mucosal satellite lesions, nonsyndromic melanotic macules, Addison disease, and the café au lait spots seen in hereditary neurofibromatosis type 1 and polyostotic fibrous dysplasia.

Microscopic features

Basal cells will show brown intracytoplasmic pigment. The pigment will be in a linear fashion along the basement membrane. Macrophages with intracytoplasmic melanin will be seen in the lamina propria.

Suggested course of action

Undiagnosed cases should be referred to an internist or gastroenterologist for evaluation and workup. Dental care can proceed as required.

Treatment

The polyps are followed and removed if symptoms develop or malignant transformation is suspected. There is no treatment required for the oral melanotic macules.

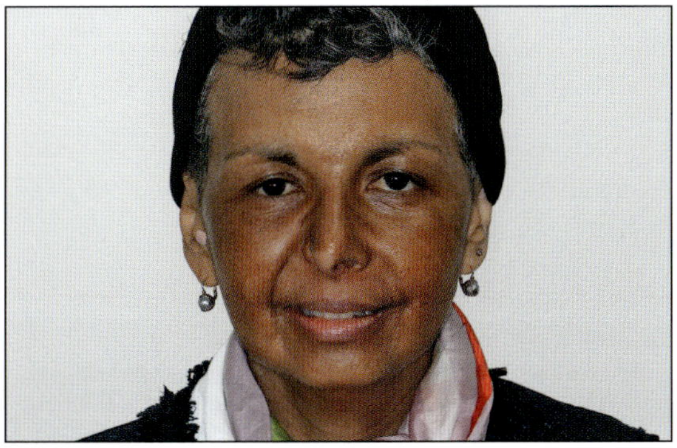

► Thin, somewhat bronzed woman with Addison disease (adrenal cortical insufficiency).

Addison Disease

Nature of disease

A deficiency in the adrenal cortex that is most often idiopathic or autoimmune but that may be caused by bacterial or fungal infections. Absent or lower levels of cortisol and aldosterone produce a constellation of signs and symptoms.

Predilections

Mature adults are affected, with a slight predilection for women. No racial predilection is known.

Clinical features

Most individuals will be thin, with bronzed oral mucosa and skin resembling a suntan. Oral melanotic macules are often present. There will be a tendency toward weakness, cold intolerance, and hypotension. Less commonly, a tendency for nausea and diarrhea may occur. Note that the bronzing of the skin relates to the depressed cortisol levels inherent in adrenal cortical insufficiency; the pituitary attempts to respond by overproducing adrenal corticotropic hormone (ACTH), but a portion of the ACTH chemistry duplicates melanocyte-stimulating hormone (MSH) to cause an overproduction of melanin.

Radiographic presentation

None.

Differential diagnosis

Melanotic macules and bronzing of the skin may also be seen in Peutz-Jeghers syndrome and hereditary neurofibromatosis type 1. Mild cases of Addison disease may be confused with a suntan or unrelated melanotic macules.

Microscopic features

An accumulation of intracytoplasmic melanin in basal cells and the lamina propria of oral mucosa and the papillary dermis of skin will be seen.

Suggested course of action

Refer to an endocrinologist for evaluation and request recommendations for dental care. Long appointments should be avoided if possible. Surgical or stressful procedures will require steroid supplementation during and after the procedure.

Treatment

Appropriate levels of corticosteroid are maintained, and an increase in dosage is provided to cover surgical procedures and/or physiologic stresses.

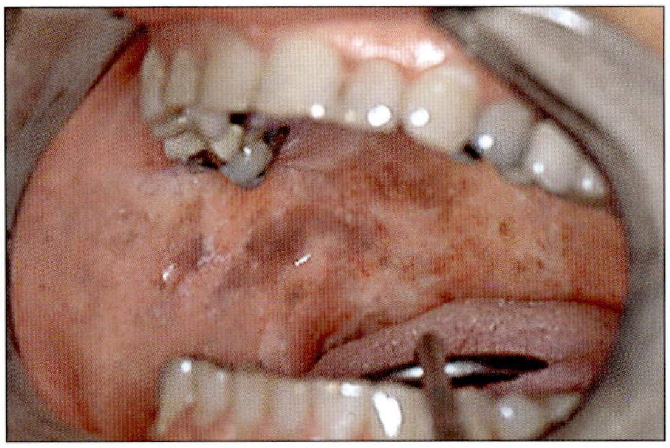

► Generalized bronzed oral mucosa in a patient with hemochromatosis. Hyperpigmented areas are the result of cigar smoking, known as "smoker's melanosis."

Hemochromatosis

Nature of disease

A hereditary or acquired excess absorption of iron resulting in accumulations of iron stores throughout the body. The hereditary form is more common and is autosomal recessive. The acquired form usually results from repeated transfusions for chronic anemic states.

Predilections

Although the genetic abnormality is present at birth, signs and symptoms do not appear until age 40 years or later. There is no known sex or racial predilection. However, men are noted to develop symptoms sooner because of female blood loss and iron loss from menstruation.

Clinical features

The oral mucosa as well as the skin will be gray to bronze in color. Hepatomegaly progressing to a nonpalpable liver from cirrhosis may be present as well as signs of insulin-dependent diabetes (ie, foot and leg ulcers, delayed healing, thirst, etc), fatigue, weakness, and abdominal and joint pain.

Radiographic presentation

None.

Differential diagnosis

Addison disease will also impart a generalized bronzed skin appearance and a concomitant similar effect on the oral mucosa.

Microscopic features

Specimens are rarely taken, but the oral mucosa may show collections of hemosiderin from hemolysis as well as iron deposits identified with an iron stain.

Suggested course of action

Suspected cases should be referred to an endocrinologist or internist for workup. Restorative dentistry is safe to accomplish. Surgical procedures must wait until after the hemochromatosis, particularly the diabetes component, is controlled with treatment.

Treatment

Each of the secondary components (ie, diabetes, liver cirrhosis, joint pain/destruction, etc) is treated individually. The iron overload is chelated with deferoxamine (Desferal, Novartis).

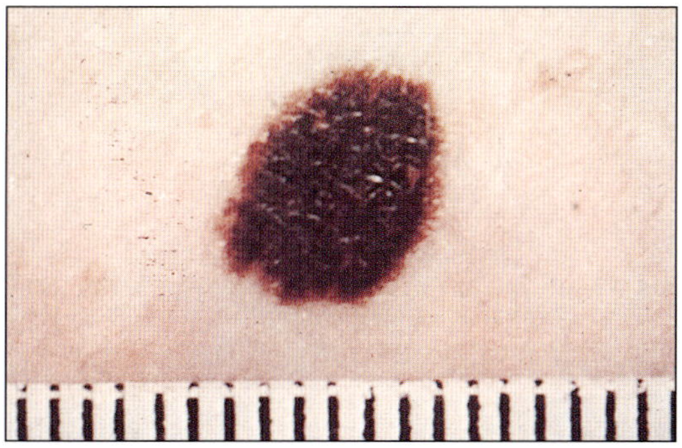

► Junctional nevus.

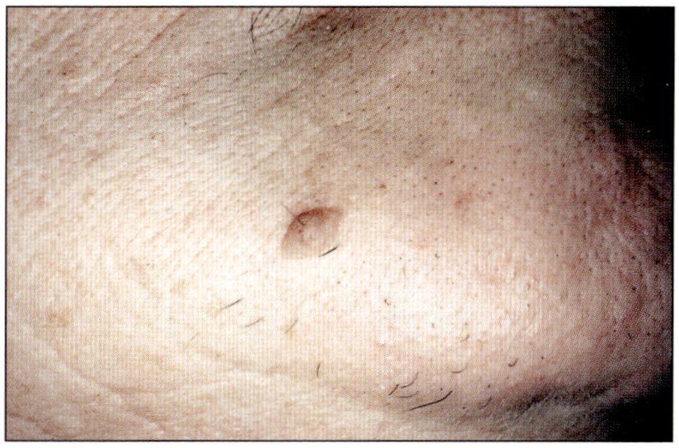

► Compound nevus.

Melanocytic Nevi

Nature of disease

Benign collections of nevus cells that may be derived from neural crest melanocytic precursors or from melanocytes.

Predilections

Oral nevi are very rare. Almost all nevi are on the skin and are very common. About 1% of newborns have a nevus, with the peak numbers occurring around puberty. White individuals are affected more than black individuals, and females are affected more than males.

Clinical features

There are three types of melanocytic nevi:

1. Junctional nevi present as flat or only slightly elevated, small, hairless lesions. Most arise at about 2 years of age and range from 1 to 10 mm in diameter.
2. Compound nevi are elevated and are symmetrically round or oval. Hair is often present around this nevus. As this nevus ages, its surface tends to become warty.
3. Dermal nevi will appear less dark and will be more dome shaped. Like the compound nevus, a warty surface may develop over time. Many will develop a stalk as well.

Radiographic presentation

None.

Differential diagnosis

Any nevus may appear similar to a melanoma. Other pigmented skin lesions to consider are seborrheic keratosis, actinic keratosis, pigmented basal carcinomas, and the café au lait spots of polyostotic fibrous dysplasia or hereditary neurofibromatosis type 1.

Microscopic features

1. Junctional nevi will be seen to have collections of round to oval nevus cells at the epithelium–basement membrane connective tissue junction.
2. Compound nevi will have clusters of the same round/oval nevus cells at both the epithelium–basement membrane connective tissue junction as well as further down in the connective tissue above the muscle layer.
3. Dermal nevi will have all the nevus cells in clusters within the dermis and none at the epithelial–basement membrane connective tissue junction.

⟶

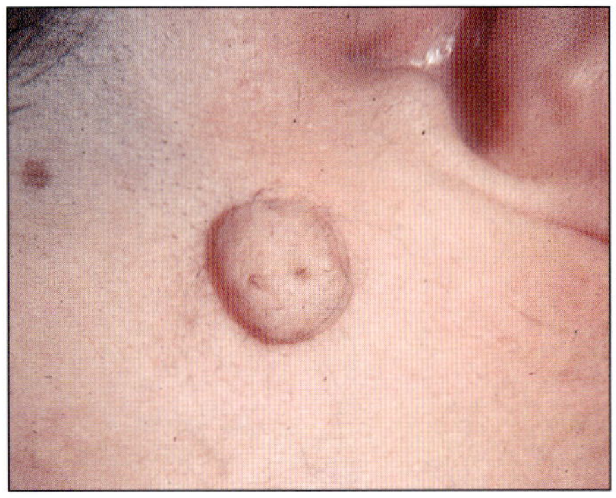

► Dermal nevus.

Melanocytic Nevi *(cont)*

Suggested course of action

Photograph with an adjacent ruler for documentation. Refer to a dermatologist for evaluation and opinion.

Treatment

Any nevus suspicious for a dysplastic nevus or for melanoma is treated with an excisional biopsy. Static nevi without suspicion for a melanoma are followed with serial examinations and photographs.

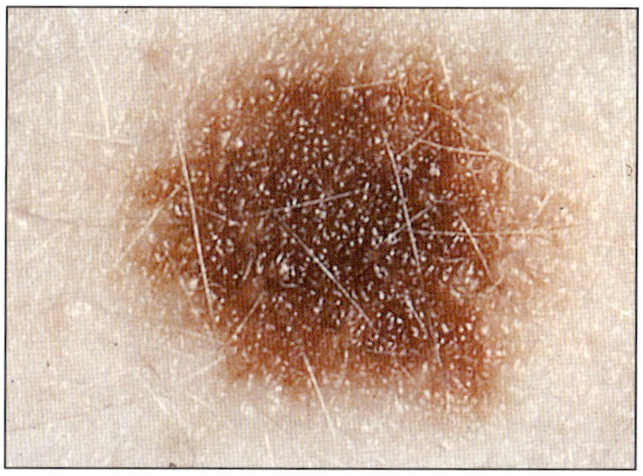

► Dysplastic nevus.

Dysplastic Nevi

Nature of disease

A dysplastic nevus is a clinically and histologically atypical nevus that represents a worrisome precursor to melanoma. They appear sporadically or may be part of an autosomal dominant inheritance known as the *dysplastic nevus syndrome*.

Predilections

White individuals and people with lighter skin are more commonly affected than darker-skinned individuals. There is a slight female predilection.

Clinical features

Dysplastic nevi will be larger and darker than most other nevi. The borders are irregular, with the pigmentation fading gradually into normal skin. The color may be variegated rather than the uniform color seen in nondysplastic nevi.

Radiographic presentation

None.

Differential diagnosis

Dysplastic nevi may resemble nondysplastic nevi on one end of the spectrum and superficial spreading melanoma on the other end of the spectrum. Other conditions that can result in brown to black skin pigmentation include hereditary neurofibromatosis type 1, polyostotic fibrous dysplasia (either the Jaffe-Lichtenstein type or the McCune-Albright type), Peutz-Jeghers syndrome, and seborrheic keratosis.

Microscopic features

Dysplastic nevi will have nests and clusters of nevus cells with pleomorphic nuclei and some mitotic figures lined up along the basement membrane.

Suggested course of action

Refer to a dermatologist for evaluation.

Treatment

Nevi that are suspicious for dysplasia are excised, observing 1.0- to 1.5-cm margins controlled with frozen sections.

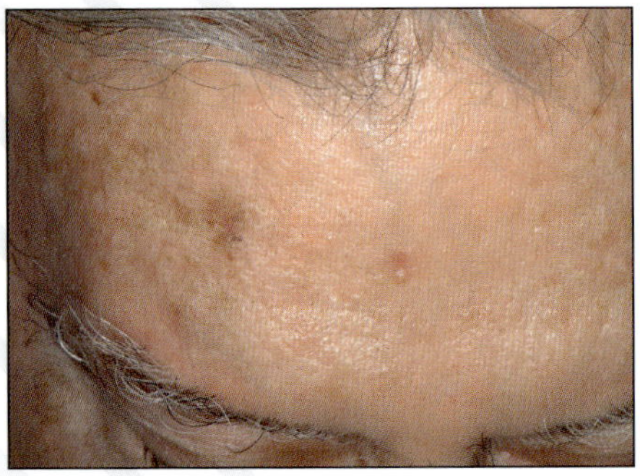

► Lentigo maligna melanoma.

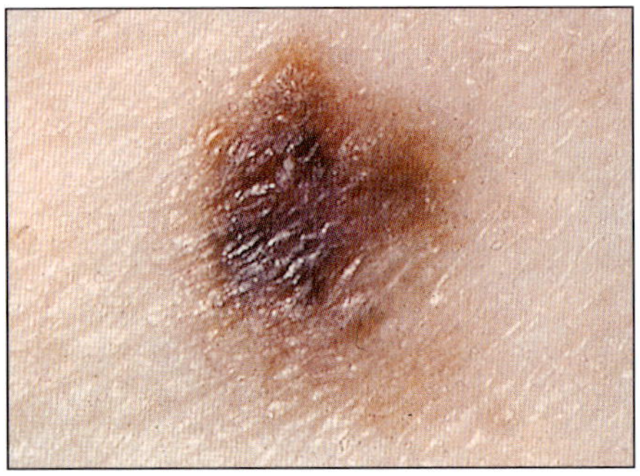

► Superficial spreading melanoma.

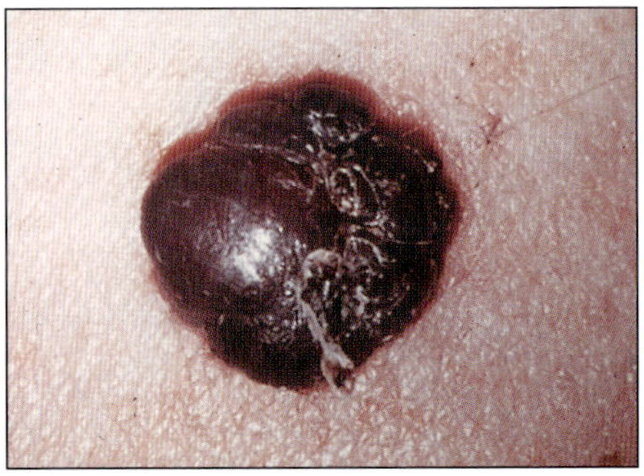

► Nodular melanoma.

Cutaneous Melanomas

Nature of disease

A malignant neoplasm arising from melanocyte precursors and noted to metastasize through small lymphatic channels and blood vessels. Most cutaneous melanomas develop de novo, but others arise from preexisting nevi or dysplastic nevus syndrome.

Predilections

An increased risk is noted from sun exposure in light-skinned individuals, particularly those with blonde or red hair and those with blue or green eyes. There is also an increased risk in those with dysplastic nevus syndrome.

Clinical features

There are four recognized types of cutaneous melanomas:

1. Lentigo maligna melanoma is common to facial skin and represents a melanoma in situ. It occurs in individuals 40 to 70 years of age.
2. Superficial spreading melanoma is common on the shoulders and upper back in both sexes and on the legs in women. The lesion will be asymmetric, slightly raised, and brown-black with irregular borders, and its color will vary and change over time. These same features (asymmetry, border irregularity, color variegation, diameter, and evolution) spell out the ABCDEs of both the lentigo maligna melanoma and the superficial spreading melanoma, allowing the clinician to distinguish melanoma from nevi.
3. Nodular melanoma is more frequent in men than women and will be seen as a blue-black to purple nodule fixed into the skin indicative of its greater depth of invasion. The surface may be ulcerated or polypoid. In some, the surface will appear more red or have a pale color, giving rise to the term *amelanotic melanoma.*
4. Acral lentiginous melanoma is a rare, peculiar melanoma seemingly unrelated to sun exposure as it occurs on the palms of the hands, soles of the feet, and in the webbing between toes. This type occurs more often in Asian and black individuals.

Radiographic presentation

None unless metastasized, in which case it will most likely show numerous soft tissue densities in each lung on a chest radiograph.

Differential diagnosis

Normal nevi and dysplastic nevi are the most important lesions to distinguish from a melanoma. However, pigmented basal cell carcinomas, keratoacanthomas, Kaposi lesions of skin, and seborrheic keratosis may also resemble a cutaneous melanoma. →

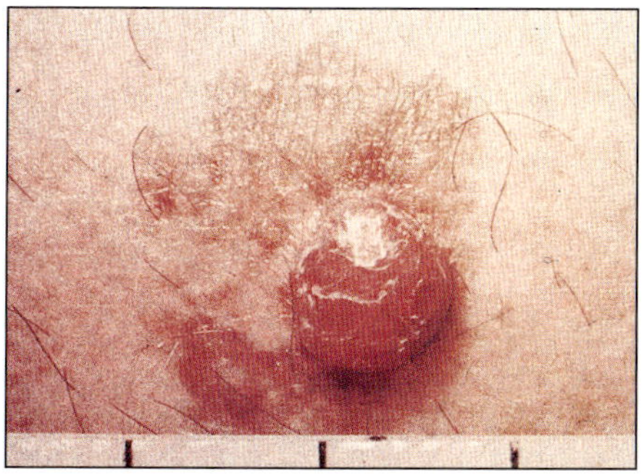

► Amelanotic melanoma.

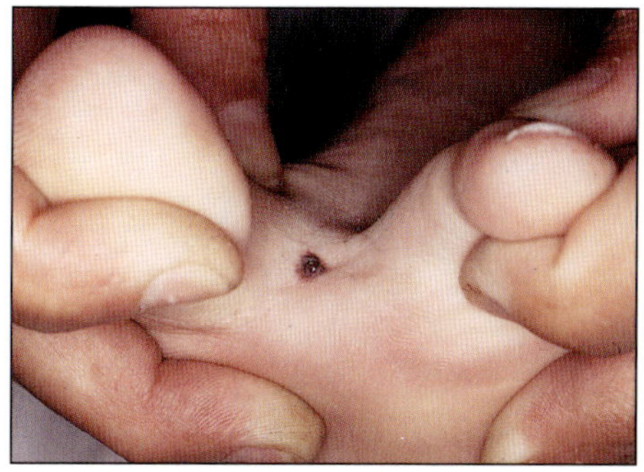

► Acral lentiginous melanoma.

Microscopic features

Melanomas can be significantly varied in their histologic appearance and can be confused with other malignancies, requiring special stains such as S100 protein or human melanoma black-45. Pathologists will assess the tumor cells and relate a depth of invasion as per Clark's levels:

- Level I: Tumor cells confined to the epidermis
- Level II: Tumor cells in the papillary dermis
- Level III: Tumor cells throughout the papillary dermis and infringing upon the reticular dermis
- Level IV: Tumor cells in the reticular dermis
- Level V: Tumor cells in the subcutaneous fat

Suggested course of action

Cases suspicious for a cutaneous melanoma in the face or neck should be referred to an oral and maxillofacial surgeon for workup and treatment. Cutaneous melanomas elsewhere should be referred to a general surgeon.

Treatment

Surgical excision is the standard treatment using the guidelines of 1.0-cm initial peripheral margins, adding another 1.0 cm of peripheral margin for each additional millimeter in depth of invasion. Chemotherapy and immune therapy continue to be researched and may be employed as an adjunct, but only limited results have been gained so far.

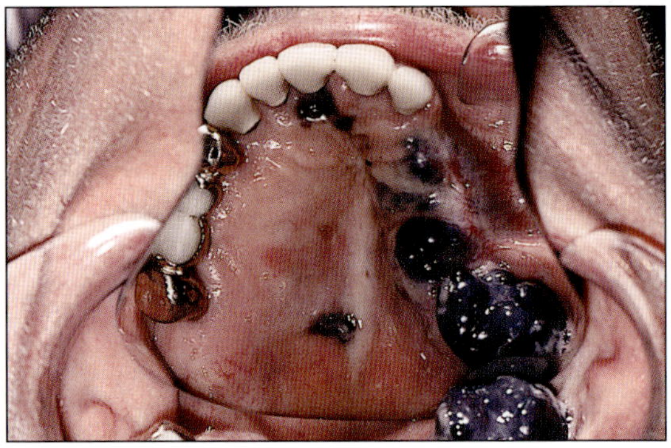

► Oral melanoma.

Oral Melanoma

Nature of disease
A de novo malignant proliferation of melanocyte precursors.

Predilections
Oral melanomas are unrelated to sun exposure or any known carcinogen. There is no known sex or racial predilection. The palate is the most common location for an oral melanoma.

Clinical features
Oral melanomas will usually appear as black, fleshy masses that may also contain some brown or blue coloration. The masses often have adjacent satellite lesions in the mucosa or the skin of the neck. Paresthesia is common, and pain may be present but is less common. Bony destruction, tooth mobility, and tooth displacement are often seen. Spread to lymph nodes in the neck may be present as well.

Radiographic presentation
Those over bone will show a destructive resorption of bone and roots of teeth. CT scans will identify a soft tissue mass infiltrating bone and adjacent tissues.

Differential diagnosis
The rapid growth, color, and destructive nature of an oral melanoma will point to its diagnosis. However, a similar presentation may be seen in some oral squamous cell carcinomas, high-grade mucoepidermoid carcinomas, Kaposi sarcoma, and rhabdomyosarcoma.

Microscopic features
Oral melanomas will have deep-staining tumor cells with numerous mitotic features. This type of melanoma will often have a more sarcomatosis pattern with spindle cells, requiring special stains to confirm the diagnosis.

Suggested course of action
Photograph for documentation of size, color, and location. Accomplish an incisional biopsy, or refer to an oral and maxillofacial surgeon for biopsy and workup.

Treatment
Oral melanomas have a poor prognosis regardless of size. Surgery observing 3.0-cm margins and bilateral neck dissection is recommended. Consultation with an oncologist for an evaluation as to the candidacy for newer-age chemotherapy or immunotherapy is also recommended.

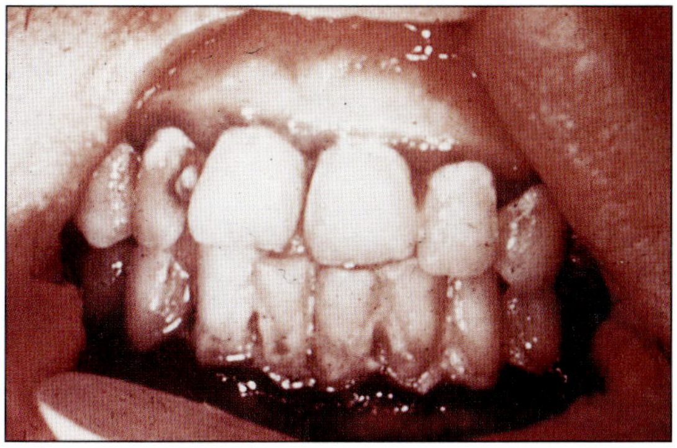

► Heavy metal pigmentation from lead poisoning.

Heavy Metal Pigmentation

Nature of disease

Uncommon today, heavy metal pigmentation resulting from substances containing lead, silver, or mercury was more common in decades past. These metals would react with bacterial sulfides to become deposited in areas of bacterial inflammation as metal sulfides. Today, the most common metal pigmentation is seen on re-entry after titanium plates or screws have been placed for fracture reduction or reconstruction. In such cases, titanium oxide deposits appearing black may be seen as well.

Predilections

No sex or racial predilection is known. It is generally seen more in adults due to their longer use of such products and/or their likelihood to have had titanium plates or screws placed.

Clinical features

The deposits of lead, silver, and mercury are most often seen as a dark band along the gingival line. Titanium oxide pigmentation is seen on re-entry where titanium plates and screws were placed and is embedded in scar tissue around the titanium plate or screw.

Radiographic presentation

None.

Differential diagnosis

The pigmentations from lead, mercury, or silver may be sufficiently dark as to resemble a melanoma. Otherwise, ischemic necrosis, hemangiomas, or lymphangiomas are considerations.

Microscopic features

Irregular metal fragments are seen within the connective tissue. In cases of concomitant inflammation, the metal fragments are within a dense inflammatory cell infiltrate.

Suggested course of action

Review the social and medical history to determine a source for systemic lead, mercury, or silver absorption. Refer the patient to an internist for evaluation.

Treatment

Discontinuation of any heavy metal ingestion. Excision of involved areas can be done if feasible. In the case of titanium oxide around titanium plates and screws, no treatment is required, but if the plate and screws are removed, the enveloping scar tissue containing the metal fragments is removed as well.

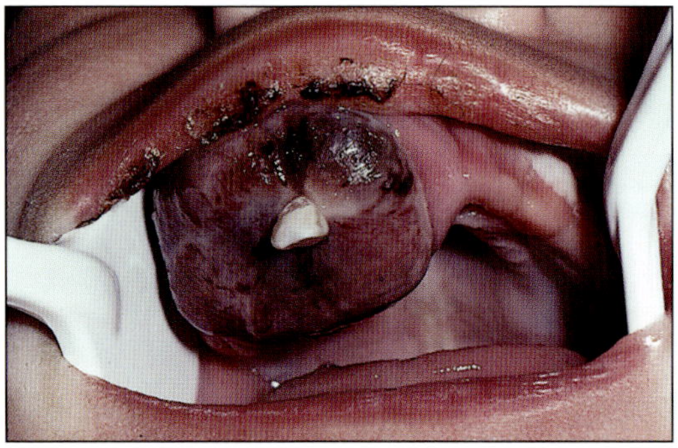

► Melanotic neuroectodermal tumor of infancy.

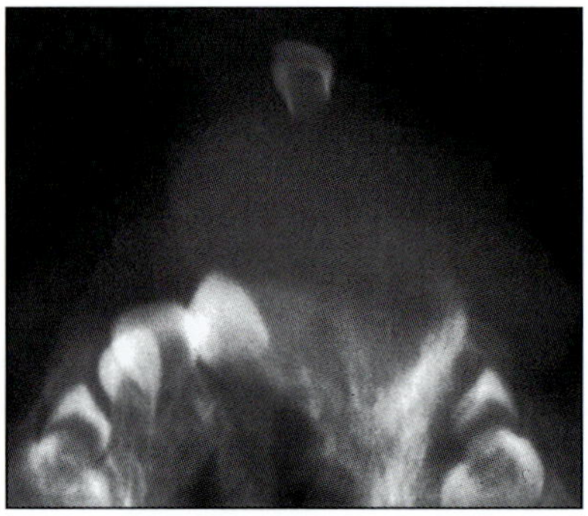

► Characteristic occlusal radiography of a melanotic neuroectodermal tumor of infancy.

Melanotic Neuroectodermal Tumor of Infancy

Nature of disease

A benign neoplasm that arises from developmental neuroectoderm.

Predilections

Most occur in the maxilla, with only rare exceptions. It is not congenital, but over 95% will develop in the first year of life. Other rare locations include the mandible, skull, and scapula. There is no known sex or racial predilection.

Clinical features

A blue-black mass with a rapid growth rate will emerge from the involved bone. In the most common location in the anterior maxilla, a single primary incisor is carried out to the periphery and is situated in the mass. This has been termed the "candle in the cupcake" appearance. The mass does not bleed and does not seem to be painful to the infant. The overlying gingiva/mucosa becomes very thinned.

Radiographic presentation

An occlusal view is usually the most practical radiograph for an infant with a mass in this location. A soft tissue destructive mass will be noted that is not well demarcated from normal bone. The radiograph will show displacement of primary teeth and tooth buds as well as the one incisor carried out to the periphery of the mass.

Differential diagnosis

The most important differential is to distinguish the benign melanotic neuroectodermal tumor of infancy from its malignant counterpart, the neuroblastoma. Other rapidly growing tumors of bluish coloration in an infant to be considered are rhabdomyosarcomas, teratogenic carcinomas, and some hemangiomas. A congenital epulis of the newborn is not a serious consideration because it is always congenital, whereas the melanotic neuroectodermal tumor of infancy is not.

Microscopic features

Two cell types within a fibrous stroma will be seen: *(1)* small round cells with dark-staining nuclei that represent neuroblasts and *(2)* larger cells containing melanin.

Suggested course of action

Obtain photographs and a high-quality occlusal radiograph. Refer to an oral and maxillofacial surgeon for further workup and definitive treatment.

Treatment

A wide local excision observing 0.5- to 1.0-cm margins is curative. In cases where a visible lesion remained after a subtotal excision, the residual tumor was observed to involute, suggesting that the melanotic neuroectodermal tumor of infancy may represent a hamartoma rather than a true neoplasm.

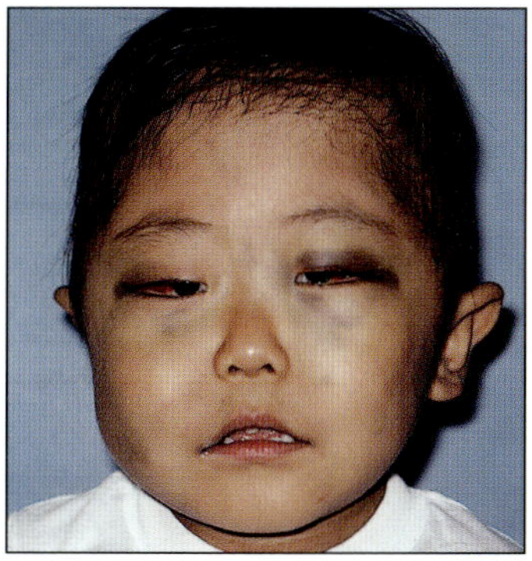

► Neuroblastoma. Multicenter tumor nodules give rise to the term "blueberry muffin baby."

Neuroblastoma

Nature of disease

A malignant tumor of neural crest cells that originate in the mantle layer around the developing spinal cord. It represents the malignant counterpart of the benign melanotic neuroectodermal tumor of infancy.

Predilections

Most (75%) appear by the age of 2 years. It represents the third most common childhood malignancy. There is no known sex or racial predilection.

Clinical features

Neuroblastomas are almost always multifocal. The maxilla, skull, femur, and humerus are the more common sites of occurrence. The tumor forms masses and infiltrations often without a significant mass effect, which, due to their bluish appearance, will appear like ecchymosis or a battered child. The multifocal skin lesions with their blue color have given rise to the term "blueberry muffin baby."

Radiographic presentation

Plain radiographs will note a bony destructive mass with irregular borders. A CT scan will identify a lobulated mass infiltrating adjacent bone and soft tissues.

Differential diagnosis

The multifocal presentation is distinctive. However, a similar picture may present from a rhabdomyosarcoma, Ewing sarcoma, or retinoblastoma.

Microscopic features

Collections of small, round, dark-staining cells with frequent mitotic figures are seen separated by a thin fibrovascular stroma.

Suggested course of action

Refer to a pediatric oncologist.

Treatment

Stage I and stage II tumors are usually treated with surgery alone, observing 2.0-cm margins. Stage III and stage IV tumors are treated by surgery followed by radiation and chemotherapy.

10

Lesions of the Facial Skin and Oral Mucosa

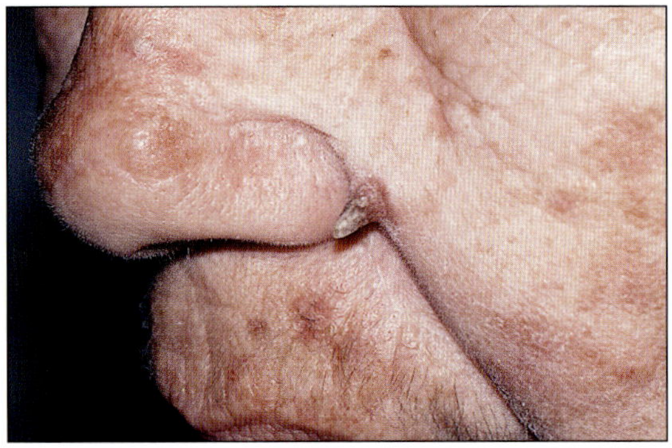

► Multiple actinic keratosis lesions and a central "cutaneous horn," which is an exophytic form of a skin squamous cell carcinoma.

Actinic Keratosis

Nature of disease

A premalignant epithelial dysplasia of the skin due to the ultraviolet B band of radiation from long-term sun exposure.

Predilections

Adults with long-term sun exposure. It mostly occurs in fair-skinned individuals with blonde or red hair and blue or green eyes. It is very rare in darker-skinned individuals. It occurs more in men than in women because outdoor careers are more common for men.

Clinical features

The skin is often atrophic and may have a surface peel or crust. The skin may be hypopigmented or even hyperpigmented. It is not painful, and there is no true ulceration or induration.

Radiographic presentation

None.

Differential diagnosis

Actinic keratosis represents a premalignant epithelial dysplasia that can progress to a basal cell carcinoma, a skin squamous cell carcinoma, or a keratoacanthoma. Early phases of these three entities require consideration. A melanoma in situ also bears consideration.

Microscopic features

The skin epithelium will show varying degrees of dysplasia mostly toward severe dysplasia/carcinoma in situ. The basement membrane will be intact, but the underlying dermis will often be less cellular with disorganized, gray-staining collagen referred to as *solar elastosis*. Inflammation in the dermis may also be present.

Suggested course of action

Refer to an oral and maxillofacial surgeon or a dermatologist for examination and treatment.

Treatment

Many practitioners begin treatment using 2% 5-fluorouracil cream together with a steroid cream. This often controls or resolves the clinical lesion. Those that progress require either Mohs chemosurgery or a local excision controlled with frozen sections.

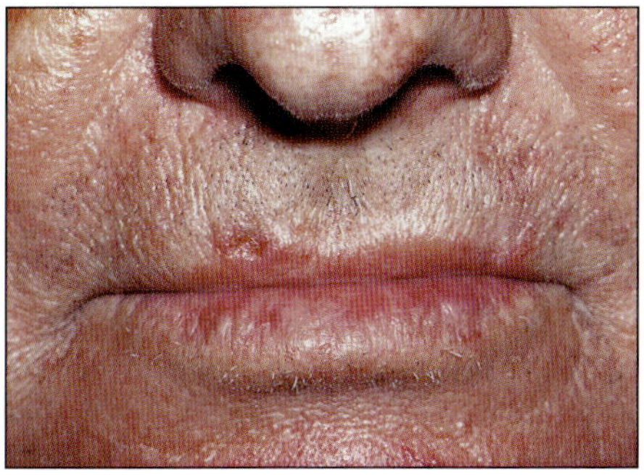

► Noduloulcerative type of basal cell carcinoma.

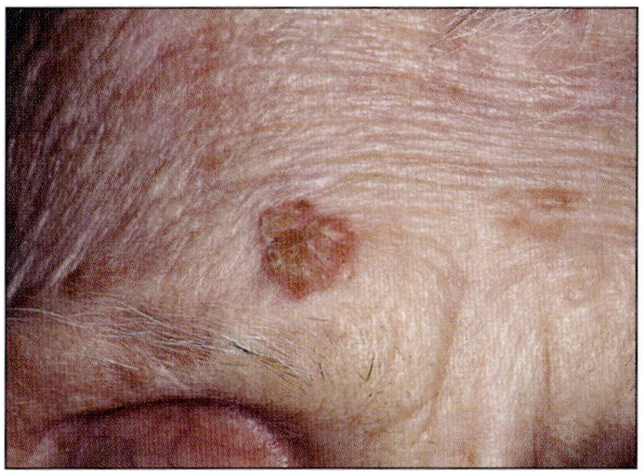

► Papulopearly type of basal cell carcinoma.

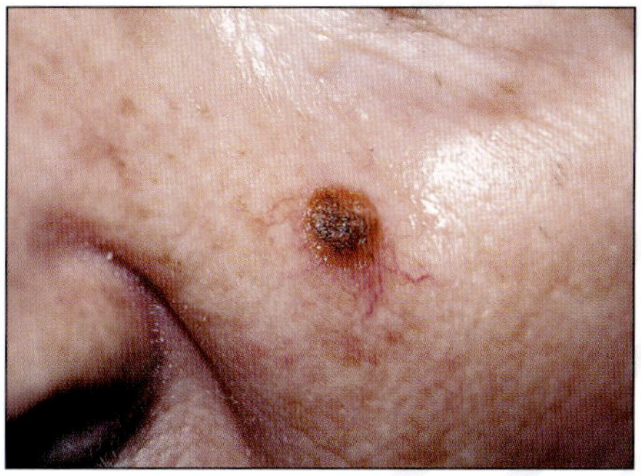

► Pigmented type of basal cell carcinoma.

Basal Cell Carcinoma

Nature of disease

A malignant transformation of the stem cells at the basement membrane of skin that retain basal cell features.

Predilections

Seen mostly in sun-exposed areas in individuals with long-term sun exposure. It mostly affects adults with fair skin, blonde or red hair, and blue or green eyes. It is very rare in darker-skinned individuals. Less commonly, basal cell carcinomas will appear in children and young adults related to a specific syndrome (ie, basal cell nevus syndrome). Note: The basal cell nevi/carcinomas in basal cell nevus syndrome will appear microscopically as a basal cell carcinoma but are smaller and have a different biologic potential. They are mostly indolent.

Clinical features

Basal cell carcinomas from sun exposure have been described with five clinical appearances:

1. Noduloulcerative: A shallow ulcer with irregular borders mimicking an animal bite called the "rodent ulcer."
2. Papulopearly: A raised skin mass with a pale surface often with small lobulations. May also be called *cystic type*.
3. Pigmented: A papillary mass with dots or areas of melanin pigmentation.
4. Sclerosing or morphoeic type: A flat and pale but somewhat erythematous lesion with irregular borders.
5. Superficial type: Flat or slightly raised scaly lesion with regular borders.

Radiographic presentation

None.

Differential diagnosis

In the sun-exposed individual, a skin squamous cell carcinoma, a keratoacanthoma, and a melanoma should be considered. A small lesion without ulceration may mimic actinic keratosis.

Microscopic features

Nests and islands of dark-staining epithelial cells will be seen growing into the dermis. An inflammatory infiltrate is frequently associated with these islands. Keratin pearls are not present, but cystic breakdown within the islands may be seen. →

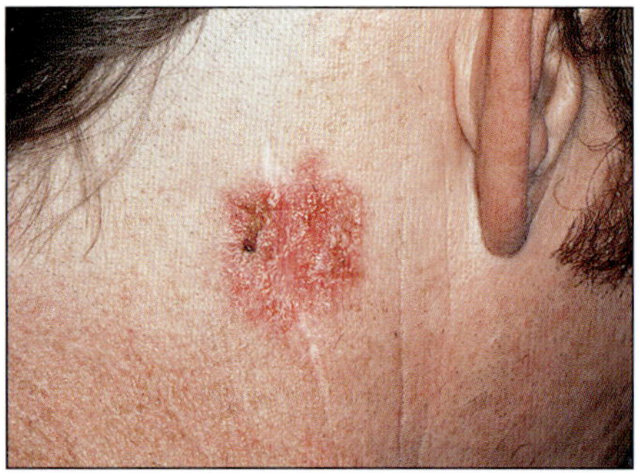

► Sclerosing or morphoeic type of basal cell carcinoma.

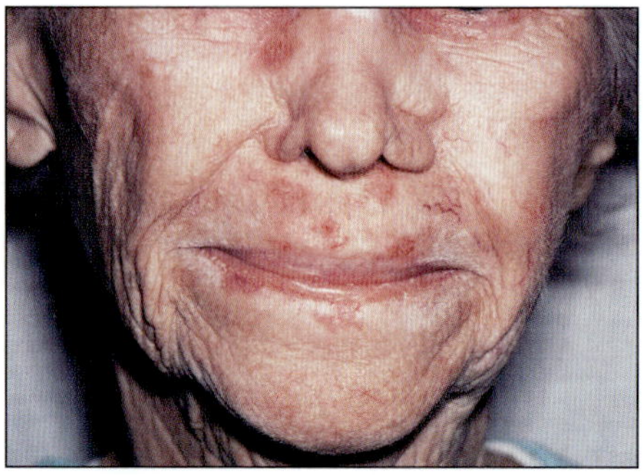

► Superficial type of basal cell carcinoma.

Basal Cell Carcinoma *(cont)*

Suggested course of action

Refer to an oral and maxillofacial surgeon, a Mohs chemosurgeon, or a dermatologist.

Treatment

Either Mohs chemosurgery or a local excision observing 0.5-cm margins controlled with frozen sections. Note: Local excisions and Mohs chemosurgery–related defects often require local flap reconstruction. Small lesions are often treated with cryotherapy or electrodesiccation.

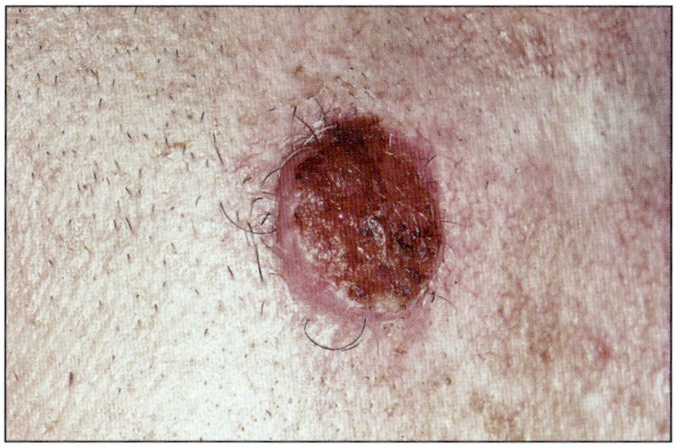

► Skin squamous cell carcinoma.

Skin Squamous Cell Carcinoma

Nature of disease

A malignant transformation of the stem cells at the basement membrane of skin that progresses to a partial squamous differentiation.

Predilections

Seen mostly in sun-exposed areas in individuals with long-term sun exposure. It mostly affects adults with fair skin, blonde or red hair, and blue or green eyes. It is very rare in darker-skinned individuals. It occurs more in men than in women because outdoor careers are more common for men.

Clinical features

The clinical appearance varies from an open ulcer with central necrosis and elevated edges to an exophytic mass with a brown to black, rough surface texture. Most are nonpainful. Lymphadenopathy is only seen in longstanding lesions.

Radiographic presentation

None.

Differential diagnosis

Keratoacanthomas, basal cell carcinomas, and nodular melanoma can present in an identical fashion.

Microscopic features

Nests and islands of pleomorphic cells infiltrating the dermis. Keratin pearls may be seen and are common. The cells will be more spindle shaped and have less nuclear staining than those in a basal cell carcinoma. An inflammatory infiltrate is usually associated with the infiltrating islands.

Suggested course of action

Refer to an oral and maxillofacial surgeon, a Mohs chemosurgeon, or a dermatologist.

Treatment

Either Mohs chemosurgery or a local excision observing 1.0-cm margins controlled with frozen sections. Note: Local excisions and Mohs chemosurgery–related defects often require local flap reconstruction.

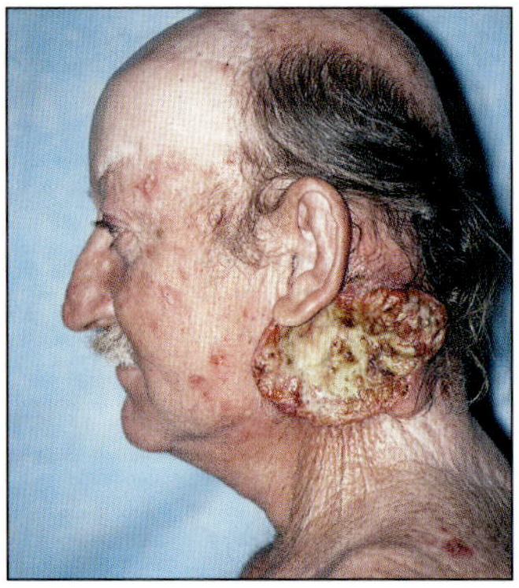

► Skin basosquamous cell carcinoma.

Skin Basosquamous Cell Carcinoma

Nature of disease

A malignant transformation of the stem cells at the basement membrane of skin that progresses to a partial squamous and basal cell differentiation.

Predilections

Seen mostly in sun-exposed areas in individuals with long-term sun exposure. It mostly affects adults with fair skin, blonde or red hair, and blue or green eyes. It is very rare in darker-skinned individuals. It occurs more in men than in women because outdoor careers are more common for men.

Clinical features

Basosquamous cell carcinomas of skin tend to be larger, more ulcerative, and more infiltrating than other skin squamous cell carcinomas. Some will appear with necrotic centers and evidence of deep invasion into bone.

Radiographic presentation

If bone invasion occurs, facial bone radiographs will show an irregular, moth-eaten appearance and surface erosion of the involved bone.

Differential diagnosis

Basosquamous cell carcinomas will appear like a more aggressive form of other skin squamous cell carcinomas, as well as some basal cell carcinomas, keratoacanthomas, and nodular melanomas.

Microscopic features

Sections will show nests and islands of infiltrating pleomorphic cells exhibiting keratin pearls and intercellular bridges adjacent to similar areas of darker-staining cells without intercellular bridges or keratin pearls. The infiltrating cells are often seen within muscle fibers and into bone. An inflammatory infiltrate frequently accompanies the tumor islands.

Suggested course of action

Refer to an oral and maxillofacial surgeon or a dermatologist.

Treatment

The size and degree of infiltration of basosquamous cell carcinoma usually mitigate against Mohs chemosurgery. Extensive local excision observing 1.5- to 2.0-cm margins and flap reconstruction is the most common treatment. In those cases where close or positive tumor margins are noted after surgery, radiation therapy is also used.

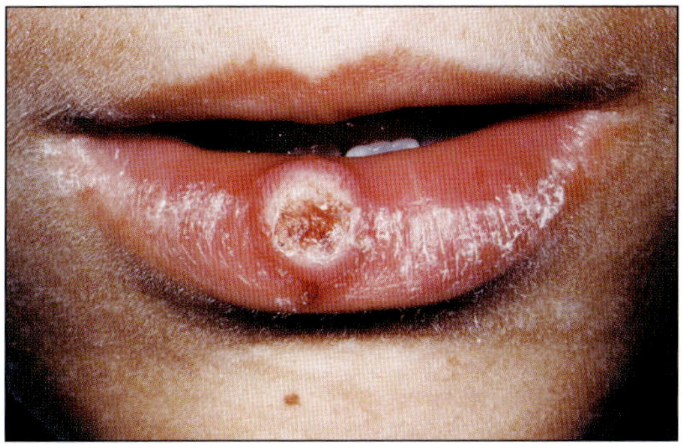

► Keratoacanthoma of the lower lip vermilion.

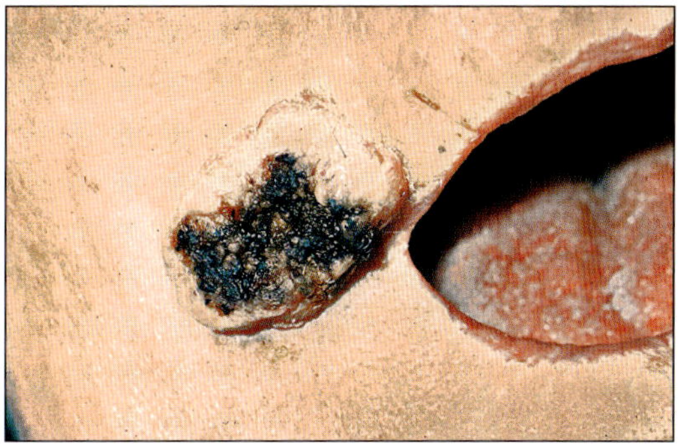

► Keratoacanthoma of the facial skin.

Keratoacanthoma

Nature of disease

A well-differentiated squamous cell carcinoma that arises from hair follicle epithelium and therefore oftentimes reproduces the 120-day hair follicle cycle.

Predilections

Mostly seen in sun-exposed areas in adults with fair skin, blonde or red hair, and blue or green eyes. It may also occur as part of the Ferguson-Smith syndrome seen in children or the Grzybowski syndrome seen in adults. No sex predilection is known. These lesions have also been known to occur on the vermillion of the lower lip.

Clinical features

Keratoacanthomas may be seen in any one of the three stages of their development:

1. Stage I: A small acnelike mass with an intact skin surface growing rapidly.
2. Stage II: A round to oval craterlike lesion with well-defined rolled edges and/or a center of brown to black keratin.
3. Stage III: Extrusion of the central keratin plug and a gradual involution of the lesion in a self-healing fashion, mimicking the exfoliation of a hair follicle after 120 days.

Note: Completion through all three stages is only seen in one-third of cases. In the remaining two-thirds of cases, the keratoacanthoma stays in either stage I or stage II, mostly stage II.

Radiographic presentation

None.

Differential diagnosis

Keratoacanthomas will appear very similar to some basal cell carcinomas, some skin squamous cell carcinomas, and some nodular melanomas.

Microscopic features

The center portion will feature a plug of eosinophilic keratin above an acanthotic layer of epithelium with minimal or no dysplasia but blunt endophytic rete pegs with an intact basement membrane, pushing downward into the dermis. The most diagnostic feature is the lesion edge, which will show adjacent normal skin epithelium abruptly invaginating to form the floor of the crater. ⟶

Keratoacanthoma *(cont)*

Suggested course of action

Refer to an oral and maxillofacial surgeon or a dermatologist.

Treatment

Many are followed in the anticipation of a spontaneous involution and self-healing. However, if no signs of an involution are apparent by 6 weeks, a local excision is accomplished, observing 0.5-cm margins. Others are excised at first presentation to rule out the other lesions on the differential diagnosis.

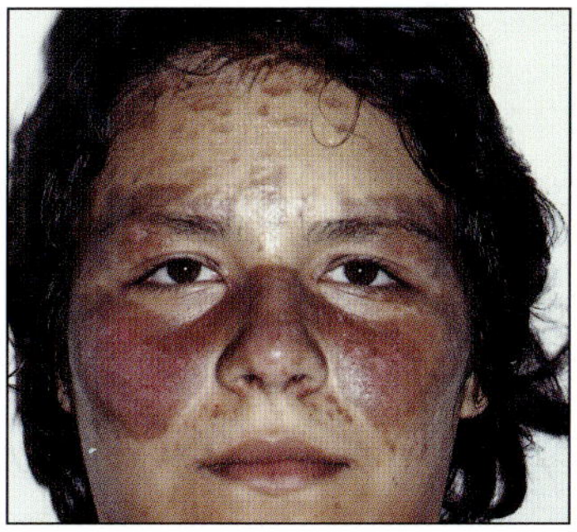

► Classic "butterfly rash" seen in some patients with systemic lupus erythematosus.

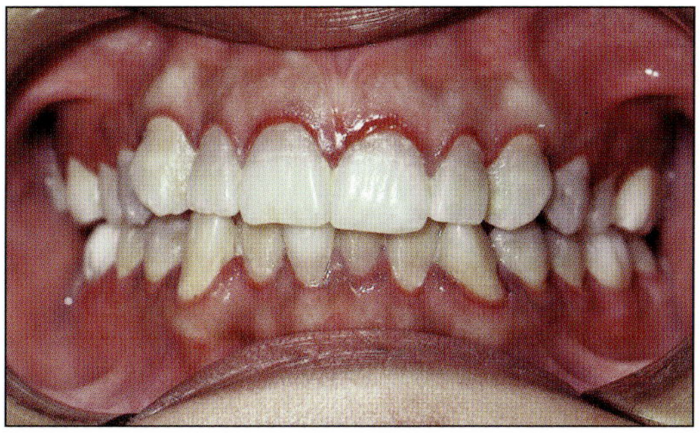

► A noninflammatory marginal gingivitis is often seen in patients with systemic lupus erythematosus.

Systemic Lupus Erythematosus

Nature of disease

An autoimmune disease that produces antigen-antibody complexes that circulate and become entrapped in most organs, stimulating an activation of the complement cascade and inflammation.

Predilections

Occurs almost exclusively in women. Most patients are between 15 and 40 years of age. There is a higher incidence in black individuals of African heritage, and yet curiously it is not found in Africa among native black Africans.

Clinical features

The clinical features can be quite variable. The most common feature is a red-purple symmetric skin lesion over the nose and cheek areas referred to as the "butterfly rash." Similar lesions may be noted at the junction of hair-bearing skin and non–hair-bearing skin. Many patients will report skin lesions erupting after sun exposure. Some skin lesions will be seen to have a wide area of pale skin with a periphery of a slightly raised erythematous band. Oral lesions will mostly appear like marginal gingivitis, but some will also include shallow red lesions on the palatal mucosa.

Radiographic presentation

None.

Differential diagnosis

The most important differential is that of drug-induced lupus erythematosus, in which a reaction to certain medications such as levothyroxine or procanamide produces a similar rash and similar symptoms to autoimmune systemic lupus erythematosus. Other diseases to consider include discoid lupus erythematosus and erythema multiforme.

Microscopic features

Relatively nonspecific collagen degeneration and fibrin deposition is seen with only a sparse amount of inflammation. However, granular deposits of immunoglobulins are seen on direct immunofluorescence.

Suggested course of action

Suspected cases should be referred to a rheumatologist for a comprehensive workup, testing, and treatment.

Treatment

Nonprogressive cases with mild symptoms are often controlled with only supportive care or with hydroxychloroquine (Plaquenil, Sanofi Winthrop) 400 mg by mouth daily. Progressive cases or cases with multiorgan involvement are treated with systemic prednisone at dosages dependent on the disease severity, to which mycophenolate (CellCept, Genentech) or cyclophosphamide (Cytoxan, Bristol-Myers Squibb) may be added or substituted.

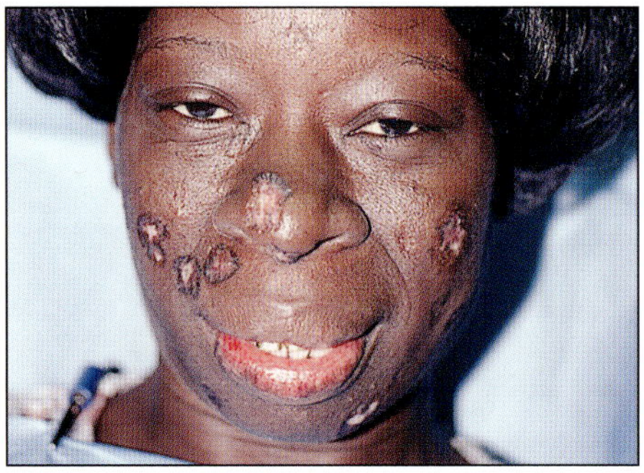

► Skin lesions of chronic cutaneous lupus erythematosus.

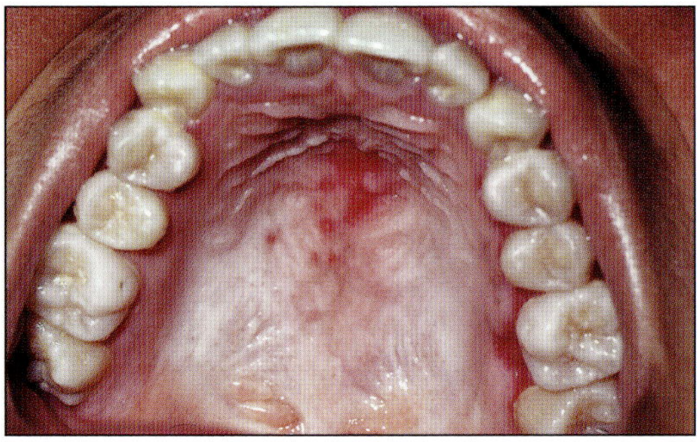

► Palatal lesions are often seen in patients with chronic cutaneous lupus erythematosus.

Chronic Cutaneous Lupus Erythematosus (Discoid Lupus Erythematosus)

Nature of disease

An autoimmune-based inflammatory disease without identifiable autoantibodies that primarily targets the skin and to a lesser extent oral mucosa with only sparse systemic and internal organ involvement.

Predilections

In contrast to systemic lupus erythematosus, there is no sex predilection. There is also no racial predilection. Occurs mostly in adults over 30 years of age.

Clinical features

Similar to systemic lupus erythematosus, a butterfly rash may be seen as well as dusky red lesions in a targetoid pattern, many within a hairline area. Oral lesions are seen as a red line across the marginal gingiva and/or shallow red ulcers on the palatal mucosa. Lesions on both skin and oral mucosa are usually asymptomatic.

Radiographic presentation

None.

Differential diagnosis

Systemic lupus erythematosus should be the first disease to be considered and ruled out by clinical criteria and laboratory testing. Other diseases that can produce disfiguring facial skin lesions include mycosis fungoides, sarcoidosis, skin tuberculosis termed *lupus vulgaris*, and even leprosy.

Microscopic features

Acanthosis and hyperkeratosis are prominent. Degeneration of basal cells with edema in the lamina propria of oral lesions and the papillary dermis of skin is seen together with a dense inflammatory infiltrate comprised primarily of lymphocytes.

Suggested course of action

Suspected cases should be referred to a rheumatologist or a dermatologist. There is no contraindication to dental care. However, tetracycline antibiotics should be used cautiously, or alternatives should be used because tetracyclines may cause a flare-up of the lesion due to their photosensitizing side effect.

Treatment

Oral lesions require no treatment, and in many cases skin lesions also require no treatment. Photosensitizing drugs such as tetracyclines, thiazide diuretics, and piroxicam should be avoided. Symptomatic skin lesions are treated with topical steroid creams such as 0.05% fluocinonide and 1% hydrocortisone cream (topical 10%). Additionally, topical immunosuppressive creams such as 0.1% tacrolimus cream (Protopic, Astellas Pharma) or 1% pimecrolimus cream (Elidel, Valeant) may be used.

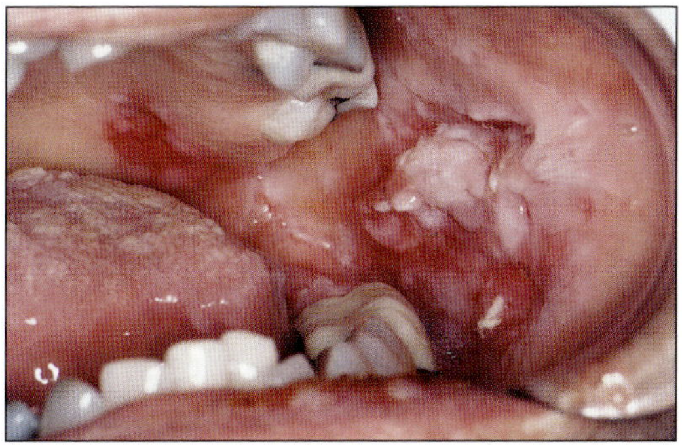

► Oral lesions of pemphigus vulgaris.

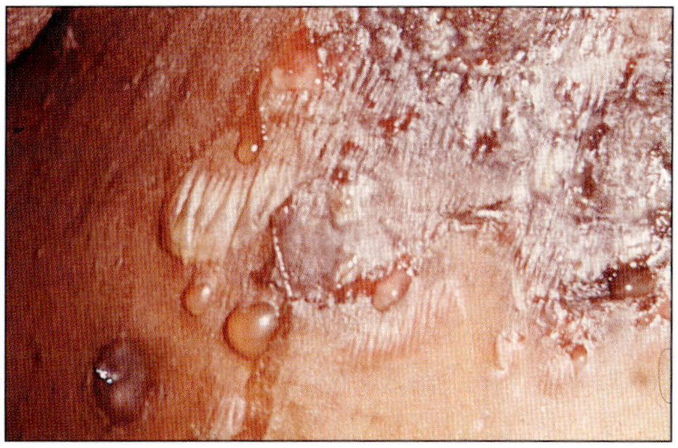

► Skin lesions of pemphigus vulgaris.

Pemphigus Vulgaris

Nature of disease

An autoimmune disease whereby autoantibodies develop against desmoglein in the desmosomes of intercellular bridges.

Predilections

May target oral mucosa only, skin only, or both skin and oral mucosa. No age, sex, or racial predilection is known.

Clinical features

Oral lesions will frequently appear with hemorrhagic crusting lesions of the lower lip vermilion and various shallow mucosal ulcers. At times, a white slough or vesicles may also be apparent. On skin, the lesions more often appear as vesicles with a peripheral erythema. Some areas of hemorrhagic crust may also be seen. The lesions in either location are significantly painful.

Radiographic presentation

None.

Differential diagnosis

Two other lesions appear with both oral and skin lesions at times: lichen planus and pemphigoid. Although erythema multiforme primarily targets skin, some will also develop a painful hemorrhagic lesion on the lower lip as is often seen in pemphigus. In children and younger adults, primary herpetic gingivostomatitis should also be considered.

Microscopic features

Routine hematoxylin and eosin–stained specimens will identify a dense lymphocytic-plasmacytic infiltrate below an intact basement membrane. The basal cells will be present and firmly attached to the basement membrane. However, most will then show a separation of the prickle cell layer from the basal cells, often referred to as a *suprabasilar split*. In biopsies of vesicles or in intact mucosa specimens, the prickle layer may be lost in the processing, leaving the basal cells positioned on the basement membrane like parallel rods above an empty space. If direct immunofluorescence is used, one will see a fluorescence within the intercellular bridge area in the prickle cell layer.

Suggested course of action

Refer to an oral and maxillofacial surgeon for biopsy or to a rheumatologist for workup and treatment.

Treatment

Pemphigus vulgaris has different degrees of severity. However, it is a serious autoimmune disease that mostly requires a structured treatment with prednisone. Refractory cases may require supplemental treatment with methotrexate, cyclophosphamide, azathioprine, or rituximab.

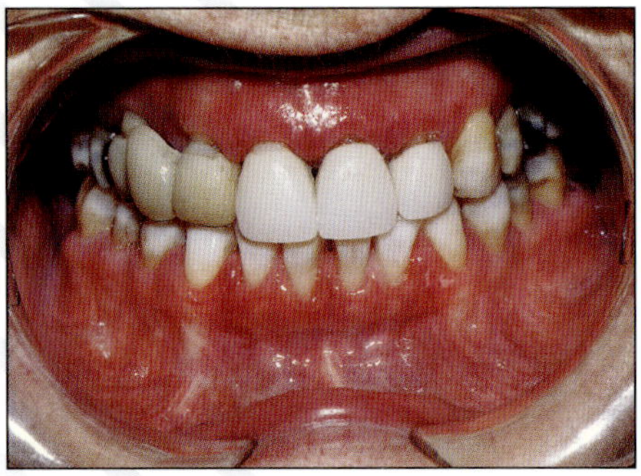

► Gingival lesions of pemphigoid.

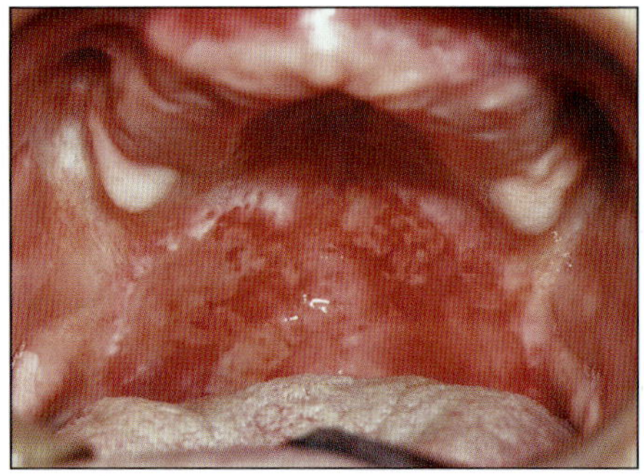

► Palatal lesions of pemphigoid.

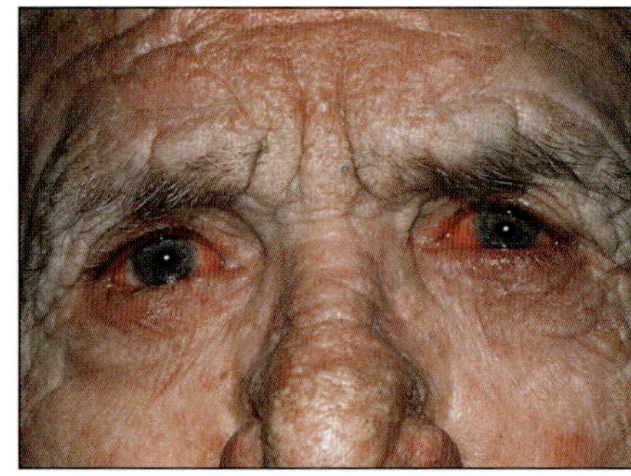

► Nonsuppurative conjunctivitis in pemphigoid.

Pemphigoid

Nature of disease

An autoimmune disease by which autoantibodies develop against various proteins within the basement membrane.

Predilections

Adults over 50 years of age. No sex or racial predilection is known. It may target oral mucosa only, ocular mucosa (conjunctiva) only, skin only, or multiple mucosal surfaces with or without concomitant skin involvement.

Clinical features

Oral and other mucosal lesions will present asymptomatic or mildly painful erythematous lesions and/or vesicles or shallow ulcers. Ocular lesions will present as a nonsuppurative conjunctivitis (red eye). Skin lesions are more likely to show vesicles surrounded by an erythematous base.

Radiographic presentation

None.

Differential diagnosis

Lichen planus and pemphigus vulgaris will more closely resemble pemphigoid than other mucosal conditions. Additionally, lichen drug eruptions and erythema multiforme should also be considered.

Microscopic features

Routine hematoxylin and eosin–stained specimens will identify a diffuse lymphocytic-plasmacytic infiltrate below an involved or split basement membrane. Most will show an incomplete longitudinal split in the basement membrane, creating a microscopic vesicle that has a portion of the basement membrane on the vesicle roof and another portion on the floor of the vesicle. If direct immunofluorescence is used, it will show a fluorescence in the basement membrane zone.

Suggested course of action

Refer to an oral and maxillofacial surgeon for biopsy or to a rheumatologist for workup.

Treatment

Mild cases may require no treatment or topical steroids. For oral lesions, 0.05% fluocinonide gel or dexamethasone elixir swish and spit is often used. Mild ocular lesions are treated with prednisone drops. Mild skin lesions are treated with 0.05% fluocinonide cream or 0.05% clobetasol cream. More extensive or severe cases are treated with systemic prednisone.

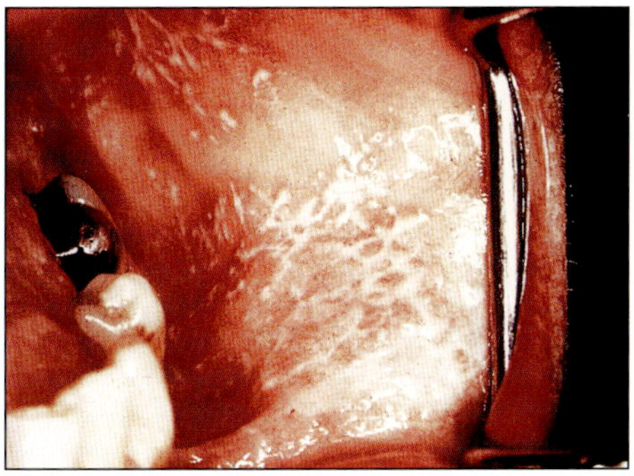

► Striaform lichen planus.

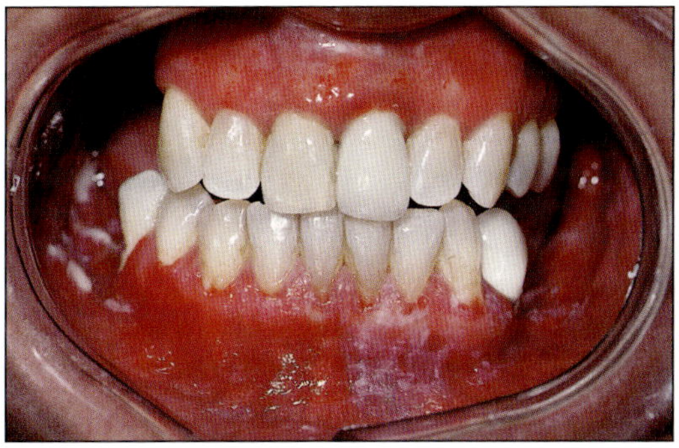

► Erosive lichen planus.

Lichen Planus

Nature of disease

An autoimmune disease whereby activated T cells attack the basement membrane area of oral mucosa and/or skin with lymphokines and other enzymes.

Predilections

Mostly adults over 30 years of age. There is no sex or racial predilection.

Clinical features

1. Oral lesions of striaform lichen planus are asymptomatic and will target the buccal mucosa. They appear as lacy white lesions that are slightly elevated.
2. Oral erosive lichen planus targets the buccal mucosa, dorsum of the tongue, and attached gingiva. The buccal mucosa and tongue lesions will often appear as broad-based erythematous ulcers with a fibrin base. The lesions will be red and white. Lesions on the attached gingiva may appear thin and atrophic. They are often friable and easily bleed. Some will appear with a white slough. Oral erosive lichen planus is painful, varying from a mild discomfort to severe pain.
3. Skin lichen planus is more pruritic than painful. Lesions will appear violaceous or red. They may be ulcerative or have an intact surface in a diffuse erythematous area.

Radiographic presentation

None.

Differential diagnosis

Pemphigus vulgaris and pemphigoid can also present with oral lesions only or oral lesions together with skin lesions. Skin lichen planus is also simulated by erythema multiforme and mycosis fungoides.

Microscopic features

Biopsy specimens will show a thickening of the prickle cell layer (acanthosis) without cellular atypia. Hyperkeratosis and a disruption of the basement membrane are also present. Jagged so-called "saw tooth" rete pegs are variably present. A primarily lymphocytic-histiocytic infiltrate absent of plasma cells is seen immediately adjacent to the basement membrane in a bandlike pattern.

Suggested course of action

Biopsy a nonulcerated area or refer to an oral and maxillofacial surgeon for biopsy. →

Lichen Planus *(cont)*

Treatment

1. Striaform lichen planus does not require treatment and may not represent the same biology as erosive or skin lichen planus. It is also not at risk for malignant transformation.
2. Erosive lichen planus requires a systemic prednisone protocol with or without adjunctive treatments such as griseofulvin, methotrexate, mycophenolate, or cyclophosphamide. Erosive lichen planus has a 1% to 3% incidence of malignant transformation over the lifetime of the disease.
3. Skin lichen planus is mostly treated with topical 0.05% fluocinonide cream or 0.05% clobetasol cream. Severe cases are often treated with the systemic prednisone protocol.

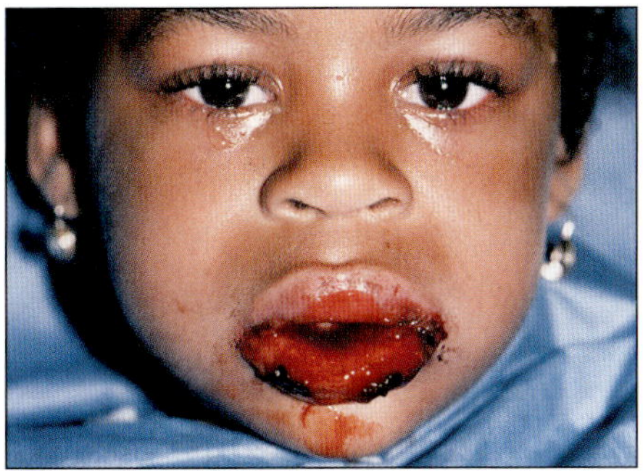

► Erythema multiforme minor.

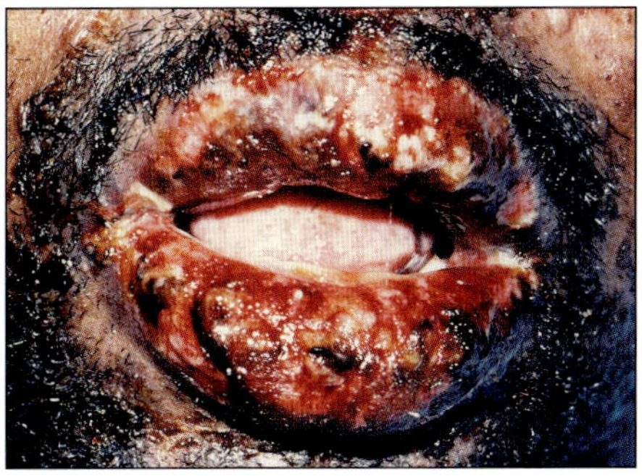

► Erythema multiforme major.

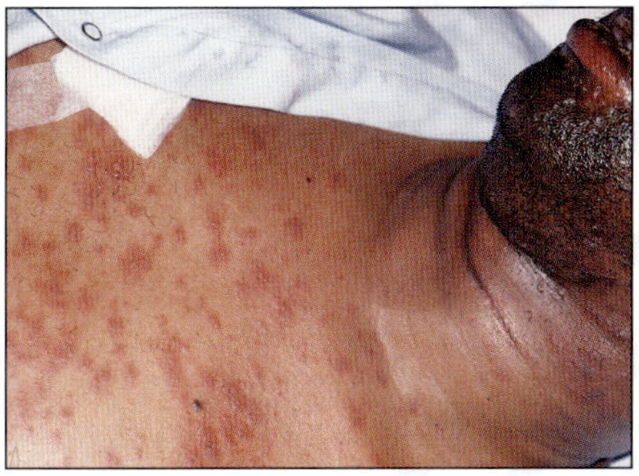

► Multiple skin lesions in erythema multiforme major.

Erythema Multiforme

Nature of disease

A rapid onset of a hypersensitivity/inflammatory reaction initiated by a trigger. The intense inflammatory reaction results in a necrosis of epithelium. In erythema multiforme minor, it is less intense and limited to skin and sometimes also includes oral mucosa, particularly the lower lip vermilion. In erythema multiforme major, the disease is much more intense and may necrose the corneas and genital skin as well as the lip vermilion. The trigger is commonly a drug but may also be sun exposure, an infection elsewhere in the body, or any physiologic stress.

Predilections

No age, sex, or racial predilection is known.

Clinical features

- Erythema multiforme minor will begin as mildly uncomfortable red-brown skin lesions, which will progress to a targetlike appearance within 24 hours. If the vermilion is involved, these lesions will be more painful than the skin lesions and will appear hemorrhagic and crusting.
- Erythema multiforme major will have an explosive onset of a greater number of more painful skin and lip lesions, photophobia, and corneal ulcerations. The skin over the genitals often develops large necrotic ulcers.

Radiographic presentation

None.

Differential diagnosis

Erythema multiforme minor will resemble pemphigus vulgaris, erosive lichen planus where both skin and oral lesions are present, and lichenoid drug eruptions. Erythema multiforme major is somewhat distinctive; only toxic epidermal necrolysis, paraneoplastic pemphigus, and necrotizing fasciitis may appear in a similar fashion.

Microscopic features

Early lesions will show vacuolation of basal cells and an intense lymphocytic infiltrate. As it progresses, epithelial necrosis will be prominent. →

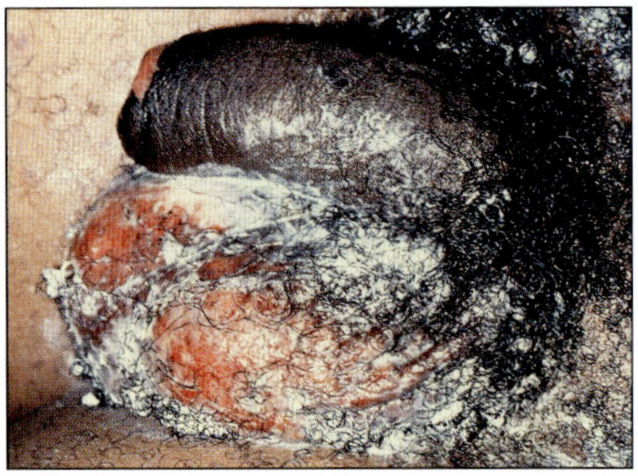

► Scrotal skin necrosis in erythema multiforme major.

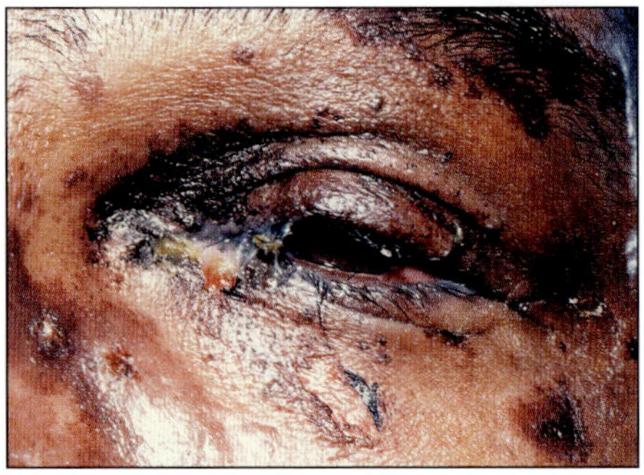

► Corneal necrosis in erythema multiforme major.

Erythema Multiforme *(cont)*

Suggested course of action

Withdraw any suspected inciting drug/medication. Refer to an internal medicine specialist or an infectious disease specialist.

Treatment

Erythema multiforme minor is treated by withdrawing possible offending drugs or situations together with hydration and rest. Erythema multiforme major is usually treated in a burn unit with topical antibacterial silver preparations for the skin lesions, intravenous fluids and electrolytes, high-dose corticosteroids, pain management, and staphylococcal-sensitive antibiotics if needed.

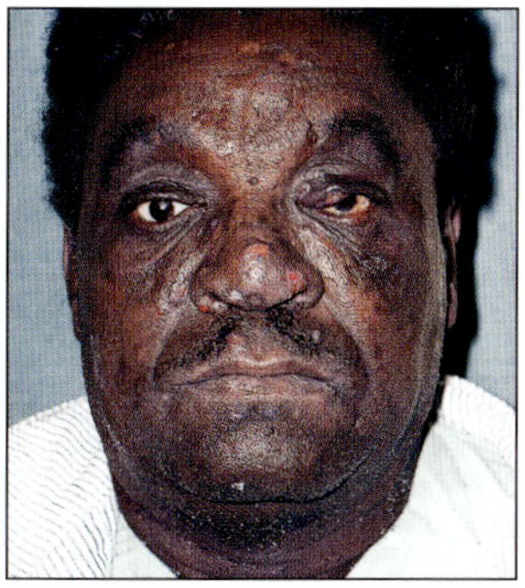

► Facial lesions of mycosis fungoides.

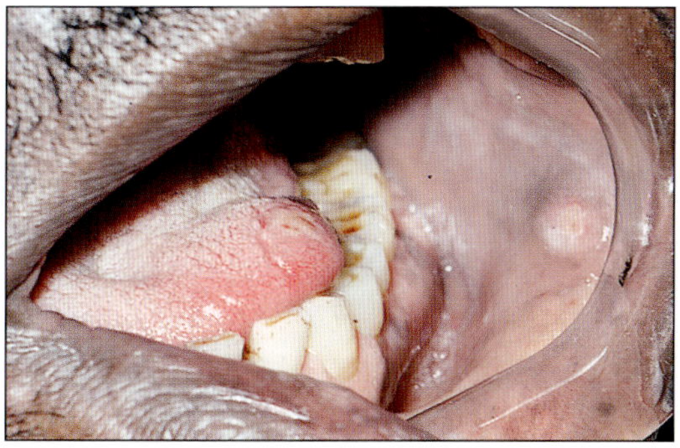

► Oral lesions of mycosis fungoides.

Mycosis Fungoides

Nature of disease

A T-cell lymphoma involving the peripheral lymphatic channels in its initial stages and then progressing to involve the peripheral blood, bone marrow, and lymph nodes.

Predilections

Older adults. No sex or racial predilection is known.

Clinical features

Mycosis fungoides presents in any one of four stages. Stage I is the erythrodermic stage in which large red-white plaques appear on the skin and lacy white striaform areas may appear on the oral mucosa. The skin lesions cause an itching sensation (urticaria). The oral lesions are usually asymptomatic. Stage II is the plaque stage in which the red-white lesions are seen to exfoliate skin into superficial ulcerations and scarring occurs. Oral striaform lesions are also found in this stage. Stage III is the tumor stage in which lymph node enlargements become evident due to a collection of the malignant T cells within lymph nodes. Stage IV is referred to as the *Sézary syndrome* in which an aggressive systemic proliferation of malignant T cells causes significant leukocytosis, fatigue, weight loss, etc, leading to death.

Radiographic presentation

None.

Differential diagnosis

Stage I and stage II mycosis fungoides will bear a close resemblance to the skin lesions of psoriasis, drug allergies, and lichen planus of skin supported by the finding of lacy striaform oral mucosal lesions. Involvement of the facial skin may appear similar to discoid lupus or even leprosy. Stage III will present with lymph node enlargement plus significant skin scarring suggestive of other lymphomas.

Microscopic features

In stage I mycosis fungoides, lymphocytes with irregular nuclei invade the epithelium above the basement membrane. As it progresses to stage II, the lymphocytic infiltrate becomes more dense and extends into the reticular dermis. The epithelium will also show aggregates of large T cells with a convoluted nucleus called *Sézary cells* forming an intraepithelial abscess referred to as a *Pautrier microabscess.* In stage III, a very dense infiltrate of malignant T cells is seen throughout the dermis as well as collecting within lymph nodes. →

Mycosis Fungoides *(cont)*

Suggested course of action

Because the initial stages will seem like a skin disease, referral to a dermatologist is recommended. If the patient is already diagnosed with mycosis fungoides, supportive dental care and dental prophylaxis is helpful.

Treatment

Mycosis fungoides is not curable. However, treatment can improve the pain and itching of the skin lesions, and systemic chemotherapy can maintain a decent quality of life and prolong life as well. Skin lesions are usually treated with topical 0.05% fluocinonide cream or 0.25% desoximetasone cream, while the tumor is treated with selective chemotherapy agents and radiotherapy.

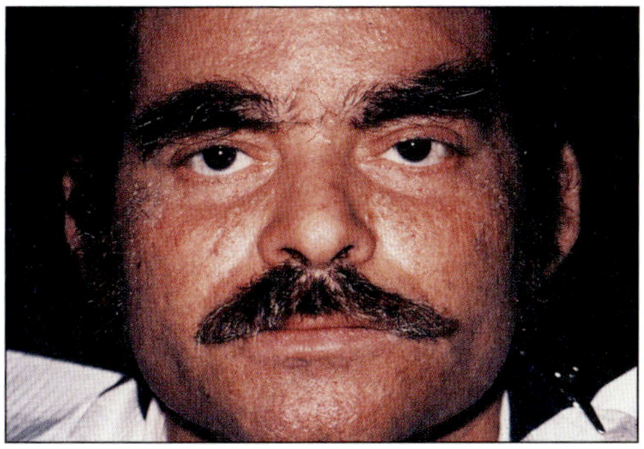

► Facial lesions of keratosis follicularis.

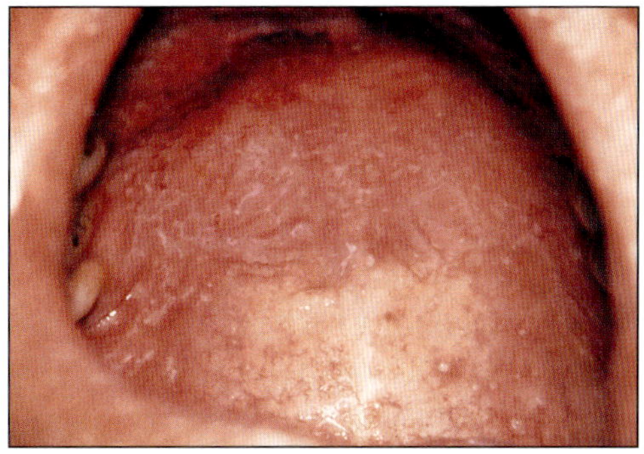

► Oral lesions of keratosis follicularis.

Keratosis Follicularis (Darier-White Disease)

Nature of disease

An inherited autosomal dominant trait that causes a defect in the gene that regulates keratin production and the maturation of epithelial cells.

Predilections

Clinically first seen in late childhood and the early teen years. There is no sex or racial predilection.

Clinical features

Early cases will show papules over the face, chest, and back and less commonly on the oral mucosa. As the individual matures, the papules become skinny and brown and then black and produce a distinctive foul odor. Mature oral lesions will be seen as closely grouped papules, giving the mucosa a cobblestone appearance.

Radiographic presentation

None.

Differential diagnosis

Pachyonychia congenita, aggressive acanthosis nigricans, and the palmar and plantar hyperkeratosis finding in Papillon-Lefèvre syndrome are the few conditions in which such dramatic skin hyperkeratosis occurs.

Microscopic features

Acanthosis and prominent hyperkeratosis often forming a villous-like appearance accompany a suprabasilar split similar to that seen in pemphigus. Within the area of the split, rounded epithelial cells with a dark basophilic nucleus surrounded by a pale halo, known as *corps ronds*, are seen.

Suggested course of action

Suspected cases should be referred to a dermatologist.

Treatment

There is no curative treatment. However, isotretinoin (Accutane, Roche) 0.5 to 2.0 mg/kg daily given in two doses reduces the number and size of papules. Additional frequent cleansing with chlorhexidine or 6% salicylic acid can control the excessive keratin and foul odor.

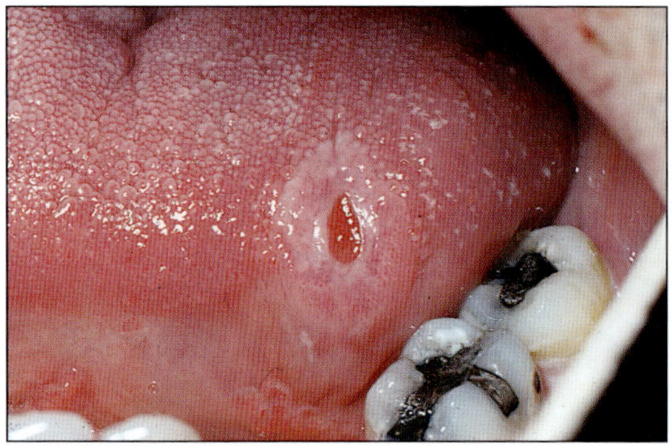

► Chancre of primary syphilis.

Primary Syphilis (Chancre)

Nature of disease

A specific sexually transmitted infection due to *Treponema pallidum*. Primary syphilis is the first stage of the disease, represented as an ulcer known as a *chancre*. If untreated, it will progress to secondary syphilis (a systemic skin and/or oral mucosal eruption) and tertiary syphilis (a widespread involvement of destructive lesions and multiorgan involvement) (see chapter 5).

Predilections

Acquired syphilis is more common in adult men. No racial predilection is known.

Clinical features

The chancre is a localized, only mildly tender, clean ulcer at the point of inoculation. The ulcer is usually found in the genital area but may also appear on the tongue and/or lips. Regional lymphadenopathy may accompany the chancre.

Radiographic presentation

None.

Differential diagnosis

An oral chancre will appear similar to a traumatic ulcer, a squamous cell carcinoma, or an oral fungal lesion of histoplasmosis or coccidioidomycosis.

Microscopic features

Characterized by a proliferative endarteritis as seen by swelling and proliferation of endothelial cells with a dense perivascular infiltration of plasma cells.

Suggested course of action

Recognition of an oral chancre requires a referral to an infectious disease specialist.

Treatment

Treated with 1.2 to 2.4 million units of benzathine penicillin delivered intramuscularly in one dose. For penicillin-allergic patients, oral doxycycline 100 mg twice daily by mouth or erythromycin 500 mg four times daily for 14 days is effective.

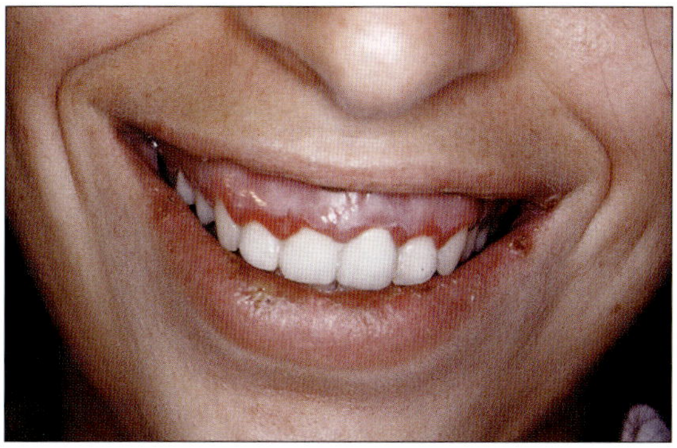

► Primary herpetic gingivostomatitis.

Primary Herpetic Gingivostomatitis

Nature of disease

A painful viral infection of the gingiva and oral mucosa caused by herpes simplex virus 1 (HSV-1), which enters the gingiva/oral mucosa via a direct airborne water-droplet vector.

Predilections

Mostly seen in children and young adults. No sex or racial predilection is known.

Clinical features

The individual will present with painful vesicular ulcerative lesions on the gingiva and oral mucosa. The person will often be drooling, and a noticeable foul odor will be present. Although the lesions will start out to be vesicular, they soon rupture, producing a necrotic fibrin-based ulcer and the thick, foul-smelling exudate.

Radiographic presentation

None.

Differential diagnosis

Painful gingival/oral mucosal lesions in children and young adults may also be seen in acute necrotizing ulcerative periodontitis, pemphigus, erosive lichen planus, and erythema multiforme if targetoid skin lesions are also present.

Microscopic features

Biopsies representative of herpes lesions must be taken in the vesicular stage before rupture. The floor of the vesicle will show a ballooning degeneration of cells with large nuclei that have irregular contours and chromatin displaced to the periphery. The connective tissue beneath the vesicle will show an intense nonspecific inflammatory infiltrate of predominantly neutrophils.

Suggested course of action

Assure parents and patients that primary herpetic gingivostomatitis is a local viral infection that will resolve within 10 days due to patient-synthesized antiviral antibodies produced in response to the infection. If tolerated or with anesthesia, a gentle lavage with 3% hydrogen peroxide, saline, or 0.12% chlorhexidine may provide some relief. Otherwise, supportive care with antipyretics, hydration, and a bland diet help somewhat. If secondary bacterial infection is suspected, phenoxymethylpenicillin or doxycycline in weight-adjusted doses can also be used.

Treatment

The methods noted above are all that is usually required for this self-limiting disease. In severe or prolonged cases, valacyclovir 15 mg/kg three times daily can shorten the course and reduce symptoms.

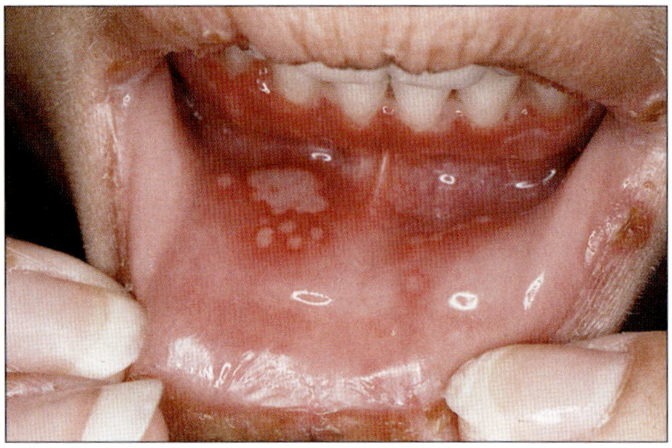

► Recurrent herpes lesions.

Recurrent Herpes

Nature of disease

A reactivation and migration of herpes simplex virus 1 (HSV-1) from the gasserion ganglion to the periphery, where it proliferates and infects the local epithelium around nerve endings, producing blisters that burst into ulcers.

Predilections

Has a predilection for the lower lip vermilion at the vermilion skin junction and to a lesser extent the lateral border of the tongue and the palatal mucosa. Occurs mostly in adults and has no sex or racial predilection. Recurrent herpes lesions are known to be more common in immunosuppressed individuals (eg, transplant patients, HIV patients, patients on immunosuppressive drugs).

Clinical features

Lesions may be preceded by a burning or itching sensation in the area to be involved (prodrome). This is followed by vesicles that will rupture into painful ulcers known as "cold sores." They are often triggered by sun exposure, physical or psychologic stress, cold temperatures, or infections elsewhere in the body.

Radiographic presentation

None.

Differential diagnosis

A single or multiple painful vesicles and/or ulcerations on the lower lip or other areas of the oral mucosa may also be seen in pemphigus, erosive lichen planus, herpes zoster (possibly as a component of Ramsay Hunt syndrome), and erythema multiforme if skin lesions are also present.

Microscopic features

Recurrent herpes lesions will appear identical to those in primary herpetic gingivostomatitis—that is, ballooning degeneration of epithelial cells at the floor of any vesicle and somewhat in the adjacent epithelium. The cells will appear to have swollen nuclei that have an irregular contour with the disrupted chromatin marginated at the periphery. The connective tissue beneath the vesicle will likely show a nonspecific inflammatory process rich in neutrophils. ⟶

Suggested course of action

With single or mild lesions, this self-limiting disease requires no action. In cases of multiple or more painful and bothersome lesions, topical agents can be used, such a penciclovir 1% cream (Zovirax, GlaxoSmithKline). Prevention protocols for the patient with repeated outbreaks are best referred to an infectious disease specialist or to practitioners in oral medicine or oral and maxillofacial surgery who are known to treat recurrent herpes patients.

Treatment

In those cases of frequent or more severe and functionally impairing outbreaks, oral acyclovir 200 mg five times daily starting at the beginning of an outbreak and continuing for 10 days or valacyclovir (Valtrex, GlaxoSmithKline) 1,000 mg three times daily for 7 days is effective in aborting or limiting the course.

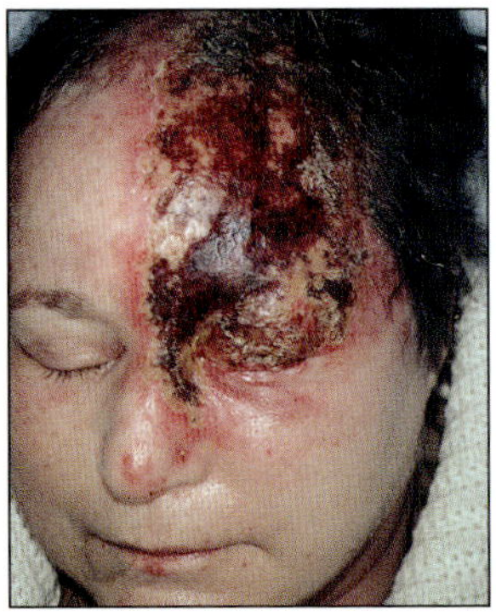

► Herpes zoster of the ophthalmic division of the trigeminal nerve.

Herpes Zoster (Shingles)

Nature of disease

A reactivation of the latent varicella zoster virus (VZV) from a resolved chickenpox infection during childhood. Dormant VZV in ganglia become activated and migrate down a nerve sheath to infect epithelial cells at the terminal nerve endings. Note: When a herpes zoster infection involves more than one cranial nerve distribution (ie, trigeminal nerve plus facial nerve, vagus nerve, or glossopharyngeal nerve), it is termed *Ramsay Hunt syndrome*.

Predilections

Adults with a history of childhood chickenpox. There is no sex or racial predilection, but it is seen somewhat more commonly in unvaccinated individuals with an immune status alteration such as lymphomas, HIV infection, or leukemia and those on immunosuppressive drugs and other chemotherapies. The chest wall is the most common site, followed by the ophthalmic division of the trigeminal nerve.

Clinical features

A prodrome of itching and mild pain often precedes the emergence of more painful vesicles and pustules over a known nerve distribution. The skin becomes necrotic and develops a surface crust. Pain becomes progressively more intense, and the individual frequently experiences episodic bursts of pain. In the oral cavity, bone beneath lesions often becomes exposed. In the fully developed herpes zoster, a distinct midline demarcation is seen.

Radiographic presentation

Despite exposure of bone at times, radiographic features are not usually seen. As the herpes zoster resolves and the exposed surface bone becomes resorbed and covered by granulation tissue, a surface irregularity may be seen on a cone beam CT scan.

Differential diagnosis

Herpes zoster is clinically distinctive. In mild cases of only oral involvement, a herpes simplex infection or a focal candidiasis may be considered.

Microscopic features

The skin and oral lesions will show ballooning degeneration of epithelial cells with swollen nuclei, disrupted chromatin, and intranucelar inclusion bodies. In the ganglion of the involved nerve distribution, ganglion cells will be swollen with intranuclear inclusion bodies. Some large neurons may be seen to become necrotic, and the ganglion itself will be infiltrated by lymphocytes, plasma cells, and macrophages. →

Suggested course of action

Suspected cases should be referred to an infectious disease specialist.

Treatment

Because herpes zoster is a serious disease known to frequently result in sequelae such as postherpetic neuralgia, encephalitis, and severe scarring, it is treated intensely. Local wound care and antibiotics to treat secondary bacterial skin or mucosal infections supplement antiviral treatment with either acyclovir 800 mg five times daily, famciclovir 500 mg three times daily, or valacyclovir 1 g three times daily for 10 days. Carbamazepine 200 mg four times daily or gabapentin 600 mg twice daily is used to treat herpes zoster pain as well as postherpetic neuralgia. Frequently, prednisone is added to the antiviral treatment to reduce the skin and mucosal necrosis.

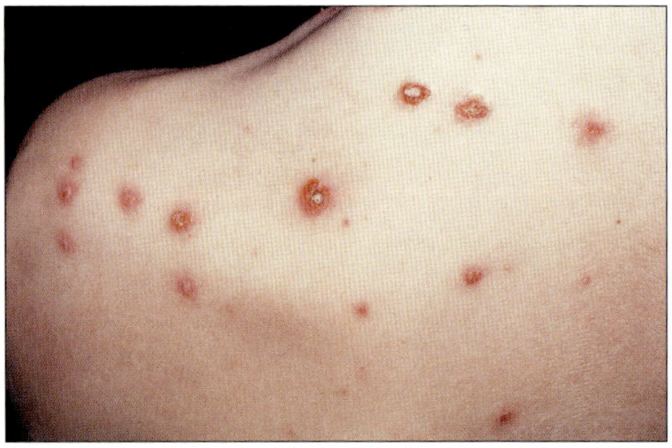

► Painful pustules with a red periphery seen in chickenpox.

Chickenpox (Varicella)

Nature of disease

A transmissible childhood skin infection that may also uncommonly form oral lesions caused by a DNA virus known as the *varicella zoster virus* (VZV).

Predilections

Children between the ages of 4 and 10 years are most commonly affected. There is no sex or racial predilection. Lesions develop mostly on the trunk and facial skin.

Clinical features

Painful red pustules develop on the trunk and facial skin 5 to 10 days after exposure to the virus via water droplet contact. Chills, fever, malaise, and headache are common. The child is often irritable due to the constant pain. In later stages, the lesions will develop a crust before healing.

Radiographic presentation

None.

Differential diagnosis

Other painful childhood diseases should be considered such as rubeola (measles), rubella (German measles), and hand, foot, and mouth disease. Additionally, erythema multiforme (particularly erythema multiforme major, also known as *Stevens-Johnson syndrome*) should be considered.

Microscopic features

Biopsy specimens are rarely taken. However, those that are taken show an identical picture to that seen in herpes simplex infections—that is, ballooning degeneration of epithelial cells with disrupted nuclei and chromatin marginated to the periphery of the nuclear membrane. The surrounding connective tissue will be seen to have a nonspecific inflammatory response with neutrophils predominating.

Suggested course of action

Nonvaccinated individuals (other patients, staff, etc) should be isolated from the infected child and should avoid direct contact. Only true dental emergencies should be treated during the course of infection, using barrier precautions, and all instruments should be separated for immediate sterilization. Disposable gowns should be used if possible; otherwise, any gowns used during treatment should be removed and replaced with fresh ones before other patients are seen.

Treatment

No treatment is required for this self-limiting disease other than supportive care. However, for immunocompromised individuals and women in the third trimester of pregnancy, intravenous acyclovir 30 mg/kg daily over 10 days or intravenous foscarnet (Foscavir, AstraZeneca) 20 mg/kg as a loading dose followed by 120 mg/kg three times daily for 2 weeks is often used.

Herpangina

Nature of disease

A viral infection caused by coxsackieviruses A and B. It will develop rapidly, producing a sore throat (dysphagia) and high fever after direct water-droplet/saliva contamination.

Predilections

Occurs almost exclusively in children under the age of 10 years. No sex or racial predilection is known. It affects the pharynx posterior to the anterior tonsillar pillars.

Clinical features

The child will be obtunded and have a fever of 103°F to 105°F. The pharynx will have 1- to 2-mm gray-white vesicles, producing the symptom of dysphagia. Pharyngeal and soft palate petechiae are frequently seen as well. Ulcers are less commonly seen.

Radiographic presentation

None.

Differential diagnosis

Pharyngeal lesions with dysphagia and fever with no skin lesions may also be seen in streptococcal pharyngitis, tonsillitis, and, although very rarely seen today due to vaccinations, diphtheria.

Microscopic features

Lesions are rarely biopsied. However, those that are biopsied show intraepithelial vesicles with a submucosal mixed inflammatory infiltrate.

Suggested course of action

Suspected cases should be referred to an infectious disease specialist or to the patient's primary care provider.

Treatment

No specific treatment is required other than antipyretics, hydration, analgesics, and rest. If a streptococcal pharyngitis cannot be ruled out or occurs as a secondary infection, phenoxymethylpenicillin 250 mg four times daily for 10 days is prescribed. For the penicillin-allergic child, erythromycin ethyl succinate 200 to 400 mg four times daily for 10 days is prescribed.

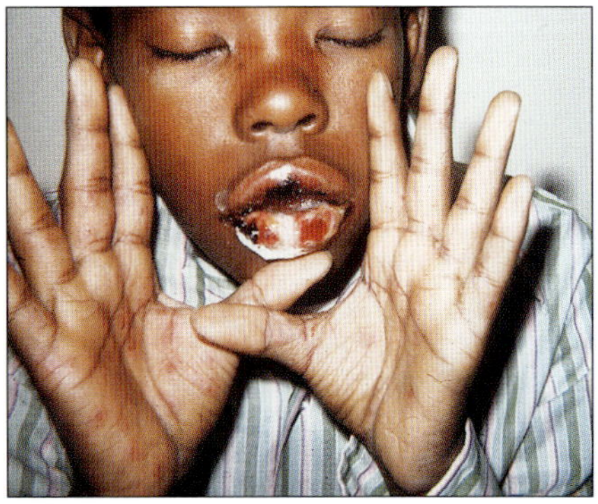

► Lesions on the hands and mouth seen in hand, foot, and mouth disease.

Hand, Foot, and Mouth Disease

Nature of disease

A viral infection caused by coxsackievirus A16, so named after Coxsackie, New York, where the virus was first identified. It is transmitted by either airborne water droplets or oral-fecal spread. The virus seems to proliferate better in areas of cooler temperature, thus focusing its systemic spread to the hands, feet, and mouth.

Predilections

Mostly affects children under 5 years of age. It occurs more frequently during the summer months. There is no sex or racial predilection.

Clinical features

Children will be seen to have oral vesicles early in the course. However, most often by the time they are seen by a practitioner, the vesicles have ruptured to form yellow fibropurulent ulcers that are only mildly painful. The skin of the hands and feet will more likely show vesicles due to their greater epithelial layer thickness. These will eventually rupture to form a targetlike lesion.

Radiographic presentation

None.

Differential diagnosis

Children with mildly symptomatic oral as well as skin lesions may also be seen in erythema multiforme minor, varicella (chickenpox), rubeola (measles), and rubella (German measles).

Microscopic features

Epithelial and subepithelial vesicles are seen together with ballooning degeneration of the epithelium and a dense inflammatory infiltrate in the reticular dermis and submucosa predominantly consisting of neutrophils.

Suggested course of action

Suspected cases should be referred to an infectious disease specialist or the patient's primary care physician.

Treatment

No specific treatment is required beyond supportive care for this self-limiting disease in which symptoms and lesions will resolve within 2 weeks.

Impetigo

Nature of disease

A staphylococcal skin infection that forms vesicles and crusting ulcers of the skin. It is transmitted by direct skin-to-skin contact usually via contamination of fingers by touching active lesions.

Predilections

Mostly occurs in children and young teenagers. No sex or racial predilection is known. Lesions concentrate around the perioral skin and vermilion but do not involve the oral mucosa.

Clinical features

Pruritic and painful lesions around the perioral skin begin as vesicles and soon burst to form a crust-covered sore.

Radiographic presentation

None.

Differential diagnosis

Skin lesions may resemble erythema multiforme minor, pemphigus, recurrent herpes, and contact dermatitis.

Microscopic features

Intraepithelial vesicles containing neutrophils are seen initially. As vesicles rupture, an ulcer with a mixed inflammatory infiltrate will be seen in the dermis.

Suggested course of action

Defer elective dental care. Treat dental emergencies with barrier protection for all staff and the direct provider. Treat skin lesions with topical bacitracin or 2% mupirocin ointment. Refractory cases should be referred to an infectious disease specialist.

Treatment

Topical antibacterial ointments are usually effective within 5 to 7 days. Extensive or refractory cases may require oral antibiotics directed against staphylococci.

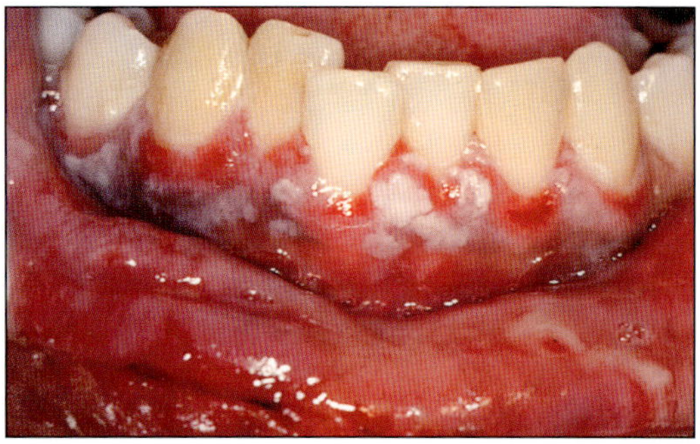

► Oral lesions of paraneoplastic pemphigus. (Courtesy of Dr L. R. Eversole.)

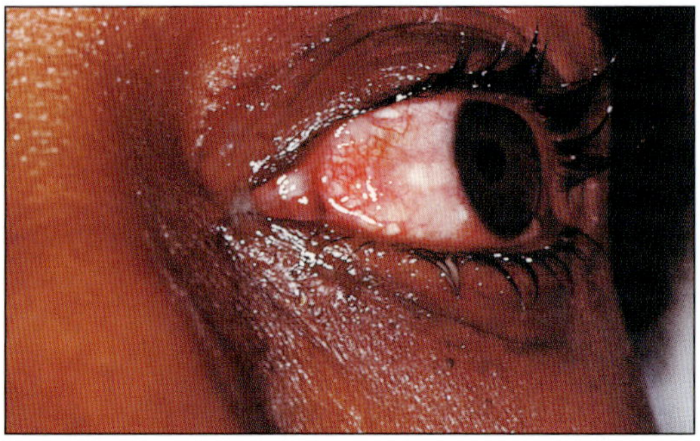

► Ocular lesions of paraneoplastic pemphigus. (Courtesy of Dr L. R. Eversole.)

Paraneoplastic Pemphigus

Nature of disease

A rare, painful eruption of skin and oral mucosal lesions in an advanced cancer patient. It is hypothesized that the cancer secretes similar proteins to normal desmoplakins that incite an overproduction of interleukin-6, producing an abnormal number of antibodies.

Predilections

Mostly occurs in patients with leukemia, Hodgkin lymphoma, and non-Hodgkin lymphoma not responsive to anticancer treatment. Less commonly occurs with other cancers. No age, sex, or racial predilection is known.

Clinical features

A somewhat rapid onset of very painful vesicles and ulcers on skin and/or oral mucosa. The ulcers will be exudative and bleed easily.

Radiographic presentation

None other than that identifying the promoting cancer.

Differential diagnosis

The painful and rapid onset of skin lesions will suggest erythema multiforme or toxic epidermal necrolysis.

Microscopic features

Similar to pemphigus vulgaris, acantholysis, epithelial necrosis, and suprabasilar separation are seen together with an intense lymphocytic infiltrate in the submucosa.

Suggested course of action

Defer all but emergency dental care. Recognize that this phenomenon suggests a possible near-terminal event. Refer to the patient's oncologist.

Treatment

Oncologists may try various new or previously used chemotherapy agents. However, death usually follows.

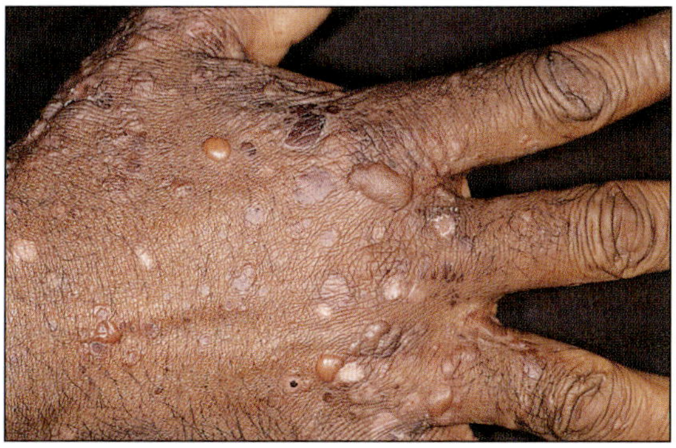

► Epidermolysis bullosa acquisita skin lesions on the hand. (Reprinted from Callen JP et al, *Color Atlas of Dermatology*, with permission from WB Saunders Co.)

Epidermolysis Bullosa Acquisita

Nature of disease

A B cell/immunoglobulin G antibody–mediated autoimmune disease that targets type VII collagen at the lower portion of the basement membrane. Three types exist:

- Type I: A noninflammatory type that occurs around pressure points on skin or from minor trauma
- Type II: A general inflammatory type that occurs on skin with pruritis (itching)
- Type III: A mucosal type that is mildly painful and may involve the oral, vaginal, and ocular mucosa.

Predilections

Occurs mostly in mature or elderly adults. No sex or racial predilection is known. Note: This acquired form should not be confused with several hereditary forms that target children. Those hereditary forms are much more severe and are due to genetic defects in the basement membrane.

Clinical features

Skin vesicles and/or bullae develop and then rupture to form a scar. Therefore, vesicles and scar areas will coincide.

Radiographic presentation

None.

Differential diagnosis

In the adult population, epidermolysis bullosa acquisita may appear similar to pemphigoid with skin lesions, pemphigus vulgaris, and the rare linear immunoglobulin A disease.

Microscopic features

Using a skin biopsy treated with salt, a characteristic split will be seen within the basement membrane. If direct immunofluorescence is then used, autoantibodies will be seen on the base of the split. The dermis will be seen to contain a mixed inflammatory infiltrate.

Suggested course of action

Refer to a dermatologist or a rheumatologist.

Treatment

Treatment responses are minimal. However, treatment with systemic prednisone, azathioprine or dapsone, rituximab, or mycophenolate have been useful in some cases.

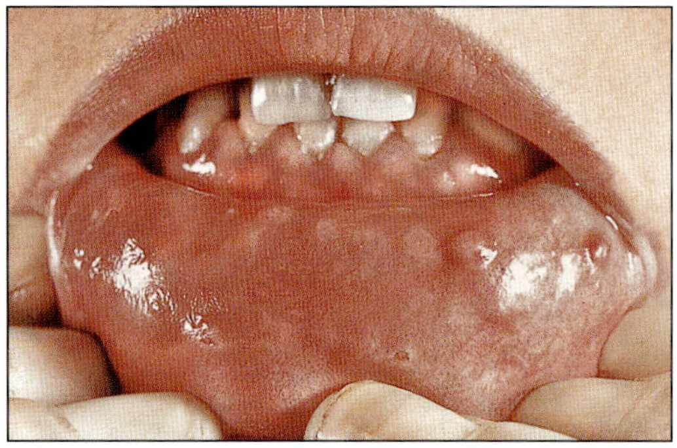

► Dermatitis herpetiformis lesions of the oral mucosa.

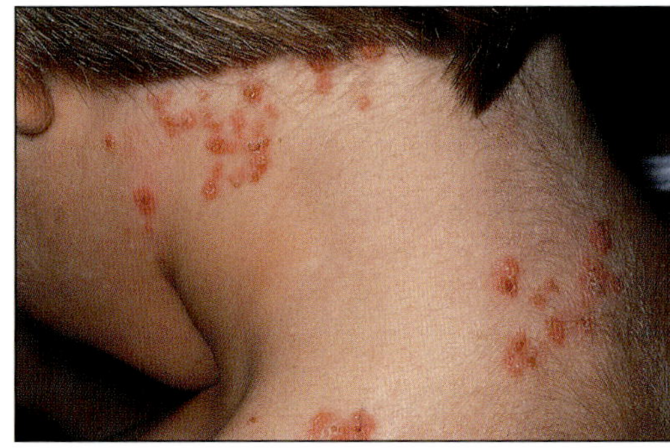

► Dermatitis herpetiformis lesions of the skin.

Dermatitis Herpetiformis

Nature of disease

A primary skin disease in which a gluten hypersensitivity causes papules and vesicles to form on skin. The skin lesions are very pruritic. Oral lesions are rare and mostly appear on the palatal and/or buccal mucosa.

Predilections

No age, sex, or racial predilection is known.

Clinical features

Pruritic red papules and vesicles will be seen more on the back of the neck, scalp, elbows, and buttocks than in other places. Oral lesions will appear as tender submucosal nodules.

Radiographic presentation

None.

Differential diagnosis

The pruritic nature of the skin lesions as well as their appearance will suggest psoriasis, skin lichen planus, and the erythrodermic stage of mycosis fungoides.

Microscopic features

Early lesions will be seen to have a collection of neutrophils in the tips of the skin's dermal papillae. These will progress to form microabscesses, with the infiltration of eosinophils to mix with the neutrophils.

Suggested course of action

If lesions are recognized and associated with a gluten-containing diet, refer the patient to a gastroenterologist for workup and management. Lesions are not transmissible. Dental care can proceed as tolerated.

Treatment

A gluten-free diet will manage the enteropathy that accompanies dermatitis herpetiformis. The skin lesions respond well to dapsone 100 mg/day or to sulfadiazine 500 mg twice daily.

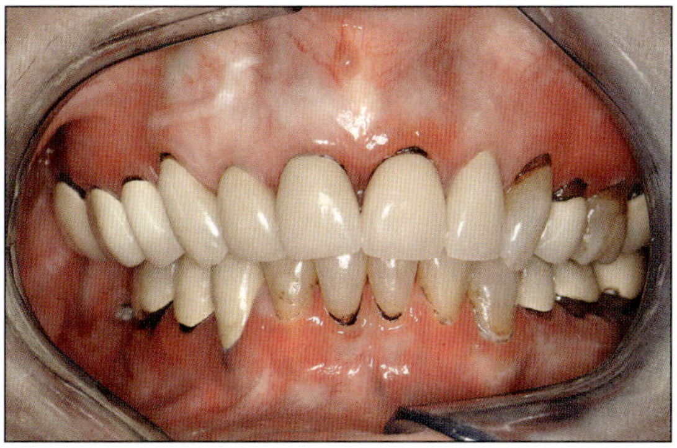

► Plasma cell gingivitis from cinnamon spice.

Contact Stomatitis

Nature of disease

There are three types of contact stomatitis:

1. Drug toxicity such as is seen in an aspirin burn or from certain spices.
2. A T cell–mediated stomatitis in which a topical drug is absorbed through the mucosa and becomes bound to Langerhans cells, which process the antigen to a T cell, which secretes enzymes termed *lymphokines* to injure local tissue. The usual agents are lipsticks, other cosmetics, and the dyes in oral medications.
3. A B cell–mediated stomatitis in which the agent is processed by Langerhans cells to antibody-producing B lymphocytes. These specific antibodies injure local tissue. This occurs when certain flavoring agents are added to toothpastes and/or mouthwash, particularly cinnamon and mint flavoring.

Predilections

No age, sex, or racial predilection is known.

Clinical features

The mucosa will have a diffuse, mildly swollen appearance. The mucosa will be tender to palpation. It will generally be localized to one area.

Radiographic presentation

None.

Differential diagnosis

The tender erythematous oral mucosa will suggest a mild form of erosive lichen planus, pemphigus vulgaris, or pemphigoid.

Microscopic features

A diffuse infiltration of lymphocytes and plasma cells will be seen in both the lamina propria and deeper layers of the mucosa. The surface epithelium will be intact without intraepithelial vesicles.

Suggested course of action

Attempt to identify and withdraw the offending agent. If it is a constant medication required by the patient, refer to the prescribing physician with a note about your findings.

Treatment

Identification of the offending topical agent and its discontinuation. If it is a required medication such as levothyroxine or an antihypertensive medication, the dye color of the pill is suspected, and either an identical daily dose is provided via other dosages/pills or alternative medications are prescribed.

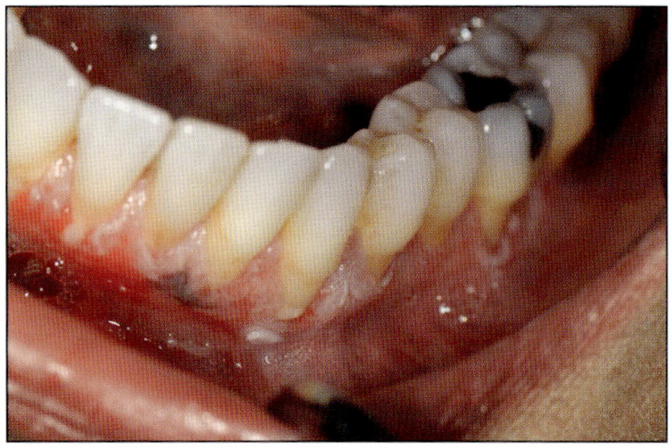

► Pyostomatitis vegetans.

Pyostomatitis Vegetans

Nature of disease

An intense, necrotizing focal inflammatory response forming pustules and exudates related to inflammatory bowel disease and ulcerative colitis.

Predilections

Mostly occurs in adults over 40 years of age, with a slight female predilection. No racial predilection is known.

Clinical features

An intense oral exudative and polypoid response seen on the labial mucosa, gingiva, and tongue. Pain is less severe than the clinical picture will suggest.

Radiographic presentation

None.

Differential diagnosis

Lesions may be similar to verrucous carcinoma or squamous cell carcinoma but also may appear similar to secondarily infected pemphigus, often referred to as *pemphigus vegetans*, or to paraneoplastic pemphigus. Severe erosive lichen planus may also appear similar.

Microscopic features

A polypoid proliferation of the epithelium sometimes with ulceration is seen over a connective tissue with microabscesses filled will a collection of eosinophils and some neutrophils.

Suggested course of action

Consult with a gastroenterologist to coordinate treatment. Inform him or her that oral lesions frequently become infected with anaerobic bacteria and that penicillin-metronidazole or doxycycline-metronidazole may be of benefit.

Treatment

Treatment is coordinated with a gastroenterologist, who may treat the patient with prednisone and/or infliximab (Remicade, Janssen), which is an anti–tumor necrosis factor alpha drug. Oral antibiotics as recommended above will complement the effectiveness of the ulcerative colitis/enteritis treatment on the oral mucosa.

Cyclic Neutropenia

Nature of disease

A very rare autosomal dominant defect in the *EAL-2* gene of neutrophils. The *EAL-2* gene codes for the protein ELANE, which prepares neutrophils to respond to infection. It is variably active in this condition every 21 days and lasts for only 3 to 5 days. This predisposes individuals to new infections and exacerbations of chronic, low-grade infections.

Predilections

It begins in childhood and persists throughout life, with no sex or racial predilection.

Clinical features

The oral mucosa will present with white fibrin-based lesions 0.5 to 1.5 mm in diameter. Some will resemble aphthous ulcers and others gingivitis or gingival abscess. Most lesions are painful and are found on the nonkeratinized mucosa at the ventral surface of the tongue and labial mucosa.

Radiographic presentation

None. It has long been anticipated that periodontal bone loss should accompany cyclic neutropenia. However, due to the paucity of cases, this is not confirmed, and due to the short duration of cyclic neutropenia, it has not been observed beyond that expected from the patient's level of plaque control.

Differential diagnosis

Oral lesions with a fibrin base are also seen in aphthous stomatitis, Behçet disease, agranulocytosis, and in adults with Wegener granulomatosis.

Microscopic features

Ulcers will have an eosinophilic coagulum of necrotic collagen and a fibrin base with chronic inflammatory cells and will be absent of neutrophils.

Suggested course of action

Suspicious cases should be referred to a hematologist for workup and confirmation. It is also reasonable to treat oral ulcers initially with antibiotics of the penicillin type or tetracycline type.

Treatment

There is no cure for cyclic neutropenia. The patient's physician should closely follow the patient for signs of pneumonia or renal infection, treating with antibiotics as necessary. The potential for oral lesions should also be followed closely; as exacerbations occur, these lesions should be treated with antibiotics and local measures.

11

Exposed Bone Pathologies

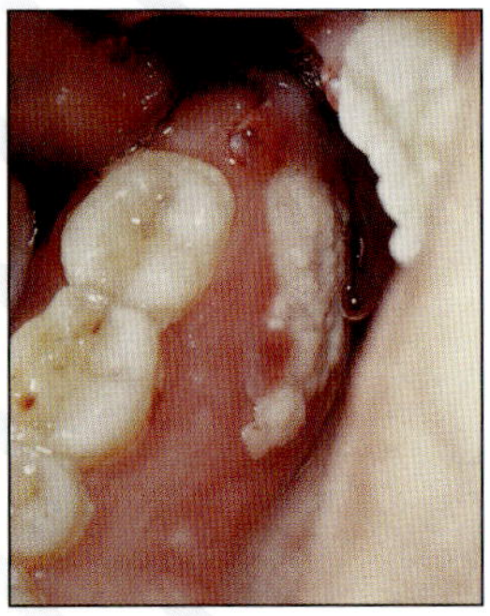

► Stage I ORN.

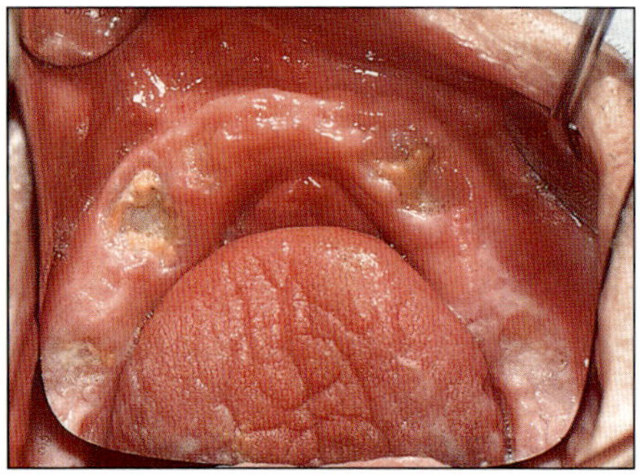

► Stage II ORN.

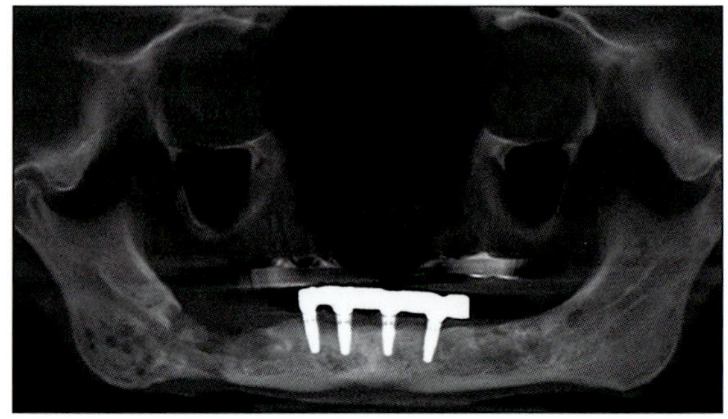

► Stage III ORN.

Osteoradionecrosis (ORN)

Nature of disease

Radiation-induced cell death and impairment of cell renewal of blood vessels and local progenitor cells, creating hypoxic, hypocellular, and hypovascular (three H's) tissue and bone necrosis.

Predilections

Occurs in bone that has received >6,000 cGy of radiotherapy. A higher risk is associated with doses >7,000 cGy, intensity-modulated radiotherapy, interstitial radiotherapy, and radiation given concomitantly with chemotherapy or hyperthermia therapy. Occurs mostly in the mandible (97%) and rarely in the maxilla (3%) but has occurred in nearly all other skeletal areas as well.

Clinical features

Exposed, often discolored (white or brown) bone. It may be seen with localized inflammation and/or pus due to secondary infection and may develop a cutaneous fistula, maxillary sinusitis, or a pathologic fracture. Significant xerostomia, loss of facial hair, skin tightness, trismus, and radiation telangiectasia are also often seen together with ORN.

ORN is staged clinically as follows:

- Stage I: Small area of exposed bone that heals with hyperbaric oxygen
- Stage II: Areas of exposed bone that fail to respond to hyperbaric oxygen
- Stage III: Patients with either *(1)* osteolysis to the inferior border, *(2)* involvement of the maxillary sinus, *(3)* cutaneously exposed bone, or *(4)* pathologic fracture

Radiographic presentation

Radiographs occasionally appear normal but more often show unhealed outlines of extraction sockets, mottled bone, irregular radiolucencies, and/or a pathologic fracture.

Differential diagnosis

Most cases are clinically evident with a concomitant history of radiotherapy and the clinical features of radiation damage to the skin and oral mucosa. Other diseases that can present with exposed bone include drug-induced osteonecrosis, osteopetrosis, florid cemento-osseous dysplasia, and the rare case of "phossy jaw" today. However, the clinician must also be alert for residual or recurrent carcinoma.

Microscopic features

Necrotic bone, marrow, and soft tissue fibrosis. Inflammatory cells may be seen if secondarily infected.

→

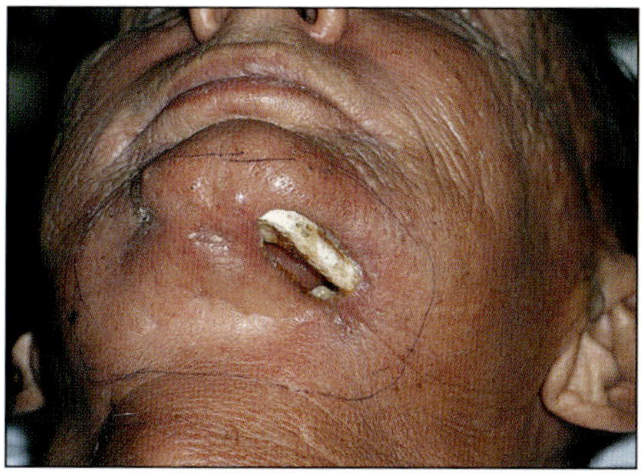

► Stage III ORN.

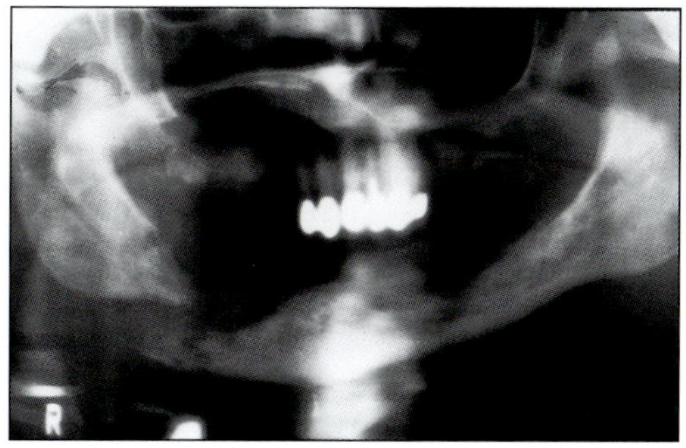

► Stage III ORN.

Suggested course of action

For radiated patients without clinical ORN:

1. Dental prophylaxis and plaque-control education.
2. Fluoride carriers with prescribed 0.4% stannous fluoride.
3. Restorative dentistry, crowns, and root canal therapy as indicated with the intent of preventing tooth extractions.
4. Well-made dental prostheses as indicated.
5. If tooth extractions, implants, or periodontal osseous surgery is required, refer to a hyperbaric medicine facility for the standard 20/10 hyperbaric oxygen protocol.

For radiated patients with clinical ORN:

1. Refer for evaluation by an oral and maxillofacial surgeon.
2. Treat other areas and teeth as indicated in the aforementioned list.

Treatment

For patients contraindicated for surgery, palliation using the standard 30/10 protocol of hyperbaric oxygen along with an intermittent course of antibiotics (eg, penicillin VK 500 mg four times daily or doxycycline 100 mg once daily) is useful to reduce episodes of secondary infection and slow the progress of bone necrosis. Curative treatment requires the 30/10 protocol of hyperbaric oxygen together with resective surgery, stabilization of the mandible with a titanium plate, and most often a soft tissue flap. In the maxilla, resection of the necrotic bone is accomplished with flap placement or an obturator prosthesis. Note: The protocol to treat clinically developed osteoradionecrosis requires additional sessions of hyperbaric oxygen (30/10) because of the advanced nature of overt necrotic bone and the more damaging effects on the soft tissues that produced the dead bone.

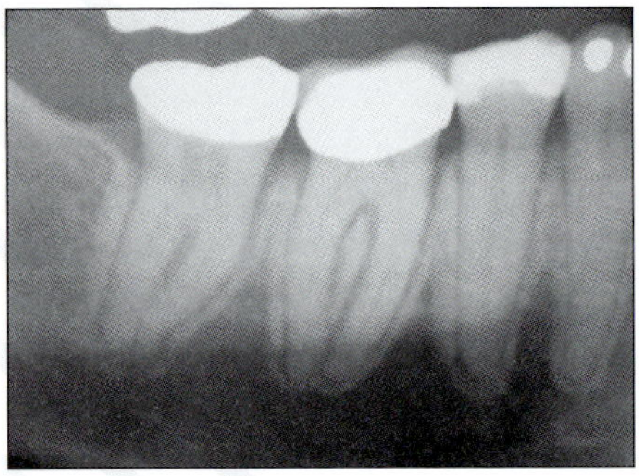

► Stage 0 DIONJ.

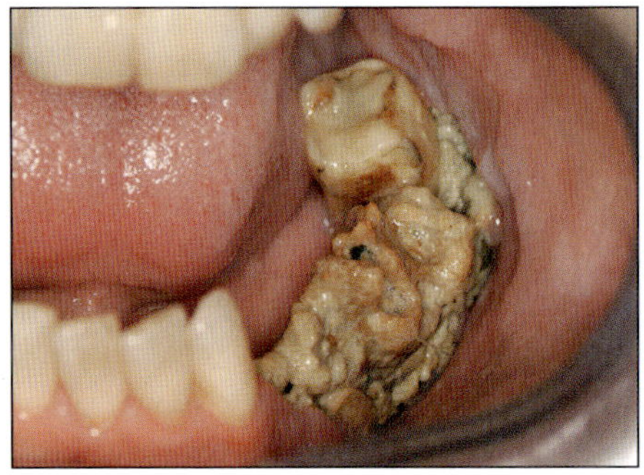

► Stage I DIONJ.

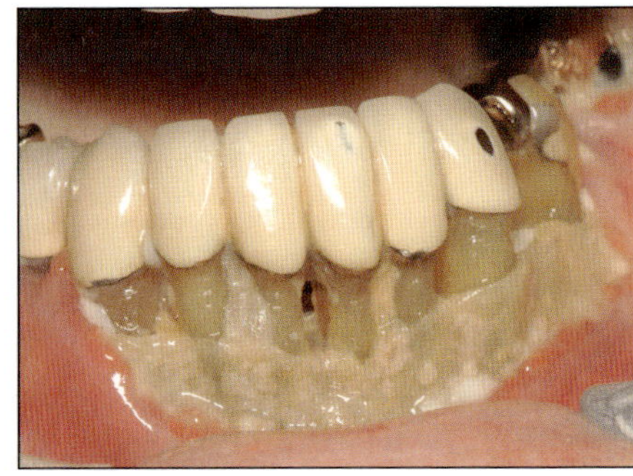

► Stage II DIONJ.

Drug-Induced Osteonecrosis of the Jaws (DIONJ)

Nature of disease

A side effect of drugs used to treat or prevent osteoporosis or to limit bone resorption and hypercalcemia in cancer patients. Drugs that cause DIONJ are either antiresorptive (ie, they impair and kill osteoclasts, thus preventing bone renewal) or significantly anti-angiogenic (they prevent new capillaries from forming, resulting in bone necrosis).

Predilections

Adult women treated for osteoporosis or the prevention of osteoporosis (rarely, adult men as well), patients treated for cancer metastasis (ie, breast, lung, prostate, or kidney cancer or multiple myeloma), and cancer patients who are treated with chemotherapy agents that cause osteoporosis as their own side effect.

Clinical features

Exposed necrotic bone in the mouth. Some exposures will be subtle through a fistula or via the periodontium. Others may be widespread with large areas of exposed bone. The exposed bone is not painful by itself but becomes painful when colonized or secondarily infected. Therefore, drainage and cutaneous fistulas may also be present.

DIONJ is staged according to its extent and severity:

- Stage 0: No clinically exposed bone but radiographic evidence of sclerosis of the lamina dura, a diffuse intramedullary sclerosis, or a mixed sclerotic/lytic picture, particularly if seen affecting the lingual cortex.
- Stage I: One quadrant of exposed bone.
- Stage II: Two quadrants of exposed bone.
- Stage III: Three or four quadrants of exposed bone, osteolysis to the inferior border, a pathologic fracture, or maxillary sinus extension.

Radiographic presentation

Early signs will show a sclerosis of the lamina dura and a widened periodontal ligament space. Further along, a diffuse intramedullary sclerosis may be seen, followed by osteolysis with sequestra or a pathologic fracture. Cone beam CT scans will frequently identify fragmentation and lysis focused on the lingual cortex.

Differential diagnosis

Exposed bone together with a history of receiving the drugs known to cause DIONJ is a straightforward diagnosis. However, osteoradionecrosis and osteopetrosis can also commonly result in exposed bone. Other diseases that uncommonly result in exposed bone are suppurative osteomyelitis, cemento-osseous dysplasia, and herpes zoster. →

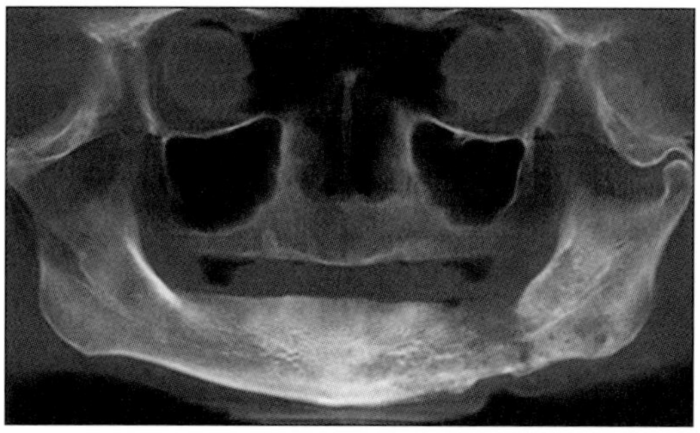

► Stage III DIONJ.

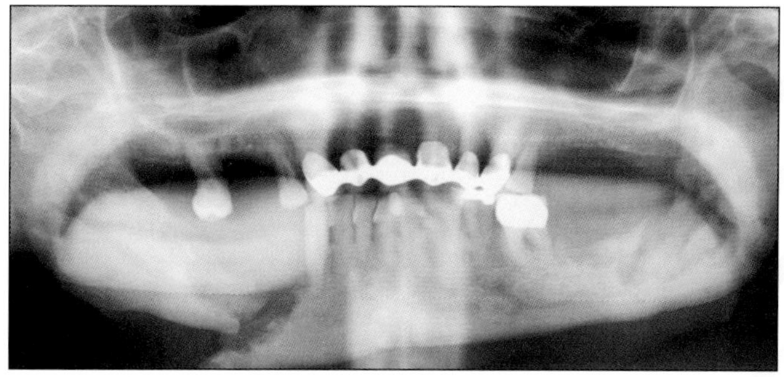

► Stage III DIONJ.

Microscopic features

Representative specimens will show necrotic bone devoid of osteoblasts and empty osteocytic lacunae. The surface may have debris and microorganisms, usually *Actinomyces*, but the marrow space will be empty without microorganisms or inflammation. In sections with secondary infection, inflammation and microorganisms may then be seen in the marrow space, but ballooned and ruptured osteoclasts as well as empty Howship lacunae will identify the specimen as DIONJ.

Suggested course of action

Perform preventive and restorative dentistry to avoid the need for later extractions or oral surgery procedures. Restorations, crowns, partial dentures, removable appliances, prophylaxis, and root canal therapy are safe to perform at all times and are recommended.

Dental procedures that pose a risk to patients on cancer drugs include extractions, periodontal surgery, apicoectomies, crown lengthening, and dental implant placements. If adult orthodontics is considered, the teeth will not move.

In the osteopenic/osteoporotic patient without cancer, all nonsurgical dental procedures are safe to perform. Invasive procedures such as extractions, dental implant placements, periodontal surgery, apicoectomies, and crown lengthening may also be conducted in these patients with minimal to no risk for osteonecrosis of the jaws provided the patient takes a drug holiday as follows:

- Alendronate: 9-month drug holiday prior to the procedure followed by a 3-month drug holiday afterward
- Risedronate: 9-month drug holiday prior to the procedure followed by a 3-month drug holiday afterward
- Ibandronate: 9-month drug holiday prior to the procedure followed by a 3-month drug holiday afterward
- Denosumab: 3-month drug holiday prior to the procedure followed by a 3-month drug holiday afterward

Note: Drug holidays should be requested of the prescribing physician.

For patients with exposed bone, refer to an oral and maxillofacial surgeon for workup and definitive management.

Treatment

DIONJ in either the cancer patient or the osteopenic/osteoporotic patient may be managed either nonsurgically for palliation or curatively, which requires surgery. In either treatment scheme, a physician-initiated drug holiday is preferred.

For palliation, treatment includes oral 0.12% chlorhexidine mouthrinse and a long-standing antibiotic regimen to control secondary infection and therefore pain. For this purpose, amoxicillin 500 mg three times daily, phenoxymethyl penicillin 500 mg four times daily, or doxycycline 100 mg once daily works well. During exacerbations or flare-ups, adding metronidazole (Flagyl, Pfizer) 500 mg three times daily but limited to 10 days usually reverses the swelling and pain.

For cure, alveolectomy or a continuity resection is required. At times, a soft tissue flap is necessary as well.

→

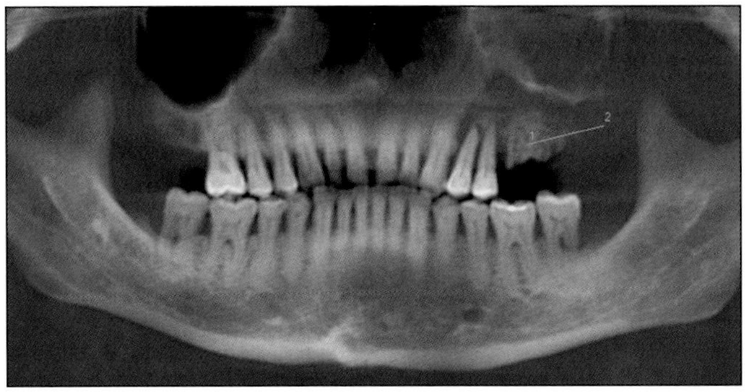

► Stage III DIONJ.

Drug-Induced Osteonecrosis of the Jaws (DIONJ) *(cont)*

Drug-related risk factors for DIONJ

Cancer drugs	
Denosumab	Very high risk
Zoledronate	Very high risk
Sunitinib	Very high risk
Pamidronate	High risk
Bevacizumab	Moderate risk
Osteopenia/osteoporosis drugs	
Alendronate	Very high risk
Denosumab	Very high risk
Risedronate	Low risk
Ibandronate	Low risk
Teriparatide	No risk
Raloxifene	No risk
Strontium ranelate	No risk
Vitamin D_3/calcium	No risk

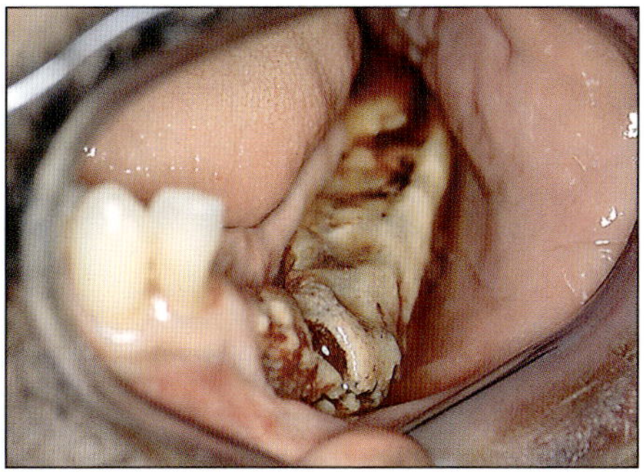

► Exposed bone in osteopetrosis.

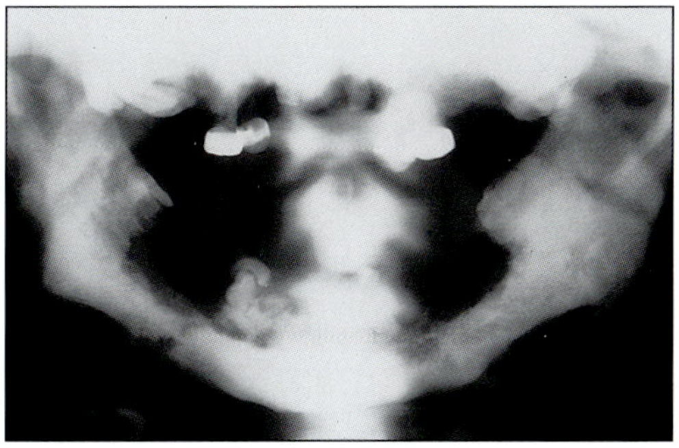

► Hyperdense sclerotic bone seen in osteopetrosis.

Osteopetrosis

Nature of disease

A rare, mostly autosomal dominant trait in which impaired bone renewal begins in utero. A genetic variation prevents osteoclast development or impairs their function, thereby preventing normal bone renewal and remodeling.

Predilections

Occurs equally in men and women who have any one of eight known genetic variations. It occurs throughout life in those affected.

Clinical features

Exposed white- or brown-colored alveolar bone similar to that seen in drug-induced osteonecrosis and osteoradionecrosis. The bone is often secondarily infected and frequently produces cutaneous fistulas and firm perioral swellings and lymphadenopathy referred to as "bumpy jaw." It involves the entire skeleton, which may cause anemia as well as long bone and vertebral fractures, but bone exposure only occurs in the jaws.

Radiographic presentation

Extremely sclerotic bone and unerupted teeth in almost all mature cases. Some will exhibit a linear pathologic fracture. Early cases show delayed or unerupted teeth, sclerosis of the lamina dura, and thickening of the cortices of all bones.

Differential diagnosis

Drug-induced osteonecrosis and osteoradionecrosis will appear very similar upon examination and can be excluded via the history. The rare case today of phossy jaw may also appear similar and should be considered if the patient has a history of working in a munitions or fireworks factory or in a poorly ventilated phosphorus mine.

Microscopic features

Necrotic bone with debris and a notable absence of osteoclasts. Inflammatory cells may be seen if secondarily infected.

→

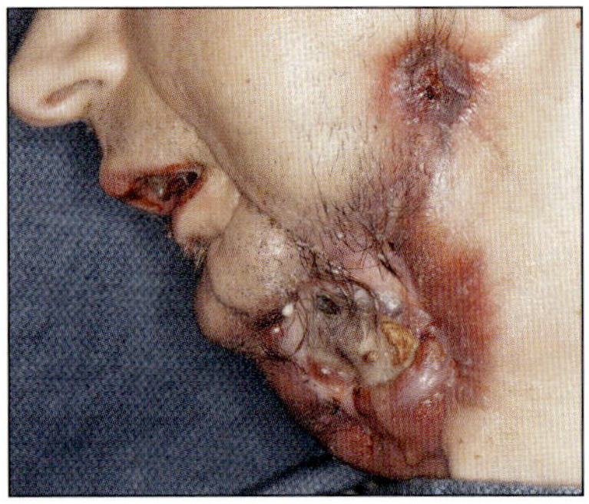

► Cutaneous exposed bone and secondary infection, a complication of a surgical attempt in osteopetrosis.

Osteopetrosis *(cont)*

Suggested course of action

Refrain from debriding the exposed bone or accomplishing a bone biopsy. Prevent the need to extract teeth with dental prophylaxis, plaque-control education, restorative dentistry, and root canal therapy as needed. Treat secondary infections with penicillin-based antibiotics or doxycycline if the patient is penicillin allergic. Refer to an oral and maxillofacial surgeon for definitive management.

Treatment

Osteopetrosis is incurable and generally results in a reduced life span. Bony surgery is avoided in any part of the skeleton, and control of secondary infections, transfusion for anemia, and calcium supplements for hypocalcemia are also part of the overall management.

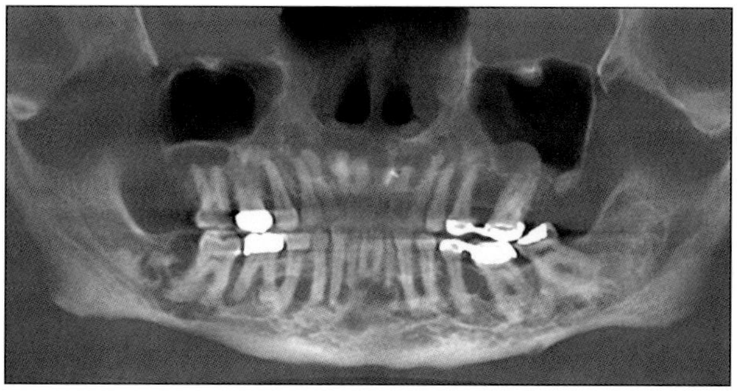

► Lytic phase of florid cemento-osseous dysplasia.

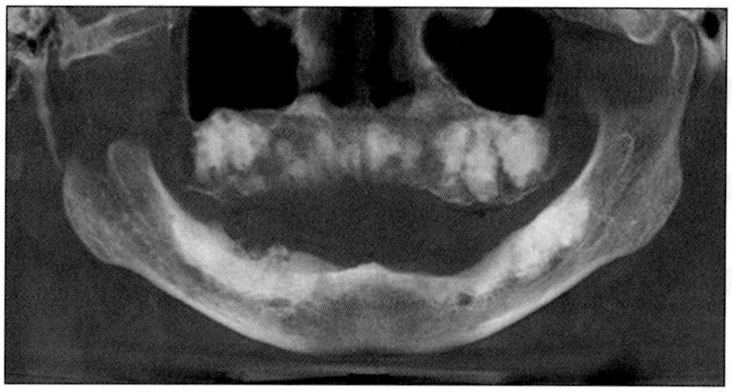

► Sclerotic phase of florid cemento-osseous dysplasia.

Florid Cemento-osseous Dysplasia

Nature of disease

A genetically driven dysmorphogenesis of the cementum–periodontal ligament–lamina dura complex.

Predilections

Almost exclusively involves adult women of black African heritage. Very rare cases may involve men.

Clinical features

Most present as an asymptomatic incidental radiographic finding. However, others may present with expansion and dull pain. Still others may present with exposed alveolar bone from a recent extraction. In those patients who report pain, the lesion is either in its initial radiolucent active phase, or secondary infection has resulted via either a pulpal route, a periodontal route, or an extraction.

Radiographic presentation

Like periapical cemental dysplasia and focal cemento-osseous dysplasia, florid cemento-osseous dysplasia may be seen in any of three phases from radiolucent to mixed radiolucent-radiopaque to nearly completely radiopaque. All four quadrants are involved in each phase, more overtly in the mandible than in the maxilla. The involvement is usually limited to the alveolar bone but on occasion may be seen to extend to the inferior border or the maxillary sinus if secondarily infected. On rare occasions, a large, round radiopaque mass is seen to grow out of an existing florid cemento-osseous dysplasia. This is usually an ossifying fibroma and may also be reported as a cemento-ossifying fibroma.

Differential diagnosis

Florid cemento-osseous dysplasia is radiographically and racially distinct so that few pathologies other than periapical cemental dysplasia, focal cemento-osseous dysplasia, and Paget disease may be considered.

Microscopic features

Dense acellular bone is prominent. In some cases, inflammatory cells are also seen as well as rare plump cells suggestive of osteoblasts (perhaps cementoblasts).

Suggested course of action

Accomplish comprehensive preventive and restorative dentistry so as to avoid extraction of teeth, which frequently creates a nonhealing extraction socket and secondary infection.

Treatment

Elective dentoalveolar surgery risks bone exposure and secondary infection and is therefore avoided if possible. In those cases of pain and/or secondary infection, surgical removal of the involved bone is necessary. Note: Bone that regenerates in such defects is normal bone. Grafts in these defects also regenerate normal bone.

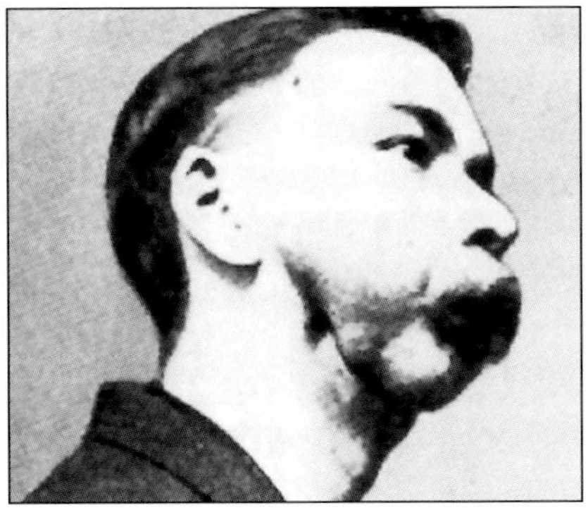

► Phossy jaw circa 1898.

Phossy Jaw

Nature of disease

Necrotic alveolar bone due to inorganic phosphorus vapors/dust being converted into a bisphosphonate by biochemical conversion in the tissues.

Predilections

Historically (1850s to 1910) seen mostly in match-factory workers exposed to phosphorus-containing vapors. Today, it is extremely rare. It is mostly seen in workers at munitions or fireworks factories as well as in a few phosphorus mine workers.

Clinical features

Exposed necrotic bone in the jaws identical to that seen in drug-induced osteonecrosis. It is painful if it becomes secondarily infected, and then it may develop oral or cutaneous fistulas.

Radiographic presentation

Maybe normal but mostly will show unremodeled extraction sockets, a diffuse alveolar bone sclerosis or osteolysis, and less commonly a pathologic fracture.

Differential diagnosis

Drug-induced osteonecrosis of the jaws, osteoradionecrosis, osteopetrosis, cemento-osseous dysplasia, and osteomyelitis are all considerations.

Microscopic features

Necrotic bone with debris.

Suggested course of action

Review for a history of exposure to phosphorus vapors or dust. Rule out a history of radiation to the jaws and the use of bisphosphonates or RANK ligand inhibitors. Refer to oral and maxillofacial surgeon for evaluation.

Treatment

Removal of the patient from the phosphorus-laden environment and antibiotics for secondary infection as palliative care. Surgical debridement of the necrotic bone is required for cure.

12

Vascular Lesions of Oral Mucosa and Skin

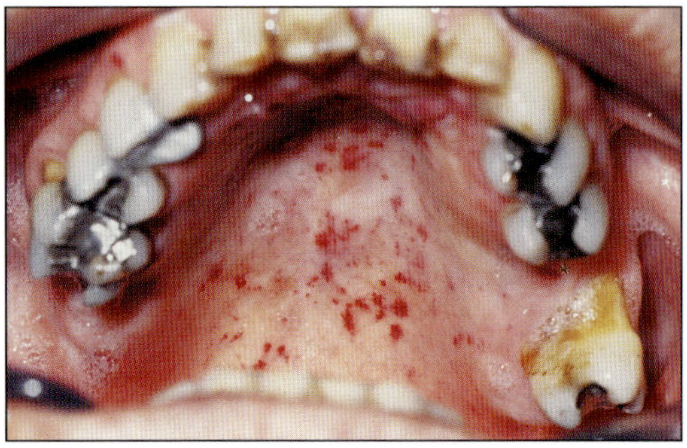

► Oral lesions of hereditary hemorrhagic telangiectasia.

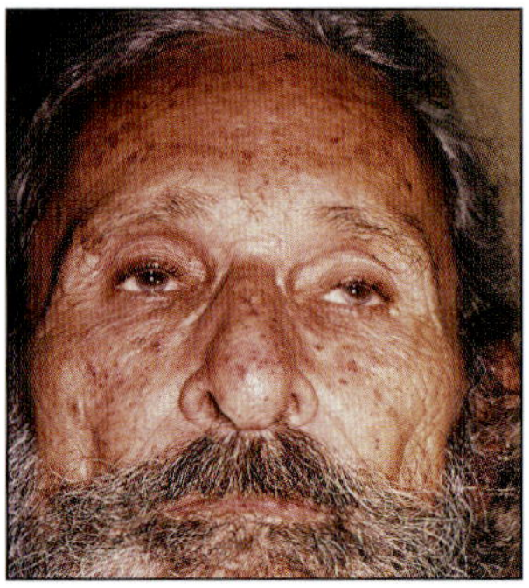

► Facial skin lesions of hereditary hemorrhagic telangiectasia.

Hereditary Hemorrhagic Telangiectasia (Osler-Weber-Rendu Syndrome)

Nature of disease

An autosomal dominant trait that causes defective endothelial interconnections within the capillaries of mucosa and skin. It results in weakened capillaries that dilate and readily bleed.

Predilections

Although genetic, it is not congenital. Clinically apparent dilated capillaries or bleeding episodes first begin in the late 30s and early 40s and progressively increase and worsen with age. White individuals are affected more frequently than black individuals. No sex predilection is known.

Clinical features

Dilated capillaries representing telangiectasias become apparent mostly on the tongue, palate, and lips. Facial and chest skin telangiectasias are frequent as well. Spontaneous nosebleeds may be the first outward sign of hereditary hemorrhagic telangiectasia as involvement of Kiesselbach's plexus in the nasal septum occurs. Severe cases of repeated bleeding episodes have resulted in anemia.

Radiographic presentation

None.

Differential diagnosis

A fully expressed case of hereditary hemorrhagic telangiectasia is distinctive. However, hereditary cherry angiomas known as *Campbell de Morgan spots* also begin at the same age. Otherwise, spider telangiectasia from liver cirrhosis will be similar as well as the telangiectasias seen in Fabry syndrome, Maffucci syndrome, and CREST syndrome.

Microscopic features

Thin-walled dilated capillaries and venules with flattened endothelial cells are the features seen on light microscopy. Electron microscope images show the gaps between endothelial cells and the absence of pericytes.

Suggested course of action

There is no contraindication to restorative dental care. However, gingival periodontal surgery and oral surgery are best accomplished with access to electrocautery, laser ablation, and/or topical hemostatic agents. Cases suspicious for hereditary hemorrhagic telangiectasia or undiagnosed cases are best referred to a hematologist for workup and decision-making about further care.

Treatment

Definitive treatment is usually not required. Areas of repeated bleeding or those causing an anemia are excised and skin-grafted, which prevents further bleeding episodes from the treated area.

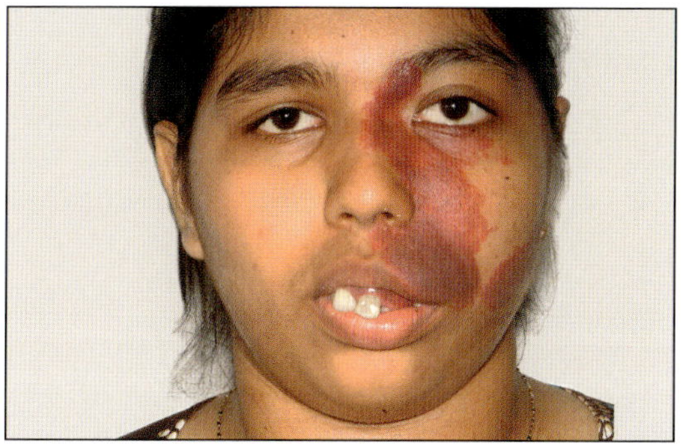

► Facial lesions of encephalotrigeminal angiomatosis.

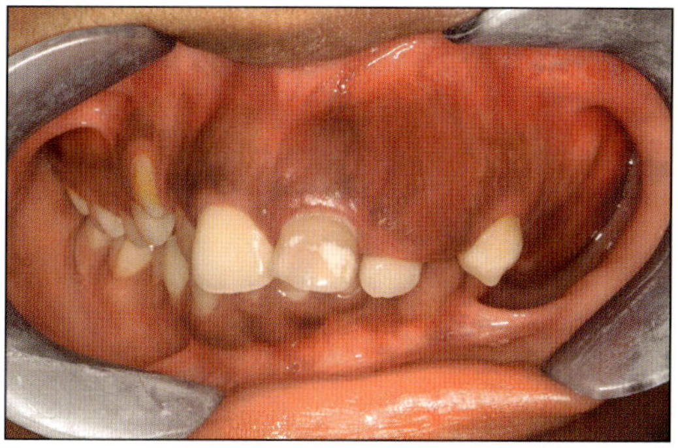

► Oral lesions of encephalotrigeminal angiomatosis.

Encephalotrigeminal Angiomatosis (Sturge-Weber Syndrome)

Nature of disease

A noninherited persistence of a vascular plexus in embryologic development. Specifically, this anomaly results from the incomplete involution of a fetal vascular plexus between the neural ectoderm destined to become brain and the mucosa/skin ectoderm. This results in a functional vascular network over the trigeminal nerve distribution and sometimes brain cortex on one side of the midline.

Predilections

Almost always unilateral, with no sex or racial predilection. The left side is favored slightly. The ophthalmic and maxillary divisions are most commonly involved together.

Clinical features

There will be a red to purple to blue discoloration of the facial skin and oral mucosa corresponding to mostly the upper two divisions of the trigeminal nerve distribution. This involvement will have a distinct cutoff at the midline. Bleeding from minor trauma can occur but is uncommon. Teeth in the area may be supererupted and the bone hyperplastic, creating a malocclusion. If the involvement includes the brain, seizures may be reported; in the very rare severe case, mental slowness has been observed.

Radiographic presentation

Plain radiographs and CT scans will often show an expanded bone with a foggy ground-glass appearance similar to that seen in fibrous dysplasia. If brain lesions are prominent, wavy calcifications corresponding to the cortical gyri may be seen.

Differential diagnosis

Capillary and cavernous hemangiomas unassociated with encephalotrigeminal angiomatosis are the more common considerations, as is the Klippel-Trenaunay-Weber syndrome, which has similar capillary bed manifestations but is usually more widespread.

Microscopic features

A normal-appearing albeit dense capillary network is seen in the dermis of skin and the submucosa of oral tissues and within bone. In calcified brain lesions, the calcifications are dystrophic concretions rather than bone.

→

Encephalotrigeminal Angiomatosis (Sturge-Weber Syndrome) *(cont)*

Suggested course of action

Undiagnosed cases should be referred to the patient's primary physician or to a neurologist for a work-up. Established cases should be referred to the patient's primary physician with a list of the oral and dental findings. Restorative dentistry is safe to perform on such patients. For corrective jaw surgery, refer to an oral and maxillofacial surgeon or an orthodontist to begin an assessment and develop a treatment plan. For cosmetic facial coloration, refer to a dermatologist.

Treatment

Those individuals with seizure disorders are treated with seizure-control medications. The few with mental slowness require special education. Many require surgical bone contouring or orthognathic surgery. Such surgery is done with good hemorrhage control, as the vessels ooze under low pressure and are controlled by cautery or topical agents. Those individuals who seek a reduction in the purple-blue discoloration may require sclerosing injections, fillers, or laser surgery.

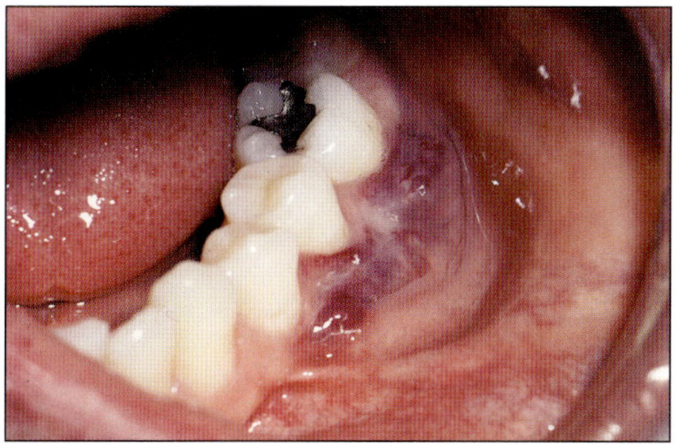

► Residual capillary hemangioma of a newborn now in the adult.

Capillary Hemangioma

Nature of disease

An overproliferation of capillaries due to overexpression of basic fibroblast growth factor within an embryonic field of capillary development.

Predilections

Rare in bone. Most commonly seen in the soft tissues of a newborn or within the first 2 years of life. Some are congenital. These are often termed *juvenile capillary hemangiomas*. Those in bone occur in older individuals.

Clinical features

In bone, most are diagnosed radiographically as the clinical picture is normal. Some will produce a mild, painless expansion.

Radiographic presentation

A multilocular radiolucency with thinned cortices and mild expansion.

Differential diagnosis

Due to its rarity in bone, lesions such as central giant cell tumors, ameloblastic fibromas, odontogenic myxomas, and odontogenic keratocysts are more realistic considerations.

Microscopic features

Very cellular lesions composed of endothelial cells forming tortuous but poorly canalized lumen.

Suggested course of action

Incisional biopsy and/or referral to an oral and maxillofacial surgeon. Note: Capillary hemangiomas will not return blood upon aspiration.

Treatment

Because capillary hemangiomas in bone are not true neoplasms with continuous growth, they are removed by enucleation and curettage.

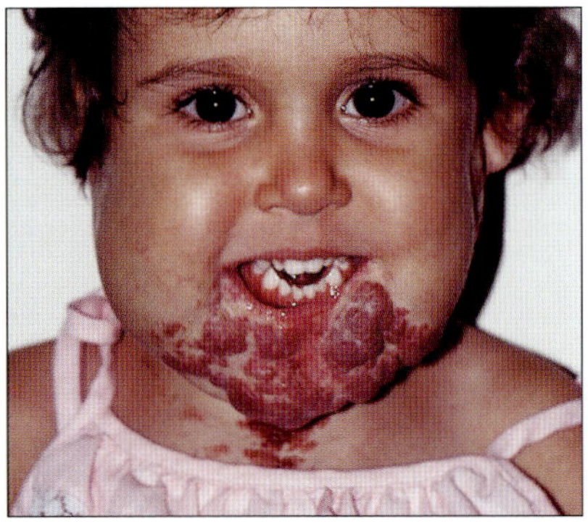

► Juvenile capillary hemangioma.

Juvenile Capillary Hemangioma

Nature of disease

A distinctive proliferation of endothelial cells around the chin, cheeks, and upper neck or in the parotid gland that begins before or shortly after birth. It is not a true neoplasm but a defect in the control of capillary regeneration within a developmental territory, often caused by the oversecretion of basic fibroblast growth factor (bFGF).

Predilections

Congenital or begins in children less than 1 year of age. There is a female predilection of 3:1. Mostly seen in white children.

Clinical features

They begin as a painless, blue, multinodular mass mostly symmetric about the midline of the chin and neck and extending to just beyond the commissures of the mouth and tapering down the midline toward the sternum. In the parotid gland, the gland will be diffusely enlarged and will have a blue discoloration. As the lesion regresses, it remains nodular but gradually becomes smaller and more pale.

Radiographic presentation

None.

Differential diagnosis

Juvenile capillary hemangiomas are clinically distinctive with few similar-appearing lesions other than a lymphangioma, which is a related lesion.

Microscopic features

Juvenile capillary hemangiomas will begin as cellular proliferations of endothelial cells forming poorly canalized blood vessels containing a few erythrocytes. As they regress, fewer endothelial cells are seen, and a fibrotic stroma develops.

Suggested course of action

Refer to centers familiar with vascular lesions. Oftentimes these lesions are overtreated, resulting in deformity.

Treatment

These lesions will spontaneously regress but may take 10 to 12 years to do so. However, the skin will be scar filled and irregular. A more rapid regression can be obtained from oral prednisone 1 mg/kg per day at 2-week intervals interrupted by 2 weeks of a drug holiday for a 3-month period. For those cases in which a 24-hour urine collection identifies an increase in bFGF, interferon alpha-2a prescribed at a dose of 1 million to 4 million units per day has been shown to induce a regression.

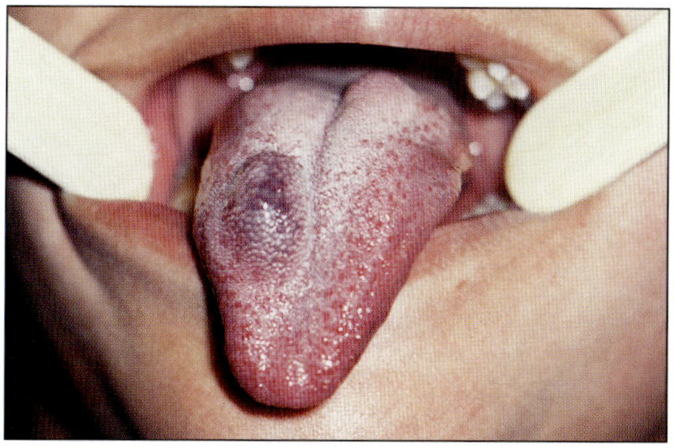

► Cavernous hemangioma of the tongue.

Cavernous Hemangioma

Nature of disease

A non-neoplastic proliferation and dilation of veins containing blood under low pressure.

Predilections

Occurs mostly in mature adults. More common in women. There is no racial predilection.

Clinical features

In bone, it will present as a mild expansion without displacement of teeth or the mandibular canal. No paresthesia or objective anesthesia is observed. In soft tissue, it will appear as a painless, blue, lobulated mass. Pulsations are usually not present. Stethoscope and Doppler examination will identify an echoing sound suggestive of venous pressure.

Radiographic presentation

A radiolucency with poorly defined borders. Displacement of teeth and/or the mandibular canal may occur but is not usually seen.

Differential diagnosis

A radiolucency with ill-defined borders should suggest an idiopathic bone cavity, a metastatic malignancy, a primary malignancy, and an osteomyelitis.

Microscopic features

Large, dilated, endothelial-lined spaces.

Suggested course of action

Aspirate. If blood is returned, refer to an oral and maxillofacial surgeon for workup.

Treatment

If Doppler sounds rule out arterial pressure, a cavernous hemangioma in bone can be curetted without significant blood loss. In soft tissue, sclerosing agents such as sodium morrhuate or sodium tetradecoyl sulfate can fibrose most lesions without surgery. Otherwise, a local excision can be accomplished with minimal bleeding.

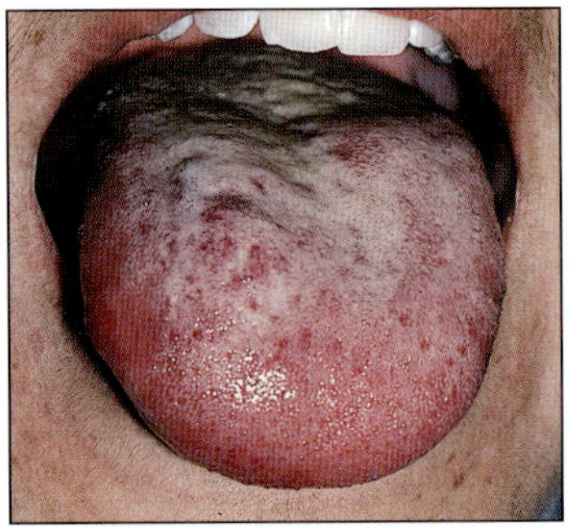

► A pulsatile arteriovenous hemangioma of the tongue.

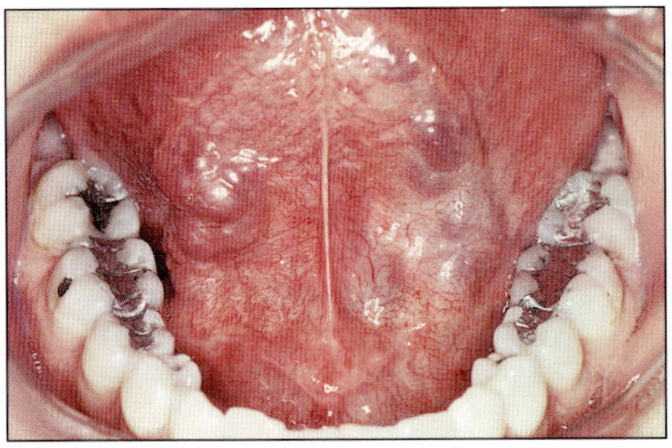

► Large, dilated sublingual veins due to an arteriovenous hemangioma in the tongue.

Arteriovenous Hemangioma

Nature of disease

A potentially life-threatening bleeding from a developmental aberration of arteries and veins. It is caused by the genetic loss of endothelial cell production of platelet-derived growth factors and transforming growth factor beta, which are required to recruit adventitial cells to support blood vessel development. The result is an expanding vascular mass under arterial pressure as the systemic vascular system matures.

Predilections

Most common in preteen and teenage girls and less common in boys of the same age.

Clinical features

Usually an expansile mass that may appear blue. It will have pulsations that may be palpable as well as arterial sounds upon stethoscope or Doppler examination. They are often brought to the attention of health care personnel in the emergency room as a severe bleeding episode.

Radiographic presentation

If the lesion involves bone as well as soft tissue, it will appear as a multilocular radiolucent lesion with mild expansion.

Differential diagnosis

Odontogenic keratocysts, odontogenic myxomas, ameloblastic fibromas, and central giant cell tumors may be considered in this age group.

Microscopic features

Large, dilated, endothelial-lined blood vessels absent of supporting adventitial cells or stroma.

Suggested course of action

Aspiration of the lesion. If blood is returned, avoid biopsy in the office. Refer to an invasive radiology center for an arteriogram and to an oral and maxillofacial surgeon to coordinate treatment.

Treatment

Embolization followed by either debridement and packing of the lesion or resection.

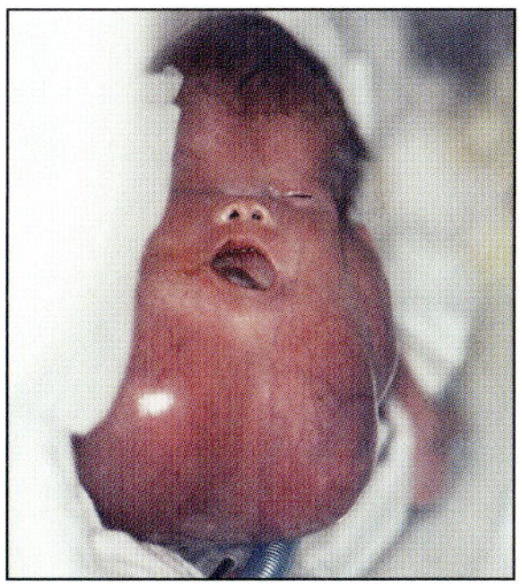

► Cervical cystic hygoma.

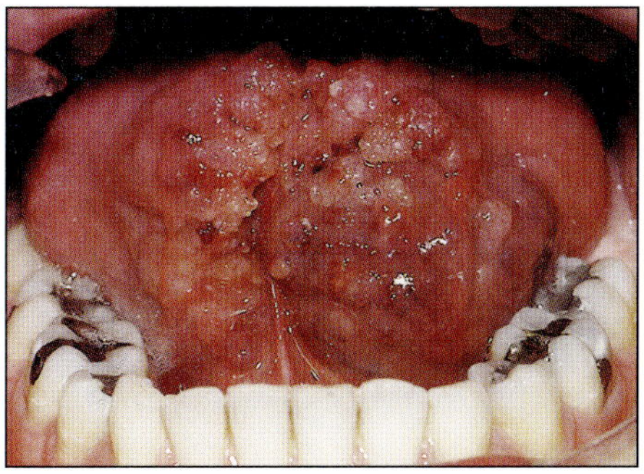

► Adult superficial type of lymphangioma.

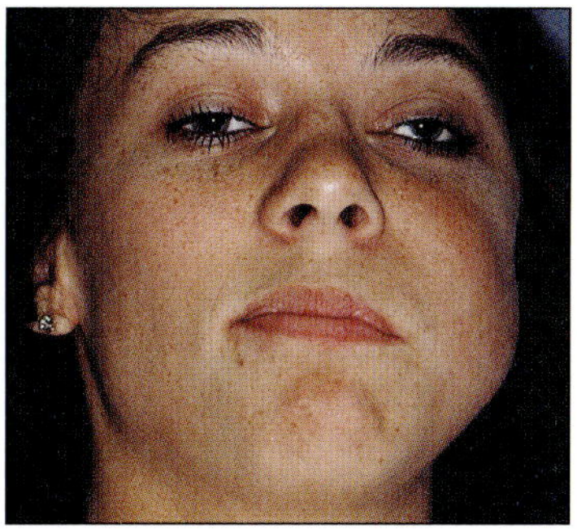

► Adult deep type of lymphangioma.

Lymphangioma

Nature of disease

A defect in the development of lymphatic channels within an embryologic field that can occur at any age and results in a dilation and a disorganized proliferation of endothelial-lined lymphatic channels.

Predilections

A strong predilection for females. White individuals are more commonly affected. One type is congenital or may develop within the first year (ie, cystic hygoma). Other types occur in adults (ie, superficial type and deep type).

Clinical features

- Cervical cystic hygoma: This type appears at birth or in early life as a large, seemingly painless, soft-textured and fluid-filled enlargement in the lateral neck. Most occur unilaterally, but some are bilateral.
- The adult superficial type: This type will appear as a mass of doughy to firm consistency with a red-brown pebbly surface that does not blanch upon pressure.
- The adult deep type: This type appears as a semisoft expansion with an intact and smooth surface.

Radiographic presentation

Lymphangiomas are not well seen on plain radiographs. They are best seen on MRI scans, which will usually identify a lobulated or irregular outline of a mass lesion with a high water content.

Differential diagnosis

The cystic hygoma type is clinically distinctive. However, it may resemble a mass from a rhabdomyosarcoma, neuroblastoma, or hemangioma. The adult superficial type may resemble a verrucous hyperplasia, verrucous carcinoma, or squamous cell carcinoma. The adult deep type may present as several deeply located benign tumors such as schwannomas, neurofibromas, and salivary gland tumors.

Microscopic features

Lymphangiomas will appear as large, empty endothelial-lined spaces with sparse or absent adventitial cells.

Suggested course of action

Refer to an oral and maxillofacial surgeon or a major medical center for workup and treatment.

Treatment

Because lymphangiomas are not true neoplasms with continual growth, most do not require treatment. Some may require debulking or a partial resection for cosmetic improvement or to remove a functional impairment.

Recommended Reading

The following list provides selected readings for several disease entities per chapter.

Chapter 2

Dyskeratosis congenita

Kelmenson DA, Hanley M. Dyskeratosis congenita. N Engl J Med 2017;376:1460.

Mason PJ, Wilson DB, Bessler M. Dyskeratosis congenita: A disease of dysfunctional telomere maintenance. Curr Mol Med 2005;5:159–170.

Nishio N, Kojima S. Recent progress in dyskeratosis congenita. Int J Hematol 2010;92:419–424.

Lichen planus

Aghbari SMH, Abushouk AI, Attia A, et al. Malignant transformation of oral lichen planus and oral lichenoid lesions: A meta-analysis of 20095 patient data. Oral Oncol 2017;68:92–102.

Fitzpatrick SG, Hirsch SA, Gordon SC. The malignant transformation of oral lichen planus and oral lichenoid lesions: A systematic review. J Am Dent Assoc 2014;145:45–56.

Van der Meij EH, Schepman KP, Van der Waal I. The possible premalignant character of oral lichen planus and oral lichenoid lesions: A prospective study. Oral Surg Oral Med Oral Pathol Oral Radiol Endod 2003;96:164–171.

Yin M, Li G, Song H, Lin S. Identifying the association between interleukin-6 and lichen planus: A meta-analysis. Biomed Rep 2017;6:571–575.

Keratosis follicularis

Halteh P, Jorizzo JL, Lipner SR. Darier disease: Candy-cane nails and hyperkeratosis papules. Postgrad Med J 2016;92:425–426.

Savignac M, Edir A, Simon M, Hovnanian A. Darier disease: A disease model of impaired calcium hemostasis in the skin. Biochim Biophys Acta 2011;1813:1111–1117.

Takagi A, Kamijo M, Ikeda S. Darier disease. J Dermatol 2016;43:275–279.

Incontinentia pigmenti

Minić S, Trpinac D, Gabriel H, Gencik M, Obradović M. Dental and oral anomalies in incontinentia pigmenti: A systematic review. Clin Oral Investig 2013;17:1–8.

Santa-Maria FD, Mariath LM, Poziomczyk CS, et al. Dental anomalies in 14 patients with IP: Clinical and radiologic analysis and review. Clin Oral Investig 2017;21:1845–1852.

Hairy leukoplakia

Khammissa RA, Fourie J, Chandran R, Lemmer J, Feller L. Epstein-Barr virus and its association with oral hairy leukoplakia: A short review. Int J Dent 2016;2016:4941783.

Moura MD, Grossman Sde M, Fonseca LM, Senna MI, Mesquita RA. Risk factors for oral hairy leukoplakia in HIV-infected adults of Brazil. J Oral Pathol Med 2006;35:321–326.

Sharma G, Oberoi SS, Vohra P, Nagpal A. Oral manifestations of HIV/AIDS in Asia: Systematic review and future research guidelines. J Clin Exp Dent 2015;7:e419–e427.

Chapter 3

Traumatic eosinophilic granuloma

Boffano P, Gallesio C, Campisi P, Roccia F. Traumatic ulcerative granuloma with stromal eosinophilia of the retromolar region. J Craniofac Surg 2009;20:2150–2152.

Chatzistamou I, Doussis-Anagnostopoulou I, Georgiou G, et al. Traumatic ulcerative granuloma with stromal eosinophilia: Report of a case and literature review. J Oral Maxillofac Surg 2012;70:349–353.

Gingival fibromatosis

Almiñana-Pastor PJ, Buitrago-Vera PJ, Alpiste-Illueca FM, Catalá-Pizarro M. Hereditary gingival fibromatosis: Characteristics and treatment approach. J Clin Exp Dent 2017;9:e599–e602.

Gawron K, Łazarz-Bartyzel K, Potempa J, Chromyszyn-Gajewska M. Gingival fibromatosis: Clinical, molecular and therapeutic issues. Orphanet J Rare Dis 2016;11:9.

Poulopoulos A, Kittas D, Sarigelou A. Current concepts on gingival fibromatosis-related symptoms. J Investig Clin Dent 2011;2:156–161.

Orofacial granulomatosis

Al-Hamad A, Porter S, Fedele S. Orofacial granulomatosis. Dermatol Clin 2015;33:433–446.

Grave B, McCullough M, Wiesenfeld D. Orofacial granulomatosis: A 20-year review. Oral Dis 2009;15:46–51.

Haaramo A, Alapulli H, Aine L, et al. Detailed follow-up study of pediatric orofacial granulomatosis patients [epub ahead of print 22 February 2017]. J Pediatr Gastroenterol Nutr doi:10.1097/MPG.0000000000001554.

Angioedema

Bernstein JA, Cremenesi P, Hoffmann TK, Hollingsworth J. Angioedema in the emergency department: A practical guide to differential diagnosis and management [epub ahead of print 13 April 2017]. Int J Emerg Med doi:10.1186/s12245-017-0141-z.

Czuka D, Veszeli N, Varga L, Prohászka Z, Farkas H. The role of the complement system in hereditary angioedema [epub ahead of print 5 June 2017]. Mol Immunol doi:10.1016/j.molimm.2017.05.020.

Javaud N, Achamlal J, Reuter PG, et al. Angioedema related to angiotensin-converting enzyme inhibitors: Attack severity, treatment, and hospital admission in a prospective multicenter study. Medicine (Baltimore) 2015;94:e1939.

Granular cell tumor

Chrysomali E, Papanicolaou SI, Dekker NP, Regezi JA. Benign neural tumors of the oral cavity: A comparative immunohistochemical study. Oral Surg Oral Med Oral Pathol Oral Radiol Endod 1997;84:381–390.

Ferreira JC, Oton-Leite AF, Guidi R, Mendonça EF. Granular cell tumor mimicking a squamous cell carcinoma of the tongue: A case report. BMC Res Notes 2017;10:14.

Freitas VS, Dos Santos JN, Oliveira MC, Santos PP, Freitas Rde A, de Souza LB. Intraoral granular cell tumors: Clinicopathologic and immunohistochemical study. Quintessence Int 2012;43:135–142.

Chapter 4

Thyroglossal tract cyst

Josephson GD, Spencer WR, Josephson JS. Thyroglossal tract cyst: The New York Eye and Ear Infirmary experience and a literature review. Ear Nose Throat J 1998;77:642–644,646–647,651.

Wampler HW, Krolls SO, Johnson RP. Thyroglossal-tract cyst. Oral Surg Oral Med Oral Pathol 1978;45:32–38.

Cat-scratch disease

Conrad DA. Treatment of cat-scratch disease. Curr Opin Pediatr 2001;13:56–59.

Nelson CA, Saha S, Mead PS. Cat-scratch disease in the United States, 2005-2013. Emerg Infect Dis 2016;22:1741–1746.

Carotid body tumor

Darouassi Y, Alaoui M, Mliha Touati M, et al. Carotid body tumors: A case series and review of the literature [epub ahead of print 3 May 2017]. Ann Vasc Surg doi:10.1016/j.avsg.2017.03.167.

Williams MD. Paragangliomas of the head and neck: An overview from diagnosis to genetics [epub ahead of print 20 March 2017]. Head Neck Pathol doi:10.1007/s12105-017-0803-4.

Dermoid cyst

Berbel P, Ostrosky A, Tosti F. Large sublingual dermoid cyst: A case of mandibular prognathism. Craniomaxillofac Trauma Reconstr 2016;9:345–348.

Jadwani S, Misra B, Kallianpur S, Bansod S. Dermoid cyst of the floor of the mouth with abundant hair: A case report. J Maxillofac Oral Surg 2009;8:388–389.

Masseteric hypertrophy

Black MJ, Schloss MD. Masseteric muscle hypertrophy. J Otolaryngol 1985;14:203–205.

Mandel L, Kaynar A. Masseteric hypertrophy. N Y State Dent J 1994;60:44–47.

Chapter 5

Cavernous sinus thrombosis

Prabhu S, Jain SK, Dal Singh V. Cavernous sinus thrombophlebitis (sans thrombosis) secondary to odontogenic fascial space infection: An uncommon complication with unusual presentation. J Maxillofac Oral Surg 2015;14(suppl 1):168–172.

Rheumatic fever

Burke RJ, Chang C. Diagnostic criteria of acute rheumatic fever. Autoimmun Rev 2014;13:503–507.

Ceylan O, Sahin DA. Acute rheumatic fever and isolated myocarditis. Int J Cardiol 2017;239:13.

Tetanus

Finkelstein P, Teisch L, Allen CJ, Ruiz G. Tetanus: A potential public health threat in times of disaster. Prehosp Disaster Med 2017;32:339–342.

World Health Organization. Tetanus vaccines: WHO position paper, February 2017—Recommendations [epub ahead of print 17 April 2017]. Vaccine doi:10.1016/j.vaccine.2017.02.034.

Histoplasmosis

Figueira JA, Camilo Júnior D, Biasoli ER, Miyahara GI, Bernabé DG. Oral ulcers associated with bone destruction as the primary manifestation of histoplasmosis in an immunocompetent patient [epub ahead of print 5 April 2017]. J Eur Acad Dermatol Venereol doi:10.1111/jdv.14257.

Muñante-Cárdenas JL, de Assis AF, Olate S, Lyrio MC, de Moraes M. Treating oral histoplasmosis in an immunocompetent patient. J Am Dent Assoc 2009;140:1373–1376.

Herpes zoster (shingles)

Dayan RR, Peleg R. Herpes zoster: Typical and atypical presentations [epub ahead of print 5 June 2017]. Postgrad Med doi:10.1080/00325481.2017.1335574.

Shah S, Singaraju S, Einstein A, Sharma A. Herpes zoster: A clinicopathologic insight. J Oral Maxillofac Pathol 2016;20:547.

Chapter 6

Primary hyperparathyroidism

Palla B, Burian E, Fliefel R, Otto S. Systematic review of oral manifestations related to hyperparathyroidism [epub ahead of print 14 June 2017]. Clin Oral Investig doi:10.1007/s00784-017-2124-0.

Pawlak W, Bohdanowicz-Pawlak A, Bolanowski M, Szymczak J, Bednarek-Tupikowska G, Luczak K. Primary hyperparathyroidism presenting as a giant cell tumor of the jaws. Neuro Endocrinol Lett 2013;34:107–110.

Rai S, Rattan V, Bhadada SK. Giant cell lesions associated with primary hyperparathyroidism. J Maxillofac Oral Surg 2015;14:930–934.

Central giant cell tumor

Pellicioli AC, Kaefer T, Martins MA, Carrard VC, Martins MD. Central giant cell lesion: Diagnosis to rehabilitation. Gen Dent 2015;63:e16–e19.

Suárez-Roa Mde L, Reveiz L, Ruíz-Godoy Rivera LM, et al. Interventions for central giant cell granuloma (CGCG) of the jaws. Cochrane Database Syst Rev 2009;(4):CD007404.

Glandular odontogenic cyst

Boffano P, Cassarino E, Zavattero E, Campisi P, Garzino-Demo P. Surgical treatment of glandular odontogenic cysts. J Craniofac Surg 2010;21:776–780.

Fowler CB, Brannon RB, Kessler HP, Castle JT, Kahn MA. Glandular odontogenic cyst: Analysis of 46 cases with special emphasis on microscopic criteria for diagnosis. Head Neck Pathol 2011;5:364–375.

Momeni Roochi M, Tavakoli I, Ghazi FM, Tavakoli A. Case series and review of glandular odontogenic cyst with emphasis on treatment modalities. J Craniomaxillofac Surg 2015;43:746–750.

Juvenile rapidly progressive periodontitis

Celenligil H, Kansu E, Eratalay K. Juvenile and rapidly progressive periodontitis. Peripheral blood lymphocyte subpopulations. J Clin Periodontol 1990;17:207–210.

Nonnenmacher C, Mutters R, de Jacoby LF. Microbiological characteristics of subgingival microbiota in adult periodontitis, localized juvenile periodontitis and rapidly progressive periodontitis subjects. Clin Microbiol Infect 2001;7:213–217.

Chapter 7

Desmoplastic ameloblastoma

Desai H, Sood R, Shah R, Cawda J, Pandya H. Desmoplastic ameloblastoma: Report of a unique case and review of literature. Indian J Dent Res 2006;17:45–49.

Kallam SR, Arutla R, Gadwalwari SS, Kubbi JR, Shylaja SR. Desmoplastic ameloblastoma: An unusual presentation. J Clin Diagn Res 2015;9:ZJ04–ZJ05.

Kishino M, Murakami S, Fukuda Y, Ishida T. Pathology of the desmoplastic ameloblastoma. J Oral Pathol Med 2001;30:35–40.

Waldron CA, el-Mofty SK. A histopathologic study of 116 ameloblastomas with special reference to the desmoplastic variant. Oral Surg Oral Med Oral Pathol 1987;63:441–451.

Gardner syndrome

Bilkay U, Erdem O, Ozek C, et al. Benign osteoma with Gardner syndrome: Review of the literature and report of a case. J Craniofac Surg 2004;15:506–509.

Brucoli M, Giarda M, Benech A. Gardner syndrome: Presurgical planning and surgical management of craniomaxillofacial osteomas. J Craniofac Surg 2011;22:946–948.

de Oliveira Ribas M, Martins WD, de Sousa MH, et al. Oral and maxillofacial manifestations of familial adenomatous polyposis (Gardner's syndrome): A report of two cases. J Contemp Dent Pract 2009;10:82–90.

Koh KJ, Park HN, Kim KA. Gardner syndrome associated with multiple osteomas, intestinal polyposis, and epidermoid cysts. Imaging Sci Dent 2016;46:267–272.

Osteosarcoma of the jaws

Baumhoer D, Brunner P, Eppenberger-Castori S, Smida J, Nathrath M, Jundt G. Osteosarcomas of the jaws differ from their peripheral counterparts and require a distinct treatment approach. Experiences from the DOESAK Registry. Oral Oncol 2014;50:147–153.

Kämmerer PW, Shabazfar N, Vorkhshori Makaoi N, Moergel M, Al-Nawas B. Clinical, therapeutic and prognostic features of osteosarcoma of the jaws: Experience of 36 cases. J Craniomaxillofac Surg 2012;40:541–548.

Lee RJ, Arshi A, Schwartz HC, Christensen RE. Characteristics and prognostic factors of osteosarcoma of the jaws: A retrospective cohort study. JAMA Otorhinolaryngol Head Neck Surg 2015;141:470–477.

Segmental odontomaxillary dysplasia

González-Arriagada WA, Vargas PA, Fuentes-Cortés R, Nasi-Toso MA, Lopes MA. Segmental odontomaxillary dysplasia: Report of 3 cases and literature review. Head Neck Pathol 2012;6:171–177.

Prusack N, Pringle G, Scotti V, Chen SY. Segmental odontomaxillary dysplasia: A case report and review of the literature. Oral Surg Oral Med Oral Pathol Oral Radiol Endod 2000;90:483–488.

Secondary hyperparathyroidism

Palla B, Burian E, Fliefel R, Otto S. Systematic review of oral manifestations related to hyperparathyroidism [epub ahead of print 14 June 2017]. Clin Oral Investig doi:10.1007/s00784-017-2124-0.

Parfitt J, Harris M, Wright JM, Kalamchi S. Tumor suppressor gene mutation in a patient with a history of hyperparathyroidism-jaw tumor syndrome and healed generalized osteitis fibrosa cystica: A case report and genetic pathophysiology review. J Oral Maxillofac Surg 2015;73:194.e1–194.e9.

Portillo MR, Rodríguez-Ortiz ME. Secondary hyperparathyroidism: Pathogenesis, diagnosis, preventive and therapeutic strategies. Rev Endocr Metab Disord 2017;18:79–95.

Chapter 8

Sialoliths

Parkar MI, Vora MM, Bhanushali DH. A large sialolith perforating the Wharton's duct: Review of the literature and a case report. J Maxillofac Oral Surg 2012;11:477–482.

Ramanojam S, Merchant Y, Bhardwaj S, Kesari A. Idiopathic sialolithiasis: Scalpel versus current trends in management. J Craniofac Surg 2017;28:e363–e364.

Osseous choristomas

Adhikari BR, Sato J, Morikawa T, et al. Osseous choristoma of the tongue: Two case reports. J Med Case Rep 2016;10:59.

Johann AC, Garcia BG, Nacif TR, de Freitas JB, do Carmo MA, Mesquita RA. Submandibular osseous choristoma. J Craniomaxillofac Surg 2006;34:57–59.

Sheridan SM. Osseous choristoma: A report of two cases. Br J Oral Maxillofac Surg 1984;22:99–102.

Traumatic myositis ossificans

Lello GE, Makek M. Traumatic myositis ossificans in masticatory muscles. J Maxillofac Surg 1986;14:231–237.

Steiner M, Gould AR, Kushner GM, Lutchka B, Flint R. Myositis ossificans traumatica of the masseter muscle: Review of the literature and report of two additional cases. Oral Surg Oral Med Oral Pathol Oral Radiol Endod 1997;84:703–707.

Myositis ossificans progressiva

Becker OE, Avelar RL, Rivero ER, et al. Myositis ossificans of the temporalis muscle. Head Neck Pathol 2016;10:340–344.

Conner GA, Duffy M. Myositis ossificans: A case report of multiple recurrences following third molar extractions and review of the literature. J Oral Maxillofac Surg 2009;67:920–926.

Jayade B, Adirajaiah S, Vadera H, Kundalaswamy G, Sattur AP, Kalkur C. Myositis ossificans in medial, lateral pterygoid, and contralateral temporalis muscles: A rare case report. Oral Surg Oral Med Oral Pathol Oral Radiol 2013;116:e261–e266.

Schiff MJ, Meara DJ. Myositis ossificans of the temporalis muscle: Case report and review of the literature. J Oral Maxillofac Surg 2013;71:1893–1898.

Tonsilloliths

Giudice M, Cristofaro MG, Fava MG, Giudice A. An unusual tonsillolithiasis in a patient with chronic obstructive sialoadenitis. Dentomaxillofac Radiol 2005;34:247–250.

Lincot J, Shotar E, Albert S, Barry B, Schouman-Claeys E, Dallaudière B. Tonsillolithiasis. Diagn Interv Imaging 2016;97:279–282.

Chapter 9

Peutz-Jeghers syndrome

Duan SX, Wang GH, Zhong J, et al. Peutz-Jeghers syndrome with intermittent upper intestinal obstruction: A case report and review of the literature. Medicine (Baltimore) 2017;96:e6538.

Kopacova M, Tacheci I, Rejchrt S, Bures J. Peutz-Jeghers syndrome: Diagnostic and therapeutic approach. World J Gastroenterol 2009;15:5397–5408.

Addison disease

Gan EH, Pearce SH. Management of endocrine disease: Regenerative therapies in autoimmune Addison's disease. Eur J Endocrinol 2017;176:R123–R135.

Napier C, Pearce SH. Current and emerging therapies for Addison's disease. Curr Opin Endocrinol Diabetes Obes 2014;21:147–153.

Nieman LK, Chanco Turner ML. Addison's disease [review]. Clin Dermatol 2006;24:276–280.

Hemochromatosis

Ulvik RJ. The liver in haemochromatosis. J Trace Elem Med Biol 2015;31:219–224.

Wallace DF. The regulation of iron absorption and homeostasis. Clin Biochem Rev 2016;37:51–62.

Oral melanoma

Chatzistefanou I, Kolokythas A, Vahtsevanos K, Antoniades K. Primary mucosal melanoma of the oral cavity: Current therapy and future directions. Oral Surg Oral Med Oral Pathol Oral Radiol 2016;122:17–27.

Hicks MJ, Flaitz CM. Oral mucosal melanoma: Epidemiology and pathobiology. Oral Oncol 2000;36:152–169.

Tlholoe MM, Khammissa RA, Bouckaert M, Altini M, Lemmer J, Feller L. Oral mucosal melanoma: Some pathobiological considerations and an illustrative report of a case. Head Neck Pathol 2015;9:127–134.

Neuroblastoma

Alvi S, Karadaghy O, Manalang M, Weatherly R. Clinical manifestations of neuroblastoma with head and neck involvement in children. Int J Pediatr Otorhinolaryngol 2017;97:157–162.

Uccella S, Ottini G, Facco C, et al. Neuroendocrine neoplasms of the head and neck and olfactory neuroblastoma. Diagnosis and classification. Pathologica 2017;109:14–30.

Chapter 10

Keratoacanthoma

Selmer J, Skov T, Spelman L, Weedon D. Squamous cell carcinoma and keratoacanthomas are biologically distinct and can be diagnosed by light microscopy: A review. Histopathology 2016;69:535–541.

Takai T. Advances in histopathological diagnosis of keratoacanthoma. J Dermatol 2017;44:304–314.

Systemic lupus erythematosus

Giannelou M, Mavragani CP. Cardiovascular disease in systemic lupus erythematosus: A comprehensive update [epub ahead of print 9 June 2017]. J Autoimmun doi:10.1016/j.jaut.2017.05.008.

Moulton VR, Suarez-Fueyo A, Meidan E, Li H, Mizui M, Tsokos GC. Pathogenesis of human systemic lupus erythematosus: A cellular perspective. Trends Mol Med 2017;23:615–635.

Chronic cutaneous lupus erythematosus (discoid lupus erythematosus)

Haber JS, Merola JF, Werth VP. Classifying discoid lupus erythematosus: Background, gaps, and difficulties. Int J Womens Dermatol 2017;3(suppl):S62–S66.

Jessop S, Whitelaw DA, Grainge MJ, Jayasekera P. Drugs for discoid lupus erythematosus [review]. Cochrane Database Syst Rev 2017;(5):CD002954.

Pemphigus vulgaris

Kayani M, Aslam AM. Bullous pemphigoid and pemphigus vulgaris. BMJ 2017;357:j2169.

Kershenovich R, Hodak E, Mimouni D. Diagnosis and classification of pemphigus and bullous pemphigoid. Autoimmun Rev 2014;13:477–481.

Sami N, Ahmed AR. Dual diagnosis of pemphigus and pemphigoid. Retrospective review of thirty cases in the literature. Dermatology 2001;202:293–301.

Herpes zoster (shingles)

Dayan RR, Peleg R. Herpes zoster: Typical and atypical presentations [epub ahead of print 5 June 2017]. Postgrad Med doi:10.1080/00325481.2017.1335574.

Shah S, Singaraju S, Einstein A, Sharma A. Herpes zoster: A clinicopathologic insight. J Oral Maxillofac Pathol 2016;20:547.

Chapter 11

Osteoradionecrosis (ORN)

Chronopoulos A, Zarra T, Ehrenfeld M, Otto S. Osteoradionecrosis of the jaws: Definition, epidemiology, staging and clinical and radiological findings. A concise review [epub ahead of print 25 June 2017]. Int Dent J doi:10.1111/idj.12318.

Gevorgyan A, Wong K, Poon I, Blanas N, Enepekides DJ, Higgins KM. Osteoradionecrosis of the mandible: A case series at a single institution. J Otolaryngol Head Neck Surg 2013;42:46.

Marx RE. Osteoradionecrosis: A new concept of its pathophysiology. J Oral Maxillofac Surg 1983;41:283–288.

Marx RE, Tursun R. Suppurative osteomyelitis, bisphosphonate induced osteonecrosis, osteoradionecrosis: A blinded histopathologic comparison and its implications for the mechanism of each disease. Int J Oral Maxillofac Surg 2012;41:283–289.

Drug-induced osteonecrosis of the jaws (DIONJ)

Marx RE. Pamidronate (Aredia) and zoledronate (Zometa) induced avascular necrosis of the jaws: A growing epidemic. J Oral Maxillofac Surg 2003;61:1115–1117.

Marx RE, Sawatari Y, Fortin M, Broumand V. Bisphosphonate-induced exposed bone (osteonecrosis/osteopetrosis) of the jaws: Risk factors, recognition, prevention, and treatment. J Oral Maxillofac Surg 2005;63:1567–1575.

Marx RE, Tursun R. Suppurative osteomyelitis, bisphosphonate induced osteonecrosis, osteoradionecrosis: A blinded histopathologic comparison and its implications for the mechanism of each disease. Int J Oral Maxillofac Surg 2012;41:283–289.

Sawatari Y, Marx RE. Bisphosphonates and bisphosphonate induced osteonecrosis. Oral Maxillofac Surg Clin North Am 2007; 19:487–498.

Osteopetrosis

Filho AM, de Castro Domingos A, de Freitas DQ, Whaites EJ. Osteopetrosis—A review and report of two cases. Oral Dis 2005;11:46–49.

Yaga U, Panta P. Osteopetrosis. N Engl J Med 2017;376:e34.

Florid cemento-osseous dysplasia

Das BK, Das SN, Gupta A, Nayak S. Florid cemento-osseous dysplasia. J Oral Maxillofac Pathol 2013;17:150.

Fenerty S, Shaw W, Verma R, et al. Florid cemento-osseous dysplasia: Review of an uncommon fibro-osseous lesion of the jaw with important clinical implications. Skeletal Radiol 2017;46:581–590.

MacDonald-Jankowski DS. Florid cemento-osseous dysplasia: A systematic review. Dentomaxillofac Radiol 2003;32:141–149.

Sarmento DJ, Monteiro BV, de Medeiros EM, da Silveira EJ. Severe florid cemento-osseous dysplasia: A case report treated conservatively and literature review. Oral Maxillofac Surg 2013;17:43–46.

Phossy jaw

Marx RE. Uncovering the cause of "phossy jaw" circa 1858 to 1906: Oral and maxillofacial surgery closed case files—Case closed. J Oral Maxillofac Surg 2008;66:2356–2363.

Chapter 12

Hereditary hemorrhagic telangiectasia (Osler-Weber-Rendu syndrome)

Grigg C, Anderson D, Earnshaw J. Diagnosis and treatment of hereditary hemorrhagic telangiectasia. Ochsner J 2017;17:157–161.

Sautter NB, Smith TL. Treatment of hereditary hemorrhagic telangiectasia. Otolaryngol Clin North Am 2016;49:639–654.

Encephalotrigeminal angiomatosis (Sturge-Weber syndrome)

Chhabria BA, Subramanium PB, Nampoothiri R, Bhalla A, Varma S. Sturge-Weber syndrome. J Clin Diagn Res 2017;11:OJ05–OJ06.

Sudarsanam A, Arden-Holmes SL. Sturge-Weber syndrome: From the past to the present. Eur J Paediatr Neurol 2014;18:257–266.

Juvenile capillary hemangioma

Ghanem AA, El Hadidi YN. Management of a life threatening bleeding following extraction of deciduous second molar related to a capillary hemangioma. Craniomaxillofac Trauma Reconstr 2017;10:166–170.

Higuera S, Gordley K, Metry DW, Stal S. Management of hemangiomas and pediatric vascular malformations. J Craniofac Surg 2006;17:783–786.

Arteriovenous hemangioma

Colletti G, Valassina D, Bertossi D, Melchiorre F, Vercellio G, Brusati R. Contemporary management of vascular malformations. J Oral Maxillofac Surg 2014;72:510–528.

Morgan P, Keller R, Patel K. Evidence-based management of vascular malformations. Facial Plast Surg 2016;32:162–176.

Lymphangioma

Colbert SD, Seager L, Haider F, Evans BT, Anand R, Brennan PA. Lymphatic malformations of the head and neck—Current concepts in management. Br J Oral Maxillofac Surg 2013;51:98–102.

Wiegand S, Eivazi B, Zimmermann AP, Sesterhann AM, Werner JA. Sclerotherapy of lymphangiomas of the head and neck. Head Neck 2011;33:1649–1655.

Zhou Q, Zheng JW, Mai HM, et al. Treatment guidelines of lymphatic malformations of the head and neck. Oral Oncol 2011;47: 1105–1109.